SIMON & SCHUSTER New York
London
Toronto
Sydney
Tokyo
Singapore

WALT BOGDANICH

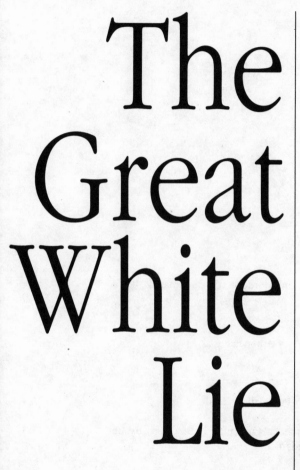

The
Great
White
Lie

How America's
hospitals betray
our trust
and endanger
our lives

SIMON & SCHUSTER
Simon & Schuster Building
Rockefeller Center
1230 Avenue of the Americas
New York, New York 10020

Designed by Karolina Harris
Manufactured in the United States of America

10 9 8 7 6 5 4 3 2 1

Library of Congress Cataloging-in-Publication data
Bogdanich, Walt.
    The great white lie : how America's hospitals betray our trust and
endanger our lives / Walt Bogdanich.
        p.   cm.
    Includes bibliographical references and index.
    1. Hospital care—United States.   2. Hospitals—United States.
I. Title.
RA981.A2B64   1991
362.1′1′0973—dc20   91-28389
                                                                CIP

ISBN: 0-671-68452-3

FOR MY PARENTS,

HELEN AND WALTER

Contents

Preface   9
Prologue: A Final Resting Place   13

ONE | CUTTING CORNERS, PLUGGING HOLES   31

1 Footprints in the Sand   33
2 Impostors   42
3 The Perfect File   53
4 "The Compelling Urgency to Ease Human
   Suffering"   65
5 The People-Pushers   85

TWO | THE NEW ETHICS   99

6 On the Threshold   101
7 Buried Secrets   111
8 Keys to the Kingdom   129
9 Sacred Heart   140
10 Candy from Strangers   158
11 Caveat Emptor   177

THREE | ABSENT WATCHDOGS

12 A Gathering of Felons
13 Midnight Fire
14 Waiting
15 Dear Ann Landers:
16 Lessons from the Grave

Epilogue: Showdown
Notes
Acknowledgments
Index

Preface

MY father was vacationing in 1985 when he suffered a heart attack. He was rushed to an unfamiliar hospital, but had the good fortune to be treated by a skilled cardiologist and attentive nurses. They saved his life. I arrived soon after his admission and found him resting comfortably in a clean, modern hospital. Its caring staff provided my distraught family with blankets and reassuring words. The cardiologist patiently explained my father's condition, answering the silliest questions over and over again without a trace of condescension.

Once my father's condition had stabilized, his doctor raised the possibility of a cardiac-bypass operation. "We do those here," he said. His words sounded so comforting. And it made a certain kind of sense to entrust with this surgery the hospital that had already saved my father's life. It seemed almost disrespectful or ungracious to spurn the hospital now that it was asking something of us—our business.

As it turned out, we decided that the operation should be done closer to home, near Chicago. Only later would we make a startling discovery: that friendly out-of-town hospital had just registered the nation's highest death rate—23 percent—among the hospitals doing 30 or more cardiac-bypass surgeries on Medicare patients. We learned this appalling fact not from the hospital but from an excellent series of articles published in Knight-Ridder newspapers.

After my father's return home, I began asking Chicago area hospitals for their bypass mortality rates. I wasn't prepared for the responses I got. One hospital told me that I could get its mortality rate from the American Medical Association. Another said it didn't keep mortality rates. Yet another said I had no right to ask for such confidential information. All were falsehoods. Feeling desperate and at a disadvantage, I stooped to asking a friendly hospital secretary to get mortality rates for her facility during her off-hours, when no one was around. A good thing I checked: patient outcomes there were poor.

Ultimately, I decided to have my father's bypass performed in Cleveland, Ohio, where, as a reporter, I knew which hospitals had successful cardiac-bypass programs. His surgery went well. Even so, there is something fundamentally wrong when a patient or a patient's family is made to feel like criminals simply for acting like sensible consumers.

Since I began this book, almost every member of my family has been hospitalized for one malady or another. I have seen up close the wonders and disappointments of hospital care. In choosing to write about the latter, rather than the former, I do not mean to denigrate the people and institutions that nobly fulfill their mission of healing. I, like so many others, have benefited from their care. But there are countless cases in which just the opposite is true. Not mere freak accidents or anomalies, such cases are the direct result of systemic health care problems of enormous proportions. The full measure of these problems will, I hope, become abundantly clear in the following pages. And in writing about them, I hope also to illuminate possible solutions.

The stories I have chosen to tell are true stories. I have not used pseudonyms, a staple of many books that report critically on the practice of medicine in this country. These are actual hospitals, doctors, and nurses whose identities are no more hidden than the names of their accusers. And although the stories told here are set in a number of cities across America, they could easily have happened in your local hospital, the place you and your family might one day go, feeling just as exposed and frightened as millions of other Americans who regularly put their lives in the hands of institutions and people they know nothing about.

The practice of medicine, we are told, requires our trust, and we give it—all too willingly. These stories reveal how often and how flagrantly that trust is violated.

Walt Bogdanich
Washington, D.C.

Prologue | A Final Resting Place

KATHRYN Hinnant began the last day of her life making love. She was 33 years old, slightly built with wide, seductive eyes. Ordinarily, she might have enjoyed lingering a bit on her day off, listening with her husband of three months to some classical music they had just discovered. But not today. There was much to be done.

Outside her warm apartment, 15 stories above the streets of Manhattan, a brisk wind made the temperature seem lower than 29 degrees—a bitter morning for those homeless people unable to claim a warm vent or a subway hideout. Now, a light snow began to fall as taxis carrying the last of the evening's revelers scooted down nearly empty streets.

For most New Yorkers, the long holiday season had ended and it was time to get on with life's routines. On this first Saturday of the new year, January 7, 1989, *The New York Times* carried a story of great interest to Kathryn Hinnant, M.D. CRISIS IN HOSPITALS, the headline warned. The accompanying article predicted no end soon to "dangerous overcrowding, long delays in care and shortages of vital staff and supplies" in area hospitals.

None would experience a rockier 1989 than the one where Dr. Hinnant worked: Bellevue Hospital Center, which houses the city's top trauma unit. One of the biggest, oldest, and most legendary hospitals in the nation, Bellevue's roots go back to 1736, when it opened on the present site of City Hall as an almshouse for the insane, the sick, orphans, and prisoners. Since moving early last century to its present location on First Avenue along the East River,

Bellevue had become a Manhattan landmark. It is here that the president of the United States would come should he suffer a medical emergency in New York, although the Secret Service would first have to clear a path through the alcoholics, psychopaths, and ripe-smelling vagrants who often clog the emergency room corridors. This chaotic yet widely praised emergency room best defined Bellevue: an open door to the most, and least, important in society. Unlike some other prestigious hospitals, Bellevue didn't close its emergency room to indigent neighbors while luring wealthy patients from overseas.

Bellevue's grandest moment arrived in 1956, when two of its doctors won the Nobel Prize for developing cardiac catheterization. More often than not, however, the hospital mirrored the plight of New York's expanding underclass: always short of money, always fighting just to survive, not get ahead. At times, Bellevue seemed to hang together like an old car, sputtering about on cannibalized parts and imagination.

Over the next twelve months, Bellevue would be threatened with the loss of accreditation for poor psychiatric care; accused of losing 124,000 syringes (the type used by drug abusers), having earlier misplaced 117,000 of them; engulfed by a noxious cloud of cleaning solvent that left 100 people stricken; forced to shut several operating rooms due to personnel shortages (delaying breast biopsies, pacemaker implants, and other elective surgeries); and ordered to pull 60 nurses off the floor at the beginning of a busy weekend holiday because of expired state registration. At one point, 60 percent of nursing slots in surgery and recovery would be vacant.

Amid this chaos lurked the daily threat of crime and violence. In 1988, nearly 1,000 felonies and 2,700 misdemeanors were committed in New York City hospitals. And those were just the ones that were reported. The new year began on a similar note when, on January 3, a feverish woman at one city hospital awoke to find a man riffling through her bedside drawer. In spirited New York fashion, she grabbed the intravenous lines tethered to her body and took off in pursuit of the bandit. She didn't catch him, but police did.

Bellevue's reputation for violence was among the worst, since its emergency room got the hard-core psychiatric cases. More guards would have helped, but being city-owned meant living in the fluid world of politics—where new facilities were supposed to be built but never were. Where equipment was promised but never delivered. In the 1870s, Boss Tweed's cronies had pilfered Bellevue cash as patients were being overrun by rats. One *Harper's Magazine* cartoon depicted Bellevue's night superintendent as a giant rodent bloated after a late-night meal of graft.

Unstable leadership had been a more recent problem. New York City's Health and Hospitals Corporation—of which Bellevue is a part—had changed presidents seven times in the 10 years ending in 1985. Bellevue, meanwhile, couldn't keep its own top executives. In November 1988, after an expensive nationwide search, Bellevue welcomed a new executive director, Richard Durbin, who arrived amid much fanfare from Texas. He lasted all of two weeks. During that time, Durbin and his wife were housed in an old, dreary, mice-infested section of the hospital that had been converted to an apartment. The new arrivals were then abandoned over the long Thanksgiving weekend, during which they ate their holiday meal at a nearby coffee shop. "I'm a lifelong New Yorker, and that would have depressed me," sympathized one Bellevue official. Days later, Bellevue's newest boss walked into his office, laid his keys on a table, and returned to Texas. "I didn't need to subject myself to that kind of life," he said later. Durbin's successor would last only two years, resigning in February 1991.

Kathryn Hinnant also had a career decision to make about Bellevue. Until recently, she hadn't thought much about family life as she aggressively pursued her career moves to New York and Washington, D.C., then back to New York again. She didn't seem bothered that friends were getting married while she remained single. The self-assured Hinnant had gone her own way ever since her high school days in an affluent bedroom community outside Columbia, South Carolina. While classmates wore fashionable jeans and sloppy shirts, Kathryn wore dresses. "We wanted to be elegant ladies," said Julianne Skinner, a high school friend.

Throughout her grueling climb to become a board-certified pathologist, Hinnant never lost her taste for elegance. As a poorly paid resident at Lenox Hill Hospital in Manhattan, she saved scrupulously to fund forays into outlet stores in search of designer clothes. Later, as if to balance out these indulgences, she worked as a volunteer dispensing food from a soup van. New York, in turn, nourished Hinnant's passion for ballet and opera.

Recently, however, Hinnant's life had taken some dramatic turns:

she had married and discovered she was pregnant. In a letter to Julianne Skinner, her friend from South Carolina, Hinnant seemed to realize that life would never be the same. Maybe it was time, she wrote, to grow up and say goodbye to the "Buzzards," a secret high school club that they had jokingly kept alive all these years. The name, chosen in a moment of loneliness, expressed their belief that buzzards, much like themselves, were really beautiful, useful creatures.

In a November 1988 visit to Columbia to celebrate her parents' 40th wedding anniversary, Hinnant had talked openly of her new dilemma: should she and her husband stay in New York, which had been so professionally, and culturally, rewarding? Or, with a baby on the way, should they opt for the safe but predictable life in her native Carolinas?

That decision, however, had not yet been made, and today, as Hinnant slipped into a two-piece red dress, she still lived in the most exciting city in the world. First, she had to put in a day's work at Bellevue, preparing slides for an upcoming lecture. From there, she planned a short hop by cab to a trendy art gallery in SoHo, where she would meet her husband at 7 P.M. After that, maybe a late dinner. Such was the life-style of a childless couple. Better enjoy it while it lasted.

And so it was that at 10:30 A.M. that January morning, Dr. Kathryn Hinnant slipped into her fur jacket, and stepped outside into a brisk winter wind.

Several blocks away at Bellevue Hospital, Steven Smith, 23, was putting on surgical scrub clothes and a stethoscope. Many young physicians working long hours often slept at the hospital. Friday night Smith had been lucky; he found a quiet place on the 22nd floor where no one disturbed him. Even during the week, the hospital's top floor was lightly traveled, housing just a few administrative offices, machines, and storage areas.

Most Bellevue workers wouldn't think of going up there, particularly at night, when its emptiness could be disquieting. Getting there wasn't easy, either. The main elevators stopped at the floor below, necessitating a switch to a cramped, slow auxiliary unit. Visitors were then greeted by a dark relic of Bellevue's past hanging ominously in the main hallway. Rescued from a nearby building before it became a homeless shelter, the heavy metal plaque read:

BELLEVUE PSYCHIATRIC HOSPITAL
CITY OF NEW YORK
JAMES J. WALKER, MAYOR

Bellevue had long been a regular, full-service hospital, but to many its name was synonymous with "nuthouse." In 1887, reporter Nellie Bly feigned lunacy and went undercover as a Bellevue patient, instructing her editor to come in after her if she didn't return in 10 days. (A wise precaution, it turned out, because otherwise the hospital would have refused to release her.) Bly's nightmarish exposé helped reform the way "alienists," as psychiatrists were sometimes called back then, treated mental illness.

Nearly a half-century later, Mayor Jimmy Walker further soiled Bellevue's reputation by saying he wouldn't send a dog to its old psychiatric ward. Although a new psych building was later built, television cop shows continued to portray Bellevue as a grim last stop for the mentally deranged. Bellevue officials have long felt cursed by the hospital's desire to help patients no one else wants. But however many miracles its trauma unit performs, the hospital remains a captive of its past, never quite managing to erase Nellie Bly's century-old legacy.

Steven Smith, however, wasn't much interested in the plaque or Bellevue's history. To him, a night on the 22nd floor wasn't intimidating at all. He had been spending a lot of time at the hospital lately, and it was nice to find a quiet place to relax and sip a beer or two. Though still a relative newcomer, Smith had learned his way around Bellevue's tunnels, quirky elevators, back stairways, eating and sleeping quarters, surgery floors, and recovery rooms. To some Bellevue workers, he had already become a familiar face. And soon, it would be time for Steven Smith to make his rounds.

Most likely, Dr. Hinnant entered Bellevue through the First Avenue entrance. Had this been a regular workday instead of a Saturday, the coffee shop behind and to her left would have resembled a commodities trading pit on a day of sudden, unexpected price swings. For many first-time visitors, the sight of wildly gesturing restaurant workers shouting orders was their first indication that Bellevue might not be exactly what they expected.

Hinnant walked down a long central hallway with signs in English, Chinese, and Spanish, eventually passing a glass-enclosed security post with the word POLICE written outside in huge letters. At the reception desk, she took a left, passing a security guard on her way to the main elevator bank. This was Bellevue's most important checkpoint since it guarded the elevators leading to patient rooms, surgery floors, and beds for prisoners and psych patients.

Hinnant took the elevator to the fourth floor, where autopsies were often performed. Like the 22nd, it was lightly traveled because there were no patient rooms. She walked south a few steps, turned right, passed through a set of swinging doors, made another right, and stopped before an orange door marked 4W41. No bigger than a large walk-in closet, it was Dr. Hinnant's office. Offices across the hall had windows and natural light. Hers did not. Even her office door, unlike the others, had no window.

The fourth-floor pathology department housed an honored discipline at Bellevue, home of the nation's first laboratory for teaching and research in pathology. Hinnant's specialty was cytopathology, the study of cells; it suited her, this quiet, meticulous detective work, searching patiently for cellular changes that might signal disease. It required a certain personality—the opposite of, say, a surgeon who aggressively attacks problems already discovered.

Hinnant worked under Dr. John Pearson, director of pathology. Like many Bellevue loyalists—and there were many—he resented criticism of the hospital by people who didn't understand how well Bellevue performed with so little money. Three months earlier, during the weekend of Hinnant's wedding, Dr. Pearson had mailed a letter to the author of a lengthy article critical of medical care inside some New York hospitals. "An extraordinary situation is developing," Pearson wrote ominously. "Revenues are frequently being reduced to levels which preclude proper functioning and it is easy to understand why some hospitals, notably those attempting to serve increasingly sick indigent populations, have extreme difficulty in achieving total compliance with the ideals of theoreticians."

Dr. Hinnant didn't have time on this particular Saturday to ponder the demands of hospital management. She had her lecture to prepare. She turned on her projector, and for the next several hours she went through slide after slide, deciding which ones to use and what to say. Between 4 and 4:30 P.M., she talked with a colleague by telephone, saying she still had work to finish. Across the hall, the last rays of light could be seen through the orange metal grating that covered the office door windows. Soon, it would be dark outside.

At some point that day, Hinnant must have decided that her office was either too warm, too stuffy, or simply too claustrophobic. Spotting a small wooden box, she moved it to prop open the door.

With a little luck, she would finish in time to meet her husband at the Penine Hart Gallery. Tonight, a French composer was to perform in concert with tape recordings hidden inside wooden sculptures of characters from Marcel Proust's *Remembrance of Things Past*. It was just the sort of thing that didn't come too often to the Carolinas.

Two floors below, Steven Smith had finished his rounds. After picking up an electrical cord, he headed up to the fourth floor. It was quiet there since no autopsies were under way. He passed one orange door after another before stopping at one office. He stepped inside, picked up two magazines (one of them *Neurosurgery*), and left.

That was it—except for one final stop. Earlier, Smith had noticed a door ajar in the west hallway. Maybe he would drop in for a visit, he thought. Turning around, he walked back to the small office door marked 4W41.

"Can I talk to you a minute?" he asked, sticking his head in the doorway.

"Yeah, but I've only got a minute," Hinnant said, noticing his doctor's garb and stethoscope.

It was the opening Smith needed. He walked into Hinnant's cubicle and smashed his fist into her face, breaking her nose. Blood splattered on the floor and nearby walls.

"Why are you doing this to me?" Hinnant cried, struggling vainly against his onslaught.

Smith didn't stop. He cracked her Adam's apple and raped and sodomized her, soaking his doctor clothes in blood. He took the electrical cord he had picked up on the second floor and wrapped it around Hinnant's slender neck. Twice her blood made his hands slip off the smooth cord. Then, finally, it was over. He listened for a heartbeat, and there was none. Kathryn Hinnant was dead.

Smith pulled off the doctor's wedding ring, then grabbed her fur coat, purse, and credit cards, and left the room. The slide projector was still running. Smith raced up to the hospital roof, dropping his stethoscope along the way. After slipping into a leather jacket, he returned to the ground floor and walked out of Bellevue.

Steven Smith was not a doctor. He was not a nurse, a medical technician, or even a hospital employee. He was a vagrant, an angry homeless man who for nearly two weeks had masqueraded as a physician at Bellevue, sleeping, eating, stealing, and, finally, raping and murdering, without being discovered or stopped.

The murder of a young, pregnant doctor in a hospital was big news even in New York. THE BEAST OF BELLEVUE, shrieked one full-page headline in the *New York Post*. THE PHANTOM OF BELLEVUE, read another. The media reported that Hinnant's husband, Eric Johnson, had waited for her at the art gallery, tried calling her, got no answer, and went home. At first, he wasn't concerned, because his wife often worked late, but as hours passed with no word from her, he began calling hospitals and police stations. Still nothing.

Finally, Johnson went to Bellevue. After persuading security to let him onto the fourth floor, he tried but failed to find his wife's tiny office. Johnson then contacted the night administrator on another floor, who accompanied him back to the fourth floor. It was nearly dawn when they found Kathryn Hinnant's body.

Several days later, three homeless men seeking a $30,000 reward told police that Steven Smith had tried to sell Hinnant's credit cards and coat at a homeless shelter on nearby Wards Island. Police raced over to the shelter, where they found Smith in the lunchroom. "I strangled her," he confessed to police. "She had on a red dress. Her hair looked nice. She looked like a real lady."

After obtaining that partial confession, police put Smith in a squad car with several officers, including the chief of detectives, for the 20-minute ride from the men's shelter to the precinct house. A little while later, Smith suddenly yelled, "Stop!" Startled officers turned to see their prisoner gesturing at something outside the window. It was Bellevue. Smith muttered a few words to no one in particular, and police continued on their way.

Months later, at a trial where Smith was convicted of murdering Hinnant, the chief detective recounted what their prize suspect had uttered that January day outside the old hospital on First Avenue: "Bellevue security sucks."

It would be easy to dismiss Kathryn Hinnant's murder as fate, a tragic misfortune not unlike many thousands of others whose victims happened to be in the wrong place at the wrong time. If only she hadn't wedged open her door, Steven Smith might never have spotted her. But those seeking a specific cause might point to a lapse in hospital security. If only the guards had patrolled the fourth floor more often. If only guards had looked more closely at everyone's identification badge. If only the hospital hadn't cut the security staff before the murder.

And what about the possible culpability of the hospital's psychiatric department? Before Steven Smith began posing as a doctor, he had been a patient in one of Bellevue's psychiatric wards. The hospital released him after deciding he was no longer a risk to himself or others. If only the people who worked in Smith's ward had recognized their former patient parading around the hospital dressed as a doctor.

Finally, there was the question of whether Bellevue's open-arms invitation to the downtrodden had gone too far. Don't treat the DTs without treating the malnutrition, the hospital's philosophy went. So Bellevue began sponsoring free meals until it had to stop because too many hungry people came. If Bellevue hadn't been so kind to the destitute, if it hadn't looked the other way when the homeless sought shelter from winter winds, maybe Kathryn Hinnant wouldn't have been murdered.

Viewed narrowly, each of these explanations had merit, but for a crime so wanton, so unfathomable, they seemed inadequate. A homeless man disguised as a doctor living and killing inside a hospital? It seemed totally absurd. But Steven Smith wasn't the only undetected boarder. After the murder, Bellevue's stepped-up security rousted another homeless man living in the hospital basement; he stayed alive by scavenging for food in patient rooms. Other intruders had previously been found sleeping inside restricted areas.

Hospitals, after all, aren't bus stations; they must maintain a delicate internal environment or else risk the spread of infection and disease among patients already near death. When you mix in the presence of the most powerful drugs on earth—not to mention the kidnapping of 85 newborn babies across the country since 1983—the control of who goes where in a hospital becomes more than just a good idea; it is required under the rules of professional accreditation and state licensure.

In a larger sense, however, Hinnant's murder was important not because a hospital broke this rule or that regulation but because it symbolized an industry that had broken down in previously unimaginable ways. Happening as it did in the final year of the 1980s, it also provided a ghastly ending to the most turbulent, disruptive 10 years in the history of American hospitals—a decade when government decided once and for all to end gluttony in America's halls of healing yet health care costs soared from 9 to almost 12 percent of the gross national product; a decade when the nation's chief health investigator said that hospital management seemed second in quality only to the scandalous savings and loan industry yet the medical community called for less government scrutiny rather than more; a decade that began with the Reagan administration pushing competition as a solution to high hospital costs, yet ended with influential corporations calling for national health insurance. Add to that the confluence of AIDS, crack abuse, uninsured patients, and personnel shortages, and no hospital emerged from the 1980s unscathed.

Even as Steven Smith wandered the hallways of Bellevue, a respected health research group called the United Hospital Fund of New York was visiting 16 New York City hospitals. In a report, the group described what it had seen as "strained," "alarming," "dangerous," "overwhelmed," "grim"—these words in the first paragraph alone. "They are almost not hospitals anymore," said Dennis Andrulis, vice president of the National Association of Public Hospitals.

By 1990, much of American society had become inured to the conditions inside its hospitals: numb to nighttime cries of babies abandoned in D.C. General Hospital by drug addicts; numb to the plight of overworked employees at Nassau County Medical Center groping through 22,000 hours a year of overtime; numb to the agony of old people discharged unhealed with no suitable place to go. By 1990, it became harder to hear the daily creaking and groaning of the nation's health care system. How many times can the word "crisis" be uttered before it loses meaning? In this environment, society found it easier to consider such previously taboo issues as health care rationing—who gets what operation, or who can pull the plug on a terminally ill patient.

"Everybody has got to die sometime," philosophized Sheila Blutstein, associate administrator of Kings Highway Hospital, after government inspectors found that nine older patients had died following poor care at Blutstein's Brooklyn facility. One victim turned blue during surgery but died because of a 70-minute delay in restoring oxygen. If that was all the state had found, Blutstein told the New York *Daily News,* then she considered that an "excellent report." She added, "There is a certain percentage of patients that are going to die no matter what you do."

Even hospital regulators weren't immune to this sort of callousness. In 1988, doctors working for the federal government made a shocking discovery at Parsons Hospital in Queens. More than half of all the patients who died there during a six-month period were victims of poor care, all of them 61 years or older. Yet there were no indictments, no professional licenses revoked. The hospital simply closed, and its employees quietly moved to other institutions around the city.

Even those New Yorkers who had grown almost blasé about medical horror stories reacted to the Hinnant murder with outrage. This, after all, was a caregiver, a young doctor, pregnant and with a full life of healing ahead of her. Even worse, the murder was only part of what became the most harrowing year that anyone can remember in New York City hospitals.

Three days before Hinnant's murder, a physician at Kings County Hospital in Brooklyn compared his emergency room to Beirut. "I worked in Beirut," he told a *New York Post* reporter. "Beirut has much better conditions." An exaggeration? Perhaps. But the doctor spoke of conditions in which 44 patients were squeezed into rooms meant for 13.

In the following weeks, area hospitals would be pushed to the brink of chaos. Ambulance crews, motors running, waited hours in hospital parking lots because there were no beds to put patients in once they left ambulance stretchers. On some days, 20 percent of the city's emergency rooms closed for lack of space. The chief of the city's rescue unit filed a criminal complaint against Montefiore Hospital in the Bronx for initially refusing to accept a sick woman.

One month after Hinnant's murder a bulky man wearing a weight-lifting belt entered North Central Bronx Hospital, screaming, "I'm going to hurt somebody!" He stabbed a security officer in the neck before police shot him. The next month, at Manhattan's Metropolitan Hospital, a security guard and a housekeeper raped a patient in the emergency room. When a supervisor charged a cover-up because the rape initially had gone uninvestigated, she was fired.

Also in Manhattan, an AIDS patient at St. Luke's Roosevelt Hospital took four hostages. Two cops mistakenly fired seven shots at each other in a hospital stairwell, and one was wounded. The hostage taker killed himself, firing two bullets into his own stomach, one into his head.

Meanwhile, the specter of a serial killer surfaced at Manhattan's Lenox Hill Hospital after two patients were stricken by a deadly muscle-relaxant drug that a would-be killer had put into their IV bags. On neighboring Long Island, a nurse was already in jail on charges that he had used the same drug to murder four patients and harm three others.

Metropolitan Hospital discovered a different drug problem: a patient was caught freebasing cocaine in his hospital bed. Patients in other New York hospitals went to the street to buy drugs, then returned to their beds.

And as if all that weren't revolting enough, the *Daily News* reported that federal and city investigators, acting on a mob informant's tip, found body parts in four tons of medical waste stored illegally in a Brooklyn warehouse. Some of that waste came from New York hospitals.

One's first reaction might be to say, Well, that's New York City, always a leader in the bizarre and unpredictable. And city hospitals did, on the surface, seem to have their own unique problem: too few hospital beds. But while hospitals blamed state regulators for creating the shortage, they didn't have enough nurses or medical personnel to properly staff the additional beds they wanted.

But staff shortages weren't unique to New York; nor were crowded emergency rooms, violence, or any of the other social problems that found a final resting place inside America's hospitals. Some AIDS patients stayed in hospitals when they were well enough to leave, because there wasn't housing for them. Drug addicts crowded hospital emergency rooms because of federal cutbacks in drug treatment programs in the 1980s. Millions of uninsured patients couldn't pay for their care.

Moreover, just as the first cases of AIDS and crack abuse began to surface and the nursing shortage intensified, hospitals were rocked as never before by federal cost controls aimed at curbing abuses in Medicare. Because Medicare, a federal program passed by Congress in 1965, paid the medical bills of elderly patients, hospitals now had a guaranteed cash flow, making it easier to borrow money for new construction projects. Indeed, Medicare helped to nurture an entirely new, for-profit, shareholder-owned hospital industry.

By 1983, however, hospitals had massively overbuilt, which in turn spawned overuse of equipment and services. Into this mess stepped the federal government with its revolutionary cost control plan called the prospective-payment system. Under this program, the federal government stopped reimbursing hospitals for the cost of treating elderly patients and started paying a predetermined fee based on a patient's diagnosis. If a hospital provided care that cost less than the set fee, it got to keep the difference. If it provided more, it had to absorb the loss. Since the federal government pays nearly 40 percent of the nation's hospital bills, the effect of the new payment plan was far-reaching. Immediately, hospitals began discharging elderly patients sooner, raising fears that doctors were providing too little care, rather than too much.

Prospective payment also exposed what happens when the government lacks a comprehensive national health care policy: it attacks one problem, only to create others. The government limited inpatient reimbursements but watched passively as hospitals boosted outpatient charges to recoup revenues. The government pressured hospitals to discharge patients who weren't acutely ill, but it missed multiple deadlines in enacting a law that eventually gave some protection to unhealed patients who ended up in shoddy nursing homes.

Statistics show only one dimension of the crisis inside America's hospitals:

- More than half of big-city hospitals have, at one time or another, been kept afloat by temporary-help agencies, whose nurses are often unfamiliar with procedures and equipment, and who lack training for their assignments. Some exhausted nurses work 24-hour shifts. Even so, one in four hospitals has had to cut services because of various staff shortages.
- In New York State alone, poor hospital care figured in the deaths of nearly 7,000 patients in just one year, according to Harvard Medical School researchers. Extrapolated to a national scale, that finding suggests that poor medical care may be linked to 80,000 deaths a year.
- Fifty-one percent of surveyed hospitals don't properly review surgeries to see whether they should have been done or were done correctly. Half don't adequately monitor treatment in intensive care or coronary care units.
- Forty percent of employee benefits managers for American companies feel that the quality of medical care is now less important as they struggle against rising costs. Eighty-nine percent of Americans say their health system could use a major overhaul. Nearly one in four Americans put off medical treatment in 1989 because of cost concerns.
- About one in seven American hospitals in 1991 was financially

"distressed," raising concern that the quality of care in those institutions might be compromised.

These numbers, however, can't even begin to convey the personal frustration of individual doctors, nurses, medical technicians, social workers, and administrators as they struggle to heal in an increasingly hostile environment.

For eight years, Nancy Henry held the hands of frightened patients at Hemet Valley Hospital in Hemet, California, seeing that they weren't forgotten by overworked nurses, and helping the elderly sort through confusing medical bills and insurance forms. Then, one day in 1989, Hemet Valley Hospital said it no longer could afford Nancy Henry or the rest of her patient services department. The hospital did, however, buy a Peugeot for its administrator, build a rooftop helipad, and speculate in real estate, according to R. W. Greene of the local *Press-Enterprise*. The Nancy Henrys of the industry don't fit into any neat statistical snapshot that medical researchers use as they debate the quality of hospital care. "The hardest part about leaving," Henry said sadly, "is that patients will no longer have that kind of help."

Statistics can't convey the anguish of Dorothy Cates, whose father was sent for burial in a pauper's grave because Jamaica Hospital in Queens had failed to tell his family not only that he had been hospitalized but that he had died nine days earlier. Nor can data capture a full life lost when social workers at St. Luke's Hospital in Newburgh, New York, failed to follow up on an apparently abused infant treated in its emergency room. Three days later the same baby died at another hospital from injuries sustained after leaving St. Luke's.

Across the country, the people who once helped make hospitals humane institutions were often the first eliminated as hospitals adjusted to the new reality of living within a tight budget. Many chose the easy cuts—the dietitians, the housekeepers, the social workers, the security guards—while investing heavily in executive salaries, marketing, new construction, and kickbacks to doctors for patient referrals. Hiring an extra employee to help families find the best posthospital care didn't bring more profit, but building a new open-heart surgery unit did bring prestige, which attracted doctors, who brought patients and profits. When Hemet Valley Hospital told Nancy Henry that it no longer needed her services, it wasn't being cruel, it was merely playing the game as others played it.

Cutting corners is a strategy not without risks, however. Some patients at Harlem Hospital choked on their own mucus because there weren't enough respiratory therapists or nurses to clear their clogged breathing tubes. Chicago's Cook County Hospital jeopardized the health of children by reusing disposable breathing tubes. Detroit Receiving Hospital provided fertile soil for a hospital-bred infection that spread to 68 patients, 22 of whom eventually died. Earlier the hospital had been cited for poor infection control stemming from sloppy housekeeping.

It will be years before anyone knows conclusively how much hospital care has suffered over the last decade, but new studies raise the possibility that federal cost controls may be killing people. Elderly patients, according to the Rand Corporation and academic researchers, are now more likely to be discharged before their medical condition stabilizes, so their chance of dying increases.

Overall, hospital care remains a crapshoot for most American families. After Arizona stopped regulating the growth of open-heart units in 1985, death rates for heart surgery rose sharply in that state as individual units got fewer patients and surgeons got less practice. Most patients lack the research tools, for example, to learn that three open-heart units in northwest Indiana had mortality rates in the late 1980s two to three times greater than some hospitals an hour away in Chicago. The federal government could provide that information to the public. It could put it in every public library. But neither President Reagan nor President Bush has done so. "We are not going to start a publicity campaign," said Thomas Morford of the federal Health Care Financing Administration.

The same stonewalling characterized Congress's 1986 decision to deny patients access to a national data bank that collects records of malpractice judgments and disciplinary actions against doctors. Hospitals were supposed to use that data bank, but budget cuts and other snafus delayed its start-up until September 1990—four years after Congress ordered that it be established.

Without access to meaningful information, patients must rely on the government to protect them from bad hospital care. Recognizing that some medical providers might cut quality in the name of competition, the government promised Medicare patients that it would protect them by setting up regional peer review organizations, called PROs, to review their care. But in one two-year period in the late 1980s, the New York State PRO—one of the nation's largest—recommended sanctions against just two physicians, even though researchers found negligence resulted in almost 7,000 hospital deaths in New York in one year. Two other huge PROs covering California and Florida have been implicated in schemes to defraud the federal government.

The era, however, was not without people who fought courageously on behalf of patients. Richard Kusserow, inspector general of the Health and Human Services Department, refused to be pressured into falsely assuring the public that no one was being harmed by the prospective-payment system. "You will never get the inspector general of this department to say there isn't a big problem out there," Kusserow said, with a passion uncharacteristic of Reagan-era regulators. After one doctor discharged a gangrenous woman scheduled for surgery because her Medicare benefits had run out, this former CIA and FBI agent didn't mute his outrage. "I'd pull his license for the balance of his mortal existence," he snapped. Sadly, budget restraints meant Kusserow had to oversee almost as many programs as he had investigators.

Greater Southeast Community Hospital showed it had a passion for its neighborhood, not just its own bottom line, when it renovated or built 600 housing units in its drug-ravaged Washington, D.C., neighborhood. "What sense does it make to cure a child of pneumonia and then send that child back to inadequate slum housing in the middle of February?" asked Thomas W. Chapman, the hospital's president.

Of course, Southeast Community will one day benefit financially from a more stable surrounding neighborhood, but by 1990 many hospitals viewed their mission more narrowly and with more immediacy. Their horizons hardly extended to the next annual report, let alone the next decade. The quickest way to financial health, they concluded, wasn't building homes for the elderly but putting up medical-office buildings for doctors, or joining them in business deals, or sometimes just giving them cash. Hospitals even had a term for it, "physician bonding." Its goal was clear: get their patients. One hospital in Monroe, Louisiana, promised a doctors' group $1 million in cash. In Minneapolis, Minnesota, it was $2.5 million. In Tonawanda, New York, doctors admitting at least 10 patients per month had "the choice of dinner for two or one round of golf at the Country Club of Buffalo."

Just as the Hinnant murder symbolized the violent 1980s, physician bonding cemented by money underscored the high ethical cost of competition. The consulting firm of Arthur D. Little called some of these arrangements not far short of bribes. "They tempt providers to turn away from choosing what is best for the health care of other people to what is financially best for themselves," the firm wrote in 1989.

Certainly, hospitals needed shrewder managers in the 1980s. They needed to be made more efficient, to do more with less. But in opening their doors to the kind of business strategies that success-fully sold chicken—in treating medical care like some product line—hospitals lost generations of goodwill. And what had they all accomplished? By 1990, the rising cost of hospital services, after slowing some, had shot up to twice the rate of inflation, prompting Bruce Vladeck, president of the United Hospital Fund, to write that health care cost controls of the 1980s were "inadequately conceived, halfheartedly implemented, and largely unsuccessful."

In *The New England Journal of Medicine,* David Kinzer, former president of the Massachusetts Hospital Association, said this about the 1980s: "The most pertinent comment I can make . . . is that I know hardly any doctors or hospital executives who are comfort-able about what has been happening in our newly competitive environment."

The story of what happened to our hospitals in their most turbu-lent decade isn't just about avarice, callousness, or stupidity. It's also about well-intentioned men and women who tried to make an unmanageable situation better. That they failed isn't an indictment of their personal shortcomings. It is an indictment of a health care and hospital system that is not really a system at all but a cobbled-together collection of policies that too often harms rather than heals. Ultimately, it is a system built upon medicine's great white lie, a myth holding that hospitals and doctors are equally good and deserving of our complete, unquestioning trust. That such a belief should still prevail in this country is as disgraceful as it is dangerous.

ONE

Cutting Corners, Plugging Holes

1 | Footprints in the Sand

IT was not a sight likely to inspire patients' confidence: a nurse in uniform passed out drunk on the front lawn of Leland Memorial Hospital in Riverdale, Maryland. At midmorning on April 28, 1988, medical personnel hoisted the crumpled body of Leelamma Mathew, R.N., onto a stretcher for a trip to the emergency room. Nurse Mathew proved resilient, if nothing else. Once inside, she revived long enough to swig another snootful of spirits from one of two liquor bottles she kept in her purse.

Mathew was no stranger to Leland Memorial Hospital. Only hours before her stuporous collapse, she had completed an eight-hour overnight shift at Leland, during which she had signed out multiple doses of the potent painkiller Demerol—sometimes called liquid heroin—without, apparently, administering it to patients. A few days earlier, Mathew had twice signed out Demerol for a patient who showed no signs of needing any pain medication. Later that shift, she suffered a grand-mal seizure at the nurse's station. On a previous shift at another institution, she was seen staggering and was accused of abandoning her patients.

None of this, however, would keep Mathew from suiting up again and again as a human lifeline to seriously ill patients. Later on the same day when she had collapsed dead drunk outside the hospital, she returned to Leland for another eight-hour shift. The hospital not only let her in, it put her to work. And twice during that shift, she again signed out Demerol with no documentation that patients had ever received it.

Leland Memorial finally concluded that it had seen enough of Mathew. No matter. She knew another job was just a telephone call away. This time, she sought employment through a shadowy, burgeoning industry that provides day labor nurses to thousands of medical facilities across America. As a nurse temp, Mathew's appalling work record disappeared like footprints in the sand. Screw up at one place, just move to another; one day here, one day there. By the time a medical facility could build a case of nursing malpractice, the offending nurse would simply disappear.

Yolanda Holland worked as an agency nurse in Maryland hospitals even though her rap sheet included a two-year prison sentence and convictions for fraud and passing bad checks. She also allegedly stole checks from patients, mishandled prescription drugs, forged the signature of her hospital nursing supervisor, and put patients' lives in danger through negligence.

Barbara Dugger's agency sent her to work in a Baltimore prison health unit. Once, while on duty at 10 A.M., she appeared unstable and intoxicated. A search of her personal belongings turned up 12 syringes, one large rubber band, pills, and 59 plastic vials of what appeared to be cocaine. She was arrested and charged with cocaine possession.

Even nurse Mathew, with the help of her agency, found work again. And once more, in August 1989, she was suspected of abusing Demerol after her employer found seven syringes of Demerol with broken seals.

In the past, hospitals could keep a wary eye on suspicious nurses and, at the very least, contain the problem. But with the rise of temp agencies, problem nurses in effect metastasized, spilling their poison into the bloodstream of the nation's hospital system.

Although many agency nurses were competent, sometimes excellent, administrators rightfully felt queasy hiring unknown and unpredictable contract laborers. But hire them they did. With one in every eight nursing jobs in hospitals vacant—one in five in New York City—agencies promised a quick fix, one less worry for administrators already facing federal cost controls, empty beds, more competition, and the onset of AIDS and crack. Temps had further appeal because hospitals didn't pay them benefits, and unlike regular employees, they did not have to be carried on the payroll when patient occupancy dropped.

But by succumbing to the quick fix, administrators soon entered a vicious circle: the more they relied on temps, the more they ignored the underlying causes of their nursing shortage, such as poor pay and overwork; and the more they ignored those causes, the more permanent staff nurses they lost, requiring more and more temps. Like a junkie with a growing habit, hospitals often found a single supplier inadequate. Soon, individual hospitals were turning to 10, 15, even 20 agencies to meet their growing demand. One midsized Florida hospital used temps to fill 140,000 work hours in 1988, while others commonly tapped contract labor for 30,000 to 40,000 hours annually.

The failure of administrators to aggressively confront the nursing shortage exposed the changing values of the hospital industry. Nurses are the bulwark of any hospital, as indispensable as a heart is to a human. Yet when new federal cost controls in 1983 encouraged hospitals to butcher their budgets—it wasn't advertising that suffered, but rather nursing care. Licensed practical nurses (LPNs) and nurse's aides had little political muscle, so they were among the first to go; nearly 125,000 of them lost their jobs from 1983 to 1987. That gussied up the bottom line, but it meant RNs had to cover for their departed coworkers at a time when they already faced sicker patients and more complex technology.

Waiting in the wings were the temp agencies. By the late 1980s, more than half of all big-city hospitals were kept afloat by temp agencies, providing everything from pharmacists to nurse's aides. The agencies could be as ephemeral as the faceless workers they provided, opening and closing like floating crap games. In Cleveland, Ohio, a new temp agency seemed to surface every couple of weeks. Florida's Palm Beach County hosted 60 agencies, more or less, depending on which month one did the counting. Free of virtually any government regulation, some set up shop with little more than a telephone and a Rolodex.

While stories of agency nurse screwups were legion inside hospitals, patients almost never knew that the nurse injecting a needle in their vein might be as much a stranger to the hospital as to them. They didn't know that the world of temporary staffing was one marked by allegations of forgeries, false billings, forced labor, theft, impostors, and poor medical care. If they were lucky, they never experienced temps who spoke no English, never had the wrong end of a thermometer inserted in them, never had their vital signs taken by a moonlighting spray-painter.

The greatest threat, however, came not from the scoundrel or the incompetent but from well-meaning, well-educated medical workers who simply were pushed beyond their endurance or dropped with no orientation into alien institutions. Hospitals don't share the conformity of McDonald's hamburger stands; they store drugs differently, call codes differently, use medical equipment differently. Temps had to know all those things and more. And when they didn't, the potential for accidents—even tragedy—was unlimited. "You need to understand that at 11 at night when you have a nursing need, [it] isn't the time to negotiate quality standards," said Peter E. Faron, a nursing director at Palm Beach Regional Hospital. "You need a nurse."

One night, about two weeks before Christmas, Chicago's Cook County Hospital experienced just that need, so it hired a temp. Far from the festive storefront displays of North Michigan Avenue in a darkened West Side neighborhood, the parents of Naymat Ahmed celebrated his birth inside Cook County Hospital. Although the baby developed a common infection, the temp nurse merely had to follow hospital protocol in administering an antibiotic. Because she didn't, the boy later suffered irreversible brain damage, and seven and a half years later could neither walk nor speak. The hospital paid a steep price for its error: an $8 million malpractice verdict. But did it clean up its act? State inspectors didn't think so. In 1989, they cited Cook County for failing to prove that it had either oriented its temp workers properly or taken the time to evaluate the temp agencies from which it obtained nurses.

Many hospitals stood guilty of the same offense, yet little has been done about it. When HHS secretary Dr. Otis Bowen formed a commission to undertake the definitive study of the nursing crisis, it reported back in late 1988 with dozens of recommendations. Not one mentioned agency nurses.

In this regulatory vacuum, patients must trust the integrity of the people who run these agencies. Their lives depend on it. Temp nurses don't just empty bedpans; they fill some of the most important jobs in the entire hospital—often in intensive care and critical care units, where nurses are the most scarce. So what actually goes on inside those agencies that play such an essential role in the health of a nation? Like most Americans, Sharon Aussler had no idea, until one summer morning she stumbled into their murky world. She was to get a lesson in life she would never forget.

• • •

It promised to be such a grand adventure. See sunny Florida. Live near the ocean, experience a life that seemed so distant and so bountiful to a single mother of three living in the dirt-poor town of Plumerville, Arkansas, population 700.

This dream of a better life visited Sharon Aussler one day in May 1987 when she picked up a copy of the *Arkansas Democrat.* She turned past stories of an airline crash in Poland and the discovery of a young woman's body with multiple stab wounds 40 miles away in sleepy Floyd, Arkansas. This morning she could not have cared less. With a sense of purpose, Aussler dug deep into the paper, not stopping until she reached the classifieds. Passing over the ads for secretaries and VCR repairmen, her eyes stopped at classified section 73. And there it was:

ATTENTION ALL NURSES
RN's & LPN's needed. RN's $16 to $18 per hour plus housing. LPN's $12.50 hour with temporary housing, free travel for all. Call 305-737-5634.

It appeared simple and small against a background of other, more impressive nursing ads, like the huge one right underneath with the long, flowing letters that promised "A Beautiful Beginning." A beautiful beginning? Are they kidding? Aussler had seen Arkansas hospitals and nursing homes make that kind of pitch before. But this little ad . . . now, that was different. Free travel for all. Even a place to stay.

Aussler welcomed any change. At age 23, her life had been marked by fitful starts and stops. She tried one year of college in Pine Bluff, Arkansas, but that didn't work out. She tried another year at the University of Central Arkansas in Conway but quit with no degree. Along the way she had three kids. Since late in her teens, however, Aussler always had a vocation to fall back on. She was a nurse, a licensed practical nurse. In past years, that would have guaranteed her a lifetime of options, but times were changing. As hospitals faced sicker patients and used more complex medical equipment, many no longer wanted LPNs, who had less formal training than registered nurses. LPNs often were relegated to depressing nursing-home care.

A wave of excitement washed over Aussler as she dialed the

number listed in the ad. At the other end of the line, she found the state of Florida and the pleasant-sounding voice of Julie Monahan, president of All Care Nursing Service.

"There's a big shortage of nurses in South Florida," Monahan explained, according to Aussler. "We're kind of close to Miami, but it's not like 'Miami Vice' or anything. We'll provide transportation once you are here, and you'll make $12.50 an hour." Monahan also promised to reimburse Aussler for her flight down and arrange a place for her to stay.

"One good thing about us," Aussler recalled Monahan saying, "is that you can pick the hours and the places you want to work. And if you find you don't like one place, you don't have to go there again." Monahan promised to send her a job application.

Aussler was hooked. She completed the application once it arrived and set about planning her move. Her two sons could stay with family in Arkansas, and her daughter could go to a sister in Illinois. If all went well, she would send money to her children, and maybe bring them down to Florida. Finally, all that remained was one last call to Monahan to arrange a few more details. With that completed, Aussler boarded a plane for Florida, the start of what she hoped would be her "beautiful beginning."

Aussler was scheduled to work in the heart of Palm Beach County. Although Palm Beach was best known as a haven for the polo set, the surrounding county had exploded in population over the last several decades. West Palm Beach, once the staging ground for its affluent neighbor, had become a major city in its own right. An influx of retirees added diversity, filling miles of condominiums that stretched south along the Atlantic in such communities as Delray Beach and Boynton Beach.

Temp agencies found Palm Beach County particularly inviting. Because residents flooded in and out depending on the season, patient loads at the dozen or so regional hospitals fluctuated widely. By helping hospitals vary staffing levels, agencies had more business than they could handle, giving rise to new agencies. Peter Faron found himself besieged by "no less than 20 or 30" agencies in his first two weeks as nursing director at Palm Beach Regional Hospital. Sometimes, it seemed, hospitals hired whoever came through the door. One area hospital, during a seven-month stretch in 1989, bought labor from 20 different agencies bearing such names as Angels in White, Expicare, High Tech Staffing, Quality Professional Nursing of South Florida, American Health Tech, Nurse Care, A Complete Health Service, Atlantic, Nurse on Call, Team Nursing, Immediate Healthcare, Olsten, and Medex.

As the purveyors of a valued and finite service, agencies became the proverbial 800-pound gorilla, sitting wherever they pleased. "Every three months there would be new prices, and there didn't seem to be any correlation between the prices that were charged and the value of the services," complained Chandler Bailey, vice president of the South Florida Hospital Association.

Agencies, meanwhile, fought one another like a horde of gold prospectors panning the same stream. Many across the country went so far as to pay bounties for nurse recruits. "Our Xmas Referral Bonus special continues!" barked one agency in an advertisement. "$200 for RNs [and] $75 for Hospital Attendants . . . This offer is limited to those referrals hired between October 1 and December 31, 1990."

Nurses from agency A tried to recruit temps from agency B by suggesting that agency B would soon go out of business. Agency B might sow dissension by saying A secretly paid certain nurses more money. Agency recruiters, however, found their biggest pigeons inside hospitals, where staff nurses tired quickly of working alongside agency nurses who earned more.

John Roylance knew firsthand how savagely the game of temp-staffing was played. One day at a Boynton Beach restaurant called the Banana Boat, he and two others began talking about how easy it would be to start an agency. From there, a plan was hatched. One participant in the meeting had a key to the temp agency where she worked. According to Roylance, she waited one night until her agency's West Palm Beach office closed; then, under cover of darkness, she went in and carted out personnel lists, employment applications, and sales packages. Afterward, Roylance said, he helped copy those documents.

That night, a new agency was born. "Being that we had [the documents], we were able to start business right away," said Roylance, who went to work for the new firm. "If you start a business, you have to go looking for nurses. We didn't have to look. I mean, we had them. Just had to dial their telephone number and say, you know, 'We'd like you to go to work.' "

As agencies mud-wrestled among themselves for greater and greater profits, complaints rolled in from doctors and patients about the quality of the labor they provided. "After they worked a shift, you would question where they got their nursing credentials," complained Sue Bradford, nursing director at Delray Community Hospital. "Physicians were concerned about what they saw—a lack of caring attitudes, lack of organization, lack of wanting to be a part [of] or even to be at the hospital."

Hospitals, on the other hand, hardly distinguished themselves in handling temps. Upon discovering an unsuitable worker, a hospital merely told the sponsoring agency not to send that person again. "We simply just took the posture that as long as it's not happening at my facility, what do I care?" confessed Peter Faron of Palm Beach Regional Hospital. This policy wasn't in the long-range interest of anyone, particularly patients.

Hospitals further tried to get around bad temps by specifically requesting people known to them as conscientious workers. Agencies eagerly promised the desired temps—even when they weren't available, a practice known as "phantom-booking." If a hospital wanted Mrs. Jones for an overnight shift and Mrs. Smith showed up at 11 P.M., the hospital had no choice but to accept her. After all, it needed a nurse. One agency official explained her company's policy this way: "They want a nurse? Give them a name. Even if you haven't filled the shift, you have to give a name so the facility thinks they have somebody coming." Usually, a body could be produced in time, but not always. "Sometimes you'd have to call 50, 60 people," said the agency official. "Sometimes you'd work till 1 [A.M.] or 2 filling a shift for an 11-to-7."

Palm Beach County residents, meanwhile, probably never pondered the dangers of a health care system that failed to screen out bad nursing until one day they read about the case of Ruth Nedermier, a well-liked, 72-year-old retired schoolteacher. In 1988, while recovering from surgery in her West Palm Beach home, Nedermier sought help from a local temp agency called Redi-Nurse. The agency sent Inger Lemont, a nurse's aide in her early 20s. Redi-Nurse did not fully check Lemont's background before sending her, nor was it legally required to do so. Consequently, neither the agency nor Nedermier knew that Inger Lemont had just gotten out of prison after her conviction for stealing $8,000 in jewelry from another elderly patient.

Lemont, true to form, would also steal from Ruth Nedermier. But that hardly seemed significant once Lemont's parents noticed a strange steamer trunk that their daughter brought home one day. Lemont gave several explanations for the trunk, which had developed a wretched stench, including one that it held wholesale meat. Finally, Lemont's father could contain his curiosity no more. With his daughter out of the house, he peeked inside the trunk. There, he found Ruth Nedermier, cut in pieces by a chain saw. Police identified the bloody mess of jagged bones by a serial number on Nedermier's artificial hip. In June 1989, Inger Lemont was sentenced to 75 years in prison for her role in the woman's murder.

Today, more than ever, people need good home nursing since hospitals, under pressure from federal cost controls, no longer allow patients to convalesce in their beds. Even so, home nursing—along with the temp agencies that provide it—continues to receive even less scrutiny than does nursing care in hospitals and nursing homes.

When Sharon Aussler arrived in Florida, she knew nothing about the rough-and-tumble world she was about to enter. As she hailed a cab to take her from the airport to Julie Monahan's All Care Nursing Service, Aussler's mind focused on how she might enjoy the upcoming Fourth of July holiday. There were beaches, sunshine, and plenty of time for relaxation. Soon, her cab turned east onto Woolbright Avenue, passing a series of ball fields, before exiting onto Seacrest Boulevard, framed by the Boynton Beach water tower on one side and a cemetery on the other. A few more blocks, and her cab pulled into a circular driveway in front of All Care's office.

Aussler said she collected $250 in travel reimbursement from Julie Monahan. She then set out to soak up her new Florida environment. On this glorious day, Aussler had no way of knowing how quickly her dream would dissolve into a blur of torment and anguish.

2 | Impostors

JULIE Monahan's round belly and casual dress cast her as an unlikely chief executive of an agency with $6 million in annual gross income. Her attire, according to an All Care customer, was your standard "flip-flops and shorts, that sort of thing." But that was dressy, at least for the office.

"Julie would hardly ever put on clothes," recalled one nurse who saw Monahan frequently at All Care's headquarters. "She was always in a long lounging gown, no bra, sitting around just like that." Monahan said she often wore a muumuu. Her short hair and ruddy complexion did little to adorn an average frame dominated by her midsection.

Her appearance, however, belied a keen business mind and a competitive edge that would make a Wall Street bond trader cower. She battled larger nationwide agencies on even terms by playing tougher and smarter. Monahan's success stemmed in part from her ability to find people of limited options. With only so many nurses in Palm Beach County, she devised a strategy of using newspaper ads to target nurses in economically depressed areas in Arkansas, Alabama, Louisiana, Tennessee, and North Carolina. She hoped that by investing up front to bring in new nurses, she would reap profits on the back end. It worked. By the late 1980s, All Care was one of the biggest agencies in Palm Beach County.

Sharon Aussler was a recruit who would depend heavily on All Care for help in adjusting to her new life in Florida. She had no car, no place to live, little money, and (initially, at least) no local friends.

All Care functioned as her umbilical cord to the world, providing at various times everything from local transportation to cheap lodging. In turn, Julie Monahan got some control over workers like Aussler.

Aussler spent her first few days in Florida relaxing in a motel. Monahan recalled that she "came off the plane asking me for a loan . . . I think I gave her $100. She wanted to party at Palm Beach." Whatever she did, Aussler found her money running low after the holiday, and she called All Care for her first assignment. She didn't wait long. An overnight shift needed filling, so All Care put Aussler to work without, she said, either testing her nursing knowledge or administering any other screening exams. The agency did, however, have her sign a contract stipulating that for three months she wouldn't work for any other agency. At the time, it probably didn't seem significant.

Aussler's first job turned out fine, but there was something about Monahan that didn't seem quite right. Soon after arriving at All Care, she was sitting with some fellow nurses when Monahan suddenly appeared. "You are here to work," Aussler said Monahan told her. "If you go to the beach, I want to know it. And I want to know exactly which beach you go to." And that was it. End of discussion.

Aussler was taken aback. It wasn't so much what she said as how she said it. This was not the same tone Monahan had used on the telephone that day in Arkansas. It was merely a hint of what was to come.

All Care had promised Aussler a place to stay, and she was in no position to turn down the offer. But if she entertained any thoughts of an apartment near the ocean with a salty breeze ruffling curtains through an open window, they quickly disappeared when she saw the reality of what awaited her. "I didn't know when I got here that we were going to be living in the back of the office," Aussler said. Instead of crashing waves, there was the rumble of high-speed freight cars on a nearby railroad track. Monahan also provided living quarters elsewhere in the city, but this is where she put Aussler— and a number of other nurses.

All Care was located in a modest one-story house in a semiresidential neighborhood several blocks from doctors' offices and Bethesda Hospital. Most nurses were given beds in a larger room, while others stayed elsewhere in the house, which included another room, a kitchen, two bathrooms, and an office that served as All Care's nerve center, filled with file cabinets, desks, and telephones. A house that an upper-middle-class family of four might find comfortable instead provided shelter for as many as 18 people at a time, according to one former All Care employee. Monahan said the most was "probably 10 or 11." Even so, that was in addition to an office staff that often labored from dawn until 1 A.M., smoking, typing, running the photocopy machine, and working the phones.

"There were four or five desks in one room," said a former office supervisor for All Care. "We were all able to smoke at our desks if we wanted to. There was a fan in the middle of the room." A microwave and a refrigerator were added nearby since going out to lunch was discouraged.

Apart from all the commotion, Aussler didn't appreciate the close living quarters. There were too many people for too few bathrooms. "You had no privacy," said one All Care nurse, who eventually moved out. "We were sharing bathrooms with men, and it was just getting wild and I couldn't handle it anymore." Personal belongings were sometimes just stored in suitcases. When All Care put in a bookshelf, Aussler claimed it for her small corner of the world, something she could control. Monahan said Aussler could have moved out anytime she wanted to.

Aussler had considerably less influence over other parts of her life. She said that although All Care had promised to help provide local transportation, such promises proved unreliable. Once, after completing a shift at a nursing home, she was picked up by an All Care driver for what she thought was a ride home. "We were in the car talking," Aussler recalled. "I thought I was going back to the house, and she pulled up at Bethesda [Hospital]. So I figured she was picking somebody else up. I said, 'Who are you waiting on?' She said, 'No, Julie said you have to work.' So I just got out of the car and went to work." Monahan subsequently said she doubted that such an incident took place. She also denied ever promising Aussler transportation.

On another occasion, Aussler had just finished an afternoon shift followed by an overnight shift. At 7 A.M., after 16 straight hours at two facilities, she anxiously awaited her ride home. It finally came— three hours later.

Aussler was plenty peeved, but her indoctrination into the world of agency nursing had only just begun. Standing up to Julie Monahan might sound simple; it was anything but. "Julie had a very, very strong personality," said John Roylance, who worked for All Care as a nursing assistant in the early 1980s. Monahan could be most generous or very nasty, he said.

Roylance recalled the time when, not wanting to be bothered at home, he unplugged his phone. Later, he heard a knock at his door. It was the police. "There's a medical emergency," the cop said. "Call your office."

"Another time she [Monahan] had me paged at a movie theater because my son answered the phone and he told her where I was," Roylance said. Monahan locked onto a target's vulnerability like an Exocet missile. Roylance believed she knew he had been put on probation for passing a bad check. So when he declined to work, he says, Monahan called his probation officer.

Yes, Monahan was tough. Yes, she was persistent. But there was another element of her personality that stood above all the rest. "There's no polite way to put it: Julie has a mouth like a longshoreman," Roylance said. "I was brought up in Hoboken [New Jersey], and I'm familiar with longshoremen."

Women in particular said they found her language intimidating. Becky Seibert, a former All Care nurse, told the story of how All Care wanted her to fill a shift even though her apartment had flooded from a broken toilet. Seibert, a former teacher, reluctantly agreed. But on the way to her assignment, her car broke down on I-95. After hitching a ride to a gas station, she said, she called Monahan to tell her she couldn't make it to work.

"We'll lose the account," Monahan pleaded.

"I'm sorry," Seibert replied.

"You stay right where you are. I'm coming to get you."

"I don't think so. You're not coming to get me. My car's broken down. I'm not going to leave my car on 95 for somebody to walk away with or drive away with."

Seibert said Monahan exploded in a string of expletives, calling her "a fucking whore, cunt, and bitch." Monahan denied ever directing abusive language at any employee, although she acknowledged that she occasionally swore. Whatever kind of language Monahan used, Seibert didn't budge. She retrieved her car, finally getting home at 11 that night. But she hadn't heard the last of All Care. When Seibert switched on her answering machine, there it was, over and over again, leaving messages at what seemed like 15-minute intervals.

Like a battered and beaten boxer, Seibert had discovered that she could indeed run, but she couldn't hide.

Although her lodging was unpleasant, Sharon Aussler didn't mind it as much as she might have under different circumstances. That was because in the beginning she spent little time there. When not working, she usually slept. When not sleeping, she worked—and there seemed to be a lot more of the latter than the former.

With hospitals spending so much money on temps (JFK Medical Center in Palm Beach County doled out $1.7 million for temp nurses in one four-month period), Monahan eagerly sought her share. In 1988, All Care filled 23,725 eight-hour nursing shifts at area hospitals. She also serviced some hospitals outside the area. About half of All Care's shifts were in nursing homes.

To meet the demand, Monahan tried to squeeze as much as possible out of her workers. And when that wasn't enough, her workers say, she squeezed some more. "We were not asked do we want to go to work, we were told we had to go to work," Aussler said.

When Aussler struck up a romance with a man outside the office, she recalled Monahan being upset. "I didn't bring you to Florida to get fucked," Aussler said she was told. "I brought you here to get work." Monahan would later deny making that comment. Aussler, who is black, said she suffered other indignities, like the time she was resting in her bed, close enough to All Care's office to hear the conversation inside.

"Where's that nigger?" Monahan asked.

"She's sleeping," an office worker replied.

"Well, she ain't fuckin' sleepin' in here today. Tell her to get her ass out of here. She ain't going to sleep in here." Later, Monahan denied that she would ever use the word "nigger." "Not unless I was talking to somebody who I was very close friends with," she said. "No, I would not use it."

Sleep, some All Care workers said, merely got in the way of money. Nurses worked 16-hour days and 20-hour days. Worse, their shifts were often consecutive—a nightmare seemingly without end.

"There were people sleepwalking, sleeptalking," Aussler said. "I was sleeping in the bathrooms in [medical] facilities, I was sleeping on the floors; anywhere I could catch a nap, I would do it. I was not the only one." Weary nurses would help each other, one watching the floor while the other slept. When Aussler finally did collapse in exhaustion at home, there always seemed to be someone kicking her bed, telling her to get up and begin the whole process all over again. "I was never Sharon, I was always a whore, or a bitch, or a slut, or a cunt," Aussler recalled. "I did not come to Florida to be treated like a dog. I came to Florida to make a life for me and my three kids . . . at least a dog can run somewhere." Sometimes Aussler would sit with her roommates and cry in frustration.

Working 80 or more hours a week took a huge toll on the nurses, not to mention their patients. Aussler said she was so tired she sometimes couldn't read a patient's medication record. And if she couldn't understand it, she did nothing, figuring no medication was better than an overdose. "I got to the point where I would skip some patients just to be done," she recalled. Sometimes she decided who got medicine and who didn't by how much work was involved. A patient on a heavy regimen of medication got nothing; one requiring only a couple of pills got them.

This informal triage system developed because agency nurses were judged, in part, on their ability to cover a certain number of patients in a certain period of time. A tired nurse who moved too slowly might not be asked to return. Aussler's conduct was guided not by nursing's noble mission but by a cold, crass assessment of her own self-interest, which she explained this way: "A patient, if he doesn't know his name, can't tell anybody if he had his medicine or not." Aussler didn't feel good about what she was doing, and she said other nurses felt the same way. "I put myself and a lot of patients in jeopardy," she said, although she doesn't know if anyone was harmed.

Hospital officials knew that temp nurses were showing up for duty exhausted from other shifts, but they felt powerless to stop it. By the time they recognized the problem, it was too late; their patients needed care, and a tired nurse was better than no nurse. Overworked temps may have been the least of their troubles, however. More than ever, hospitals and nursing homes were failing to grasp a basic truth about some temp agencies: what you see is not always reality, and what you buy is not always what you get.

Becky Seibert first heard about Monahan's temp agency through an advertisement in a New Orleans newspaper. Unlike Aussler, she had a car, so she set out for the long drive from Louisiana to southern

Florida. Although she held an out-of-state nursing license, Seibert had no Florida license. Thinking she could merely pick up credentials, she stopped in Jacksonville, only to learn she needed a physical that screened out anyone who might be seriously ill and a danger to patients in weakened conditions.

Frustrated, Seibert continued her trip to Boynton Beach. After getting lost and calling All Care for better directions, she finally arrived with the bad news that she lacked the credentials to work as a Florida nurse. But All Care, Seibert says, told her not to worry about it. Then, ignoring Seibert's status, and the fact that she had just driven into town, Seibert says All Care tried to send her out on a midnight shift.

Seibert declined on that evening but soon began working without a Florida license, she said. Seibert eventually got one, but she said other risky practices would follow.

Seibert, a licensed practical nurse, could not perform all the duties of a registered nurse. One day, about a week before Christmas in 1987, Seibert recalls, Julie Monahan came to her with an unusual request: "Can you work this evening as an RN? This nursing home needs an RN on the premises."

"But I'm not an RN. What do I do? How do I do this?"

"Just scribble 'RN' after your signature and do your job."

Seibert said Monahan discussed how to camouflage this notation. By signing a sloppy "RN," Seibert could later, if necessary, deny writing it. She practiced scribbling it several times on scratch paper. "That's fine," Monahan observed. Later, through her lawyer, Monahan would deny that she ever knowingly sent out a worker to fill a job without the proper license.

On the same day, Seibert, whose story was backed up by a former office supervisor at All Care, went out to work as an RN from 11 P.M. to 7:30 A.M. No other RN was on the premises, she recalled. If a serious problem developed on another wing, a second LPN was to call Seibert, not knowing that she, too, was only an LPN. As it turned out, the facility did have seriously ill patients that evening, so Seibert had to remain past the end of her shift until "another" RN arrived to relieve her.

One day, in a private moment, Becky Seibert confessed to Sharon Aussler about her secret life as an RN. "Sharon," she said, "you can do it. Just go in and act like you know what you're doing. I've been a nursing supervisor. There's nothing to it."

Aussler was shocked. "Becky, what are you going to do if a patient codes?" she asked. "You might have to start an IV, push medicine through the IV. We're not licensed to do that."

"I'll dial 911," Seibert said, a retort better suited to a Mel Brooks movie than a medical facility.

Eventually, Seibert said, she would pose as an RN for about half a dozen shifts in several medical facilities. As she bent the rules, she began to wonder about others who worked beside her—like the LPN who didn't seem to know how to do a simple tube feeding. It was almost as if she had never done it before, Seibert thought.

Aussler had also heard of some strange goings-on. Two LPNs besides Becky Seibert told her they had posed as RNs, Aussler said. She also suspected, although she had no specific proof, that certain individuals were posing as certified nurse's aides (CNAs). Her first tip: they could hardly speak English. "There is no way I felt they could even pass CNA school," she said. "When you say, 'Go give a bath,' and they tell you, 'Me don't speak no English.' If you're a nurse's aide, you got to know when somebody tells you go give a bath." Some CNAs merely showed up for work, grabbed a blanket, and lay down.

CNAs were supposed to do more than just clean patients. They should know how to take a patient's vital signs, such as temperature and blood pressure. Aussler, however, saw temp CNAs who could do neither. "I had a nurse's aide from All Care give me a 110 temp," she said.

All of this raised a basic question: if All Care was so bad, why did Seibert and Aussler continue working for the agency? "It was good money, more money than I ever had made in my whole life," Seibert said. When that money wasn't enough, Julie Monahan further extended her influence by advancing loans to workers. Plus, she charged workers only $40 a week for lodging.

And if the carrot didn't work, there was always the stick. "You knew if at any one point that you didn't do what you were asked to do, you wouldn't work there. You wouldn't work anywhere," Seibert said. When she moved out of All Care's office into her own apartment, thus lessening Monahan's control over her, Seibert said, she stopped getting regular work. She moved back in. When Sharon Aussler declined certain shifts, she said, her flow of assignments suddenly dried up. With a family back home that needed money, Aussler couldn't afford any interruption of income.

Aussler and Seibert also feared being sued for violating contracts that restricted their temp work to All Care. "Any law student knows that's involuntary servitude and unenforceable," said Phil Allen, a Miami lawyer representing southern Florida hospitals. Even so, it kept Aussler and others in line.

Intimidation was a more subtle form of control. Apart from Monahan's alleged use of foul language—which Aussler began returning in kind as the weeks rolled on—Aussler worried about her physical well-being. Once, she said, she heard someone talk about paying money to rough up another worker. Another time, Aussler said she answered the All Care phone and listened to someone deliver a bomb threat. Although no bomb was found, it added to the overall tension.

One thing was for sure. As soon as her three-month contract expired, Aussler wouldn't waste a second getting the hell out of there. Still, she wondered whether there wasn't some way to pay Monahan back, to help others avoid going through the same thing. Yes, she thought: maybe if she could collect enough evidence of Monahan's alleged wrongdoing, she could present it to authorities. Monahan would then get what was coming to her, she fantasized.

But no matter how much Aussler knew, it would never be the full story. Always the outsider, she never crashed Monahan's inner circle; only they knew what really went on inside that smoke-filled room packed with All Care's file cabinets and telephones. One insider who did know plenty was a high school graduate named Sheila Ripley Brubaker, who early on had caught Monahan's eye.

Sheila Brubaker came to All Care as a nurse's aide in August 1985. Several weeks after beginning work, Monahan called her into the office. "You're bright," she said. "Can you type? Would you like to work in the All Care office?" Six months later, Monahan promoted Brubaker to office supervisor. Brubaker would also become roommates with Monahan's daughter.

Brubaker was All Care's equivalent of an air traffic controller, making sure All Care workers got in and out of their assignments. It was a tense job with a demanding boss. "I had a boyfriend take me out to lunch, and I asked for an hour lunch break. [Monahan] thought I said a half hour. I got back an hour later, the allotted time, and she raised her voice at me and told me never do that again."

Brubaker didn't. In fact, she avoided going out to lunch at all, so as not to upset Monahan.

Part of Brubaker's job amounted to fitting square pegs into round holes. In the ideal world, she could draw on an unlimited supply of well-qualified temps whenever a medical facility needed extra help: a specially trained RN for critical care units, an LPN to administer basic medicines, a CNA to take vital signs. Unfortunately, the right people weren't always available. No reputable agency would send an unqualified person, but All Care did, according to Brubaker and other former employees. Monahan denied playing any role in sending out unqualified personnel.

But John Roylance, the ex–All Care employee from Hoboken, said Julie Monahan once sent him to work as an LPN. The only problem: he wasn't an LPN, or an RN, or a nurse at all. He was simply a nurse's aide. "You can go to a uniform store and buy an LPN pin and [stick] it on," Roylance explained. He said Monahan told him to buy one of those pins—a charge Monahan denied. Such subterfuge wasn't all that dangerous, he said. "Julie never sent me on a nurse case where it wasn't more than a baby-sitter job." His nursing assignments were mostly for very wealthy people who wanted a white worker. No pin was necessary for that particular qualification.

Fooling a hospital usually required more than a name tag, however. That called for a more imaginative approach, one that Bethesda Hospital accidentally uncovered. To screen out unsuitable employees, Bethesda and several other area hospitals devised a test to measure an agency nurse's knowledge of drugs and medicine. The system appeared to work fine, until Bethesda began noticing the percentage of accurate answers rising sharply. After switching to a new test, the hospital couldn't ignore a pattern of very strange answers. The responses weren't just wrong, they bore little relationship to the questions. This had never happened before. At some point, a hospital official followed a hunch and retrieved the earlier test. The answers matched. The temps had memorized answers to the wrong test.

The discovery may have come as a big surprise to Bethesda, but not to Sheila Ripley Brubaker or others inside All Care. Brubaker recalled passing the test around to All Care nurses before they went to the hospital. In fact, Brubaker remembered All Care having the medicine tests from two hospitals in addition to Bethesda. Monahan said that the tests were used only as a teaching tool, and that she had obtained the tests openly from the hospitals. And All Care wasn't the only temp agency to obtain copies of the test. At least one other coached its workers for the exams.

Although circumventing the purpose of exams could expose patients to nurses who might not be competent, it was merely a school-yard prank compared to other allegations of All Care's mischief. In attempting to meet the needs of the agency's clients, Sheila Ripley Brubaker had developed an exciting new skill: forgery. Like a master counterfeiter, she resolved to create a masterpiece.

It had a name. She called it the Perfect File.

3 | The Perfect File

IF what former All Care employees alleged was true, then the agency had more to worry about than just fooling hospitals and nursing homes. All Care also had to undergo the occasional visit from state health authorities. And that required preparation. Actually, Florida did more than other states, most of which never bothered to visit temp agencies at all. A hard-nosed regulator in Florida could indeed make life unpleasant for an errant agency.

Over the years, Florida had enacted rules to protect patients from incompetent medical personnel. Nurse's aides in certain settings must be certified as having completed educational requirements. Medical personnel must have proof that they were examined by a doctor and found in good physical health. LPNs and RNs must be properly licensed and must meet continuing education requirements. A conscientious regulator would check all those things.

That posed a dilemma for All Care, according to Brubaker. All Care needed an accurate record of the background of its employees, yet it didn't want possible violations of state rules to be discovered in the agency's own files. The solution, Brubaker said, keep two files: the unvarnished truth in one, and a scrubbed-up version—the perfect file—in the other. "The perfect file was a file that had been created," explained Brubaker. In other words, if a worker lacked an essential document, All Care forged one.

"Julie told us to create perfect files because if you didn't have a perfect file she would go out of business," Brubaker said. "She demanded that I get things in order, on time, because the state was coming in July or August or whatever month they were scheduled to come in. She would notify me months beforehand. 'Have you got all the files in order? You have to get all the files right. They've got to be perfect.' "

There was plenty to do before such visits. Brubaker recalled that Doctors Hospital, for example, specifically requested certified nurse's aides, yet she remembered instances where she had sent the hospital uncertified workers to pose as CNAs. She said Monahan told her that was okay so long as the fill-ins knew how to do vital signs. But All Care didn't necessarily pay its workers CNA wages. "I feel this one works good like a CNA," Brubaker remembered Monahan saying. "Pay her like a CNA." But for another it might be: "This one, you know, she's not worth what a CNA really makes, so pay her less."

Brubaker also recalled sending out nursing graduates who hadn't yet taken the state licensing exam to work as LPNs. "Julie said to work these people as an LPN [and] charge the insurance company or the facility LPN wages or RN wages, depending on the circumstance."

In this environment, making the perfect file required a lot of work, including a thorough knowledge of state regulations and what real certificates looked like. The process usually began with an authentic document. Brubaker, for example, admitted creating a phony CNA certificate using her own CNA credentials. First, she copied her CNA certificate, then whited out her name and her ID number. She then typed in the new name, plus a new number, the first series of digits indicating the ostensible date of issue, and the following digits for the person's Social Security number. "Put it in the copy machine again and then *voilà,* you have a CNA certificate," Brubaker said. "You put it in the person's file and it was ready for state inspection."

Brubaker said dozens of phony certificates were made, including more than two dozen false graduation certificates from different schools. Some required special modifications. One school wrote the graduate's name in heavy pencil, rather than typing it. Brubaker had to make sure the writing styles matched. At times, the process took on a production-line quality, involving two All Care workers in addition to Brubaker. "I would hand one of them a stack to be typed, tell her the name that needed to be typed and the date, whatever information needed to be typed where the whiteout had been. And most of the ones that are written I did do myself."

Perfect files also required a physical exam, so All Care made up phony ones, according to Brubaker. One morning, Brubaker said she was handed a pile of documents that were mostly blank except for a doctor's signature. "Put the names that need to be there," she was told.

Brubaker wasn't through yet. When some nurses needed current CPR cards (many hospitals required nurses to be CPR-certified), Brubaker said, All Care altered those as well. "Everything that I did at All Care Nursing was under Julie's instruction," she said. "She always knew everything that was going on." Monahan, through her lawyer, disputed that allegation.

Yet the imagination and craftsmanship and hard work that had gone into All Care's alleged forgeries went largely unappreciated. Brubaker said she was told that the inspector from Florida's Department of Health and Rehabilitation Services who visited All Care offices examined only three files—one each for an RN, an LPN, and a CNA. In the ultimate gesture of trust and goodwill, the regulator let All Care pick one of the folders.

Sharon Aussler couldn't have been happier to see the final days of her All Care contract winding down. Before she actually walked out the door, however, she reached a big decision: she would make one dramatic attempt to get even.

It was early October 1987—two nights before she was to leave—when Aussler made her move. Waiting until the office closed and the nurses were asleep, she walked into All Care's file room. It was after 1 A.M. As she stopped at the office's personnel files, her mind flashed to the stories she had heard of unqualified people being sent out on assignment. Now, she had come to copy their records. "I [knew] exactly whose cards I wanted to find," she recalled. Using the office machine, Aussler made copies, hid them, then returned to her bed and went to sleep. Later, one nurse would tell Monahan she had seen her altering and copying All Care records, but Aussler denied seeing anyone in the room that night. Two days after, at dawn, she gathered up her things, including the copied documents, and left All Care for good.

For many months, Aussler did nothing with her copies. At one point, she said, she tried to get a local television station—even "The Oprah Winfrey Show"—interested in probing All Care. Nothing happened. Then, one June day in 1988, Aussler anonymously shipped her records to the Department of Professional Regulation (DPR), the administrative arm of the Florida Board of Nursing. She later said she had turned over the documents not just for revenge but for the good of other nurses as well. "I don't want anybody to have to go through what I went through," Aussler said. "You go to nursing school to be a professional, to care for people." Working for All Care, she said, made her lose sight of that commitment.

A month or two later, Aussler called the DPR investigator, who said the state had found evidence of serious wrongdoing by Monahan. "After that," Aussler said, "I thought, Sure, it would come [out] in the papers, or her office would be closed."

The state did end up filing an administrative complaint against Julie Monahan, RN, accusing her of unprofessional conduct. In response, Monahan provided investigators with a sworn statement, in which she said her business "lends itself to a high probability of dealing with disgruntled independent contractors and the possibility of making bookkeeping errors." Monahan admitted that Becky Seibert (then known by her married name, Becky Black) "may have been incorrectly billed as an RN on three or four occasions," but, she added, that couldn't be confirmed, because certain records weren't available. Monahan also said that another LPN was possibly billed as an RN, but that the nurse in question denied working beyond her license. Above all, Monahan told investigators that she never knowingly sent an unqualified worker into the field.

On September 29, 1989—two weeks before the nursing board was to hear Monahan's case—things took a strange twist. On that date, Lisa Bassett, a senior attorney for the Department of Professional Regulation, wrote a cryptic memo to the chief of investigative services: "I have a feeling Ms. Monahan is going to falsely testify in her informal hearing." Bassett did not elaborate, nor did she offer any evidence backing her belief. Later, Bassett, as well as Monahan's lawyer, declined to discuss the comment.

At any rate, on October 12, 1989, at the Howard Johnson Downtown Hotel in Orlando, Julie Monahan, RN, came forward to plead her case before a meeting of the Florida Board of Nursing. The complaint included the serious allegation that Monahan "on numerous occasions . . . placed persons in positions for which they were not qualified." Once the hearing began, however, the state quickly dropped this allegation for lack of evidence. That left only billing errors.

Monahan's lawyer, Donald Orlovsky, began her defense by pointing out that she did business with more than 100 hospitals and
nursing homes and employed 500 nurses. With that out of the way,
Orlovsky got to the point. "The background of the investigation was
initiated under precarious, at best, circumstances," he said. "It was
initiated anonymously by a disgruntled employee, we believe." He
then submitted a letter to the board from a nurse, Bessie Tikker,
which, he said, suggested that someone had altered All Care's records before delivering them to state regulators.

"I have statements from members of the community detailing their
views of Ms. Monahan as a businesswoman and her agencies,"
Orlovsky continued. "Uniformly, they regard her as honest, a person
of integrity, a person with professional significance in nursing, a
philanthropist, and a nursing teaching advocate." Orlovsky down-
played the six apparent billing errors. "The errors in question, if they
occurred, amounted to no more than $100. They took place in a
volume of business that involved 40,000 shifts."

Bonnie Phipps, an investigator with the Department of Professional Regulation, concurred that most of the people she talked
to—including officials at hospitals and nursing facilities—said
Monahan was a fine citizen.

After a few preliminaries, the following exchanges took place:

QUESTIONER: Ms. Monahan, can you tell us what you think oc-
curred in these specific six cases?
MONAHAN: I hope I don't cry.
QUESTIONER: You're doing good. Take some water.
MONAHAN: I have a letter here. Jesus, I'm sorry. [Ms. Monahan cries.]
QUESTIONER: That's all right. You're doing good.
MONAHAN: It is brought to my attention this week what happened.
I'm sorry. [Ms. Monahan cries.]
QUESTIONER: That's all right. Drink some water if you want
to . . .
MONAHAN: . . . I thought I had been framed, you know. A nurse
came in and told me, she had seen them doing it, and—I'm sorry.
God, I'm crying.
QUESTIONER: That's all right. . . . Have you worked very hard to get
where you are today?
MONAHAN: You bet.
QUESTIONER: . . . It's not beyond the scope of reality, I don't think,
to anyone sitting here that there are going to be the possibility of some
errors, and the fact is that you have undoubtedly dealt with those in

an appropriate manner or you wouldn't be held in the esteem that you are by the community.

MONAHAN: Sir, I have installed a computer and I also put everything under lock and key.

QUESTIONER: You'll love the computer.

By the hearing's end, the Florida Board of Nursing enthusiastically gave Monahan a clean bill of health. All charges were dismissed.

Meanwhile, a different and more far-reaching attack on temp agencies was quietly being mounted back in Palm Beach County. Periodically, the heads of various hospital nursing departments got together to discuss their common problems, including temp agencies that dumped low-quality workers on them while charging high rates. From these meetings sprang an idea: area hospitals could band together and say, in effect, "We won't buy any temps from agencies that don't meet our qualifications."

With the help of the South Florida Hospital Association, 10 or so hospitals solicited bids from area agencies, then selected eight as "preferred providers." All Care wasn't one of them. Agencies not selected were understandably unhappy and filed an antitrust lawsuit against the hospital association and the hospitals.

So began what promised to be a dull journey into the arcane world of antitrust law. It hardly turned out that way, however. The hospitals, recognizing their potential liability, probed aggressively into the backgrounds of the agencies. And, unlike the state of Florida's timid regulatory effort, the hospitals didn't conduct a narrow, low-budget investigation.

Spearheading the probe was the politically connected Miami law firm of Mershon, Sawyer, Johnson, Dunwody & Cole, where the late congressman Claude Pepper had hung his legal hat. According to William Dunaj, a partner in that firm, state regulators hadn't even bothered to ask hospitals for all their billing invoices so they could compare them with state licensing records. Had they done so, Dunaj said, they would have found many examples of hospitals paying for temps who they thought held certain licenses when, in fact, they didn't. One of Monahan's lawyers, Helen McAfee, said All Care committed nothing more than "some billing errors."

Armed with these leads, Mershon, Sawyer hired a private investigator named Tom Whiteman, a tenacious ex-cop, to track down former employees of All Care, as well as other agencies. He quickly hit pay dirt. With Monahan feeling the heat, her lawyers obtained sworn statements from several workers accusing Whiteman of harassing them. The most serious charge came from Bessie Tikker, the same woman who claimed to have seen Aussler altering some of All Care's records. Tikker said she saw Whiteman "inside my fenced-in yard, looking into my windows."

Whiteman denied any misconduct and said it was Monahan who had engaged in misconduct and fraud, a charge Monahan, in turn, denied. Former All Care workers told him she had engaged in "extraordinary harassment and intimidation," Whiteman said. Some feared for their lives, and one even went into hiding.

Relying on records they had obtained and Thomas Whiteman's spadework, the hospitals charged in court papers that Monahan had orchestrated a scheme—which she denied—whereby

> . . . individuals with absolutely no nursing training were recruited and . . . sent to hospitals and misrepresented to be trained health care personnel. License credentials were forged and altered and untrained persons were provided with answers to medicine tests and other skills tests, all so these individuals could avoid detection. In short, All Care, through its owner Julie Monahan, took every conceivable step to deceive hospitals . . . without the slightest regard for the welfare of the patients for whom these untrained individuals were caring.

The state of Florida, of course, had found none of this. But then, state investigators—unlike Mershon, Sawyer—never tracked down people like Becky Seibert, John Roylance, Sheila Brubaker, and others who might be willing to testify under oath that All Care had engaged in gross misconduct. The state never persuaded Sharon Aussler to come forward and publicly tell her story. The state never found the spray-painter or the construction worker or the secretary who allegedly were sent out by All Care to pose as trained nurse's aides.

The state didn't even bother to fully probe the letter—which Monahan used in her defense at her nursing board hearing—in which an unidentified woman was accused of altering All Care documents. The October 8, 1989, letter, signed by Bessie Tikker, alleged that Tikker had seen a woman, later identified as Sharon

Aussler, going through All Care files after hours. It said the suspicious woman "stated that she had asked for a loan and been refused. She was gonna make Julie Monahan pay. I observed her altering and copying records." Later, in a deposition for the antitrust lawsuit, Tikker admitted to Mershon, Sawyer that it was possible she had not written the letter herself, although she admitted signing it. She also didn't remember who might have written it, or for what reason.

Palm Beach County hospitals, meanwhile, were unamused to learn from their lawyers how easily they could be fooled by local temp agencies. "The fact of the matter is they were [being] defrauded and the system they came up with was not good enough to detect this," said William Dunaj of Mershon, Sawyer, the hospitals' law firm. "They are embarrassed." But Monahan's lawyer, Helen McAfee, said that it was Mershon, Sawyer that should be embarrassed, since it had counseled the hospital association in setting up a preferred-provider organization that allegedly violated antitrust laws. She accused the law firm of throwing "dirt" because it had neither the facts nor the law on its side.

As for Sharon Aussler, she would continue to work as a nurse, although she said she will never feel the same about her profession. "I did the right thing a long time ago to stop what was going on at All Care, and nothing happened."

As the year 1990 came to an end—a full nine months after Mershon, Sawyer filed public papers in court alleging gross misconduct by All Care—state regulators still hadn't bothered to investigate those charges. But the federal government disclosed that it was conducting an investigation of certain Palm Beach hospitals for possible violations of federal antitrust laws in their attempts to control the billing rates of temp agencies. The hospitals denied the charges.

The presence of unqualified, overworked temps in the nation's hospitals was just one noxious by-product of the nation's nursing crisis. Four of five nurses surveyed by *RN* magazine believed that the nursing shortage had put patients at risk. Not only were shortage-related incidents occurring frequently, but they often involved the sickest patients. "Ninety percent of ICU/CCU nurses report problems," *RN* wrote.

A special federal commission on nursing concluded that errors will only increase as RN work loads become "more and more unrealistic and inappropriate." One state nursing board told the HHS Secretary's Commission on Nursing that the shortage had already resulted in more drug errors, more patient falls from bed, and more substance abuse among RNs.

Patients did not have to be physically harmed by the shortage to feel its impact. "The so-called frills go by the wayside," one Dallas nurse told the *American Journal of Nursing*. "But what some people call frills are not frills. A colostomy patient needs to know how to take care of his colostomy before he goes home. A cardiac patient needs to understand the implications of her medications." Another Dallas nurse told the magazine, "I've always thought that patients deserve to get all the little extras that we're forced to cut out now: like washing their hair, or taking them out to the patios to get some fresh air, spending a little extra time with them, sitting there and listening. We have so many tasks to be done that the emotional aspects of an illness are getting pushed aside."

Patricia Murphy spoke for many nurses when she said, "The powerlessness is overwhelming out there. You write it up and you send it down to the office, and then you write it up again and send it down to the office. Eventually, you don't even have the time to write it up. They're drowning out there, seriously drowning."

Desperate hospitals have shown they will try just about anything to plug the gaps. The Elvis Presley Memorial Trauma Center in Memphis approached its nursing problem by giving staff nurses the option to work 24-hour shifts. During the first week of a two-week pay period, nurses worked one 24-hour shift and one 12-hour shift. The second week, they worked two 24-hour shifts.

Although common sense says tired nurses put patients at risk, many nurses in major cities earned extra money by working day jobs as hospital employees and night jobs as agency nurses. While many nurses volunteered to work long hours, others said they were pressured into it. Nurses at Easton Hospital in Easton, Pennsylvania, felt the need to negotiate a protective clause in their contract that allowed them to refuse overtime twice per year without being disciplined.

One risky but common stopgap measure to combat the nursing shortage was to float nurses—pull them from one section of the hospital to another. The Maryland Nurses Association said it received a stack of letters from nurses complaining that they weren't qualified for many of their assignments. In one letter, a float nurse with no critical care training said she had to care for two ICU patients who needed ventilatory assistance. "The result was a near death," the nurse wrote. "One patient developed acute respiratory distress and a code had to be called." Atlanta's Physicians and Surgeons Community Hospital tried to get away with using LPNs, rather than RNs, to handle admission assessments, according to a 1989 government report. Government inspectors also found unqualified temps working in the intensive care unit, as well as temp orientations that were short, ineffective, and poorly attended.

Ironically, floating may actually worsen a hospital's nursing shortage. When Crawford W. Long Hospital in Atlanta interviewed nurses to learn why they had resigned, half the respondents identified "inadequate orientation and supervision as their main reason for leaving."

To find more nurses, hospitals turned to scouring the globe, particularly English-speaking countries like the Philippines or Jamaica where poverty is widespread. More than 500 hospitals—roughly 10 percent of all U.S. hospitals—have actively recruited foreign nurses. About one in every four nurses in New York City's public hospitals is foreign-trained. Unfortunately for patients, foreign workers tend not to resist pressure to work dangerously long hours or fill jobs for which they aren't qualified. "Filipino nurses do double shifts, and they don't complain," said Flor de Guzman, a New Jersey RN.

Asian nurses in particular are unlikely to be assertive, since their culture doesn't encourage outspokenness. "They're very much exploited," complained one lawyer who worked for the Philippine Center for Immigrant Rights. One Filipino nurse told *Newsday* that she came to the U.S. after being recruited to work at Harlem Hospital Center in New York. Later, she discovered that she would be working for a temp agency instead. "We feel that if we complain, we will be deported," she said.

Immigration authorities in 1988 found 30 or so illegal aliens working as nurse's aides at one temp agency, according to the *Boston Business Journal*. One nursing-home director, according to the journal, said he had seen temp aides who couldn't read, including one who didn't know which end of the thermometer went under the tongue. Hospitals found that about half of their foreign nurse recruits fail RN exams. Consequently, they must either pay to further train foreign workers or use them in less important positions.

But while hospitals spent huge sums of money to recruit foreign workers, many qualified students in this country couldn't enroll in nursing programs. In 1988–1989, some 2,500 qualified students in Texas were kept out of programs by a shortage of clinical facilities and faculty, according to the American Hospital Association. The future looks bleak, the association added, because the federal government cut allocations for nurse education.

State nursing boards, meanwhile, haven't done enough to protect patients from overworked, unqualified, or otherwise dangerous nurses. Many boards are secretive and have received less media scrutiny than the state boards that police doctors. Only a small number of states even bother to collect the names of temporary-staffing agencies. In some cases, regulation has been blocked by nursing lobbies that see the agencies as bringing about an overall rise in nursing salaries. This regulatory vacuum has produced suggestions that would be funny if lives weren't at stake. "Equipment manufacturers may need to make nursing equipment easier to use since agency nurses often operate such equipment with little or no training," the consulting firm of Arthur D. Little wrote in a March 1989 report.

Detroit Receiving Hospital was all too typical of many hospitals that fail to orient their new temps adequately. In February 1990, inspectors from the Michigan Department of Public Health found that the hospital hadn't fully explained infection control policies to its temps. As it turned out, infection control—or a lack of it—was very much on the minds of hospital officials because, over the previous five months, 68 patients had developed a particular hospital-acquired infection. Twenty-two of them died; the infection was believed to be at least marginally implicated in 15 of those deaths. The source of the infection and how it spread remained unknown.

One rainy day in the fall of 1989, a spokeswoman for one of New York's premier hospitals spent five hours with a reporter reciting the virtues of her hospital. Yet she confided privately, at the end of the conversation, that she hired an agency nurse when her mother was hospitalized, because she didn't trust overworked staff nurses. It cost her several hundred dollars a shift—up front, and cash only. People who can afford it, people who know the threadbare state of the nation's nursing care, do likewise.

Yet even that provides no guarantee. In 1987, after Andy Warhol died at New York Hospital following routine gallbladder surgery, state health officials criticized the hospital for failing to supervise Warhol's private, agency-supplied nurse. The state said the nurse, subsequently barred from New York Hospital, failed to monitor the artist's condition properly.

Not everyone, of course, is rich and famous. And when they die from poor nursing care, they do so quietly, not on the front pages of America's newspapers. Dr. Michael Lansing, chief medical resident at Lincoln Hospital in the South Bronx, told *The New York Times:* "You do the best you can to treat a patient and you find there is nobody to fill the orders you are giving." One 69-year-old heart patient stayed on a stretcher in Lincoln's emergency room for three days with virtually no care. In October 1990, a fill-in nurse at Lincoln mistakenly administered drug overdoses to four patients, one of whom died. "People of the South Bronx have as much right to top-quality health care as people who live on Fifth Avenue," said Peter Slocum, a spokesman for New York State's health department. Unfortunately, as Warhol's wealthy friends discovered, it isn't so great even for them.

New York City officials know the suffering that the nursing shortage brings, yet they allow it to continue, their poor management compounding the problem. The city's callousness was expressed in the voice of Fred Winters, a spokesman for city-run hospitals. "I can't find anyone willing to publicly discuss the problem," he said. Even sadder were studies showing that hospitals, if they desired, could successfully combat their shortages through better pay and working conditions. But that would require a long-term commitment that many hospitals lack.

Nurses aren't the only hospital workers in short supply. With hospital administrators putting out fires elsewhere, these lesser-known workers don't always get the attention they deserve. Indeed, although lacking in visibility, they are every bit as important to healing as anyone else laboring in the complex setting of today's modern hospital. And no one knows that better than one large, prestigious hospital in the southern boomtown of Charlotte, North Carolina.

4 "The Compelling Urgency to Ease Human Suffering"

THE most important moment in Dillon Murphy's life was now just seconds away. It was January 30, 1988, and for nearly an hour, this father of three had been living without a heart. Soon, he would reclaim it fully mended and ready again to begin pumping blood.

So far, Murphy's coronary-bypass surgery had gone well. A week before, a heart attack almost killed him. Now, with new bypass grafts ready to provide an unobstructed flow of blood, his doctors hoped to reduce his chances of another attack. Successful surgery would mean that in a matter of months he could return to driving a truck for one of North Carolina's many furniture outlets.

Murphy had been kept alive during the operation with a heart-lung machine, which allowed surgeons to stop the heart so they could delicately cut, stitch, and repair the organ. Although the machine has helped bypass surgery become commonplace, it's a poor substitute for the real thing. The longer patients remain tethered to it, the more their key bodily functions deteriorate. The heart surgeon's creed, then, is to do what fixing is necessary but waste not a minute. If no longer a pioneering procedure, heart surgery can still be a high-wire act. When all goes well, it brings fame and prestige to institution and surgeon alike. When it doesn't, it can undermine public confidence in the entire hospital.

Patient Murphy had decided to have his bypass surgery at Charlotte Memorial Hospital and Medical Center, an 843-bed nonprofit institution whose influence extended deep into the most powerful corporate suites in Charlotte, North Carolina. As other hospitals slunk around Congress like homeless beggars cadging quarters, Charlotte Memorial had a swagger reminiscent of the industry's golden years in the 1970s. Already the city's biggest hospital, it would soon have $69 million in construction projects under way, as well as a $3 million advertising budget to powder its nose as needed.

Charlotte Memorial's heart surgery program was its biggest success story. Evidence of that would come a month after Murphy's operation, with the christening of its newly relocated Carolinas Heart Institute. Years ago, before hospitals fell under the spell of marketing wizards, it might have been just another hospital department where hearts were mended. Not now. This unit had the institute's own name emblazoned on a new, five-story building, complete with rooftop helicopter landing pad and designer-quality furniture arrangements such as one might expect to see in the office of a prospering personal-injury lawyer.

Sitting atop this heart surgery empire was Dr. Francis Robicsek, the man Murphy selected to perform his bypass procedure. Hungarian by birth, Dr. Robicsek liked to say he differed from native-born Americans only in that he had his pants on when he became a citizen. Now in his 60s, with distinctively large hands, Dr. Robicsek was described by admirers as a compassionate Renaissance man with a healthy appreciation of humor.

He was also more than a bit odd. One visitor to the doctor's house watched him pull open a drawer filled with funny-looking bags. "What are those?" the visitor asked. Motion sickness bags, he replied—from over 400 airplanes. Dr. Robicsek, when he wasn't repairing hearts, collected vomit bags.

Like Charlotte Memorial, Dr. Robicsek reaped the benefits of a thriving heart program. In 1976, he was anointed North Carolina Citizen of the Year. And just two days after Murphy's surgery, a regional business publication would send him a valentine in the form of a 1,500-word personality profile that noted: he operated on patients regardless of their ability to pay; collected medieval Dutch paintings; read eight to 10 novels a week; and held patents on more than a dozen surgical devices. He was also an archaeologist, an art historian, a free-lance photographer, and a writer.

But if life at full throttle is exhilarating, it is partly because the threat of crashing is ever present. This sense of danger is what lures certain people into becoming surgeons. An occasional crash is part of every surgeon's life, whether due to a mistake or just fate. And in

1976, fate struck Charlotte Memorial and Dr. Robicsek's heart program. Between the months of February and April, a mysterious infection invaded the bodies of 19 open-heart patients (four women and 15 men). Nearly all were found to be oozing pus from around the steel wires used to close the sternum after surgery. One victim developed a strange green drainage from her sternum that later began coming out yellow, red, then orange. Five of the 19 victims died. Seven had to have their chest bones surgically removed after a raging infection destroyed them. With no bone to protect the heart, they had their organ covered by a surgical flap from their intestinal cavity. A full year and a half after the outbreak of that infection, only five were considered completely healed.

The hospital and Dr. Robicsek did all they could to find the source of the infection, identified as *Mycobacterium chelonei,* an organism found in soil. Charlotte Memorial even called in a special investigative team from the Centers for Disease Control, but they couldn't trace it either. In the end, the hospital and the surgical team were cleared of any responsibility for the tragedy. To this day, however, the source of that infection remains a mystery.

It was an experience no one forgot easily, and it may account for Dr. Robicsek's somewhat fatalistic view of his job. Just days before the Murphy surgery, Robicsek remarked, "I'm delighted with the opening of the Carolinas Heart Institute." Then he added, "But maybe next month I'll be . . . very disappointed—when something didn't go as well as I was hoping for. You need an appropriate mixture of successes and disappointments."

On this day, January 30, 1988, as Dr. Robicsek stood in the operating room, he was 12 years removed from that infection nightmare. It was midday, and he was about to finish work on Murphy, his second and last open-heart surgery of the day. The first procedure, on William Amick, had been a little unsettling; following surgery, Amick had trouble developing a healthy heartbeat. Still, surgeons were able to dispatch him to the recovery room.

Now, it was time to restart Murphy's heart. This moment may be more symbolic than dangerous. Surgeons keep the heart healthy during surgery by pumping cardioplegic solution directly into the organ; it not only stops the heart from beating but cools it as well, thus minimizing the need for oxygen. Unless cardioplegia is induced, the heart muscle deteriorates more rapidly and becomes problematic to restart. Getting a heart to beat again is usually easy.

Sometimes, however, the process can be likened to jump-starting a car engine on a cold day, particularly when a patient stays too long on the heart-lung machine.

With the heartbeat indicator reading zero, Dr. Robicsek's team placed electrical-shock contacts on Murphy's heart. The current surged, and the operating team watched for the reaction it had seen so many times before: a heart leaping back to life. This, however, would not be one of those times. Murphy's heart wasn't responding. Again, they tried. Nothing. Something was terribly wrong. It wouldn't turn over. Dillon Murphy's heart, so neatly stitched and ready to go, just sat still.

There was time yet; Murphy hadn't been on the machine that long. But Dr. Robicsek needed to find out exactly what had gone wrong. He quickly ordered extensive blood tests, hoping that would provide a clue. After an anxious wait, the lab reported its findings: Murphy's blood had an abnormally high glucose level. Where could it have come from? Robicsek wondered. He ordered new tests on fluids used in surgery, but they turned up nothing unusual. Could it have been a bad batch of cardioplegic fluid used to cool the heart? That seemed plausible since the solution was mixed in the hospital pharmacy. With precious minutes slipping away, Robicsek's team began searching frantically through the operating room waste bins to find the used bags.

There they found them. At first glance, the transparent plastic bags appeared to have held the clear fluid used for cardioplegia. But subsequent lab tests on the contents showed that not all had contained the heart solution—three had been filled with an IV glucose solution used to nourish patients with digestive problems. Instead of inducing cardioplegia, the surgical team had been bathing Dillon Murphy's heart in sugar.

Then, another realization jolted Dr. Robicsek. The other patient, William Amick—he, too, had had problems sustaining a strong heartbeat. Was it possible that he'd also gotten the wrong solution? Hospital workers scrambled over to Amick's operating room, where again they retrieved used plastic pouches from the waste bins. Three were found to have contained cardioplegic fluid, but one had contained the IV solution.

In all his years of heart surgery, Dr. Robicsek had never seen such a mix-up. Now, he had two patients who needed rescuing. The sugar solution had damaged the hearts of Murphy and Amick by sucking water out of heart muscle cells. Could this be reversed, doctors wondered. To find a remedy, hospital personnel began calling medical schools, anyone they could think of who might have experienced such a problem. Dr. Robicsek placed Murphy on a kidney dialysis machine, hoping to cleanse his body of the excess sugar.

Meanwhile, Murphy's relatives waited and worried. The task of telling them that a problem had developed fell to Dr. Robicsek. During the crisis, he would make several trips to the waiting room. Days later, he said the entire episode was probably "the worst thing that's ever happened to me."

Murphy continued to deteriorate more rapidly than Amick. Something had to be done soon. Maybe a heart transplant; Robicsek had done that before. First, however, he had to find a suitable donor. Quickly, the hospital broadcast a nationwide appeal for a heart through the United Network for Organ Sharing (UNOS) in Richmond, Virginia. UNOS workers were specially trained for such emergencies. Immediately, they began telephoning nearly 300 transplant centers and organ procurement groups around the nation. This was no time for wasted words.

"UNOS—STAT," the workers kept repeating urgently into the telephone. Those code words carried a precise message: a patient needing a heart had less than 24 hours to live. It also instructed the centers to check their computers, linked to UNOS headquarters, for more information. At any given moment, a thousand people or more may be waiting for a heart. But because of Murphy's critical condition, his name leapfrogged to the top of the list. The next usable heart would be his.

Back in Charlotte, as day turned to night, doctors began to fear the worst. Still on the heart-lung machine, Murphy was slowly deteriorating. Besides damaging red blood cells, the machine harmed his body's ability to pass oxygen from the lung to the blood without fluids leaking back. The result was a serious condition called pulmonary edema, in which the lungs choke on excess fluids. Soon, Murphy's system would be too badly damaged to sustain the rigors of a transplant.

That moment arrived the next day, near dawn. The call they had been waiting for, announcing that a suitable heart had been found, never came. Doctors could do no more. Before his Saturday surgery, Murphy had been talkative and optimistic. Sunday morning he lay dead in the operating room. He left a wife and three children.

Dillon Murphy was 33 years old.

• • •

It was Thursday morning, February 4, when the telephone rang in the Carrboro, North Carolina, office of David R. Work, executive director of the North Carolina Board of Pharmacy. The caller was Steve Hudson, a board investigator, and did he have a story to tell. Work listened carefully as Hudson described what he had read in that morning's *Charlotte Observer:* two open-heart patients got the wrong medicine . . . one died Sunday, the other Monday . . . a pharmacist had quit . . . the hospital was Charlotte Memorial.

The more Work heard, the more excited he got. A tall, blunt-spoken man, he had been at the board for 13 years, policing thousands of pharmacies and pharmacists across the state. Work had a simple enforcement philosophy: step over the line, and you answer for it. And that meant no on-the-job training where mistakes were greeted with friendly admonishments to do better next time.

Work's pharmacy board was an obscure regulatory body, but it had a clear sense of mission: follow the clues wherever they lead. A pharmacist, professor, and lawyer by training, Work could have mined a more prosperous regulatory position, but the pharmacy board gave him something more important: freedom. "I have a strange job. I can say things other regulators can't. It's worth $10,000 in lost salary just to be able to do that."

Work found the *Observer* story intriguing, not only because of what had happened but also where. Just last year, he had had occasion to witness Charlotte Memorial's regard for state pharmacy laws. His board discovered that the pharmacy there had allowed a pharmacist to practice without a license. "The pharmacy was more interested [in] covering a shift than doing things properly," Work said. Consequently, the board formally reprimanded the hospital pharmacy. Although no one was harmed by the incident, it told Work something important about Charlotte Memorial: this was an institution to be watched.

As for the open-heart deaths, the fact that Work had to learn about them from a newspaper days after they happened pointed up the spottiness of hospital regulation. People who by law are supposed to protect patients are often the last to know when hospital mistakes kill. Charlotte Memorial had no legal obligation to report Murphy's and Amick's deaths to the pharmacy board or to state officials.

Even when hospitals were required to report harmful incidents, they didn't always do so. The U.S. General Accounting Office, for example, expressed serious concern about the failure of hospitals to report patient injuries involving medical devices. And New York State health officials accused hospitals there of violating state regulations by reporting only a small fraction of patient injury cases.

North Carolina, on the other hand, had no idea how many people died from hospital mistakes. In the perverted logic of hospital regulation, North Carolina required only that hospitals write incident reports—not also that they send them someplace. "We don't plow through all these reports," explained Ernest Phillips of the state hospital licensing agency. "We used to require them to mail all those things to us in 48 hours, but what happened is we literally got a flood of paper, an absolute flood." Now, North Carolina hospitals had only to keep incident reports in their own files—a largely worthless gesture since state inspectors didn't regularly inspect most North Carolina hospitals, and thus never saw them.

Karen Garloch, an *Observer* reporter, said she first heard of the open-heart deaths at Charlotte Memorial through an anonymous caller, who provided not only details of the incidents but something even more valuable: the names Murphy and Amick. "It had to have come from someone inside the hospital who was upset," she said.

As David Work learned more about the deaths, he became increasingly troubled by Charlotte Memorial's explanation that one hospital worker alone was responsible for the tragedy. Human error is inevitable, he realized, but well-run hospitals have an elaborate quality assurance program to catch errors before they kill. Might these deaths be rooted in the pharmacy's mismanagement, rather than in one worker's mistake? Work wondered.

Another interesting twist he noticed was that both Murphy and Amick had undergone weekend surgery. Anyone who has visited a hospital on weekends knows how activity slows markedly, as doctors, nurses, and other regular staffers leave for weekends with the family. For that reason, doctors don't like to admit patients on Friday, knowing little will be done to them until Monday. Still, illnesses don't conform to regular workweeks, so hospitals, scrambling to find weekend employees, turn frequently to temp agencies or part-time employees.

"It's generally considered inefficient to use operating suites on weekends," Work said. "When you think about it—and there's no diplomatic way to say it—many of the folks there on weekends, except the surgeons, are the second string; folks working second jobs, raising families. This isn't to say they are less capable, but maybe they aren't concentrating as much." Heart attack victims, for example, fared worse in hospitals on weekends than on weekdays, researchers found.

Cleveland Clinic, the pioneer of coronary-bypass surgery, had so many people wanting the operation that it once considered instituting weekend heart surgery. "We started looking into the ramifications of that," said Dr. Delos (Toby) Cosgrove III, one of the clinic's top heart surgeons. "You not only have to man the operating room with surgeons, nurses, anesthesiologists, perfusionists, but you also have to have the same sort of support from the blood bank, the pharmacy, nursing, and all of that." The clinic ultimately rejected the idea. "All the facilities have got to be ratcheted up another notch," Cosgrove said. The clinic decided it couldn't do elective bypass surgery on weekends without hiring more personnel.

David Work's pharmacy board, of course, had no jurisdiction over how hospitals scheduled surgery. But he was curious about what role weekend staffing at Charlotte Memorial might have played in the tragedy, along with the more obvious questions: how did the mistake occur, why didn't anyone catch it, and was the hospital telling the full story?

To get the answers he needed, Work turned the sleuthing over to Steve Hudson, an ex–street cop from Anniston, Alabama, whose occasionally halting speech and youthful appearance belied his ability as a seasoned investigator. Hudson was perfect for the job: methodical, enthusiastic, not easily ruffled. Charlotte Memorial would become the biggest case in Steve Hudson's 11 years on the pharmacy board.

A major hospital pharmacy is a world apart from the corner drugstore or discount chain. A local druggist, besides filling prescriptions, might personally sell everything from over-the-counter cold medicine to prophylactics. Chain store druggists may be spared the added task of promoting safe sex, but their basic mission remains simple: sell drugs directly to consumers, with a pinch of advice when needed.

A big hospital pharmacy, on the other hand, employs more people, compounds more drugs, and is the 24-hour command post for a vast distribution network extending throughout the institution. The pharmacy department helps to ensure that the right medicine gets to the right place in the right dose at the right time. It helps spot physicians who may be prescribing medicines incorrectly. It sees to it that outdated drugs are removed from the distribution chain. It oversees the guarding of dangerous drugs—including pure cocaine and other addictive substances—scattered across the hospital in carts, refrigerators, and transitional-storage areas.

One Raleigh hospital found itself in trouble with David Work's pharmacy board after discovering that nearly a pound of pure cocaine—with a street price of maybe $200,000—was missing from storage. Poorly managed pharmacies are rife with temptation for hospital employees susceptible to drug abuse. "Most hospitals don't report these drug thefts and drug addictions," complained one Ohio pharmacy board official. "They basically want to get rid of the problem, so the offender is pushed out, usually to another hospital, where the same thing occurs."

Catching medication errors is particularly important when patients are sick enough to have been hospitalized. A vigilant pharmacy at Clayton General Hospital near Atlanta's Hartsfield International Airport uncovered a 32 percent error rate in drug dosages ordered by the hospital's medical staff. Unfortunately, Clayton General's medical staff had not bothered to do anything about it by the time hospital regulators accidentally discovered the error rate in early 1989. Government inspectors, it turned out, had visited the hospital only because of a press report that a man had bled to death after waiting six hours for an emergency room surgeon.

Vital as hospital pharmacies are, regulators inspect them only seldom, and then not as thoroughly as they might. Even worse, when problems are found, there is little outside pressure to fix them. In 1989, the Joint Commission on Accreditation of Healthcare Organizations reported that the most common major problem it found— affecting 88 percent of its hospitals—was failure to evaluate drug usage properly, which is partly the pharmacy's responsibility.

The agency, however, rarely revoked accreditation for serious violations of any kind. In early 1989, for example, state investigators responded to complaints from disgruntled employees at Atlanta's Physicians and Surgeons Hospital and found improper training of a pharmacy student and pharmacy technician, inadequate compounding and packaging of drugs, and failure to notice that half the drugs on a recovery room crash cart were expired, as were drugs in the emergency room and other dispensing areas. Despite this, and major quality control breakdowns in other departments—including the use of unlicensed physicians—the 149-bed hospital was fully accredited at the time of the government inspection.

Even David Work's pharmacy board couldn't be counted on to catch problems of this kind in North Carolina; he no longer conducted regular inspections of hospital pharmacies. With his puny staff of four investigators, he focused on only two areas: allegations of wrongdoing, and retail pharmacists—the theory being that other government agencies monitor North Carolina's 150 or so hospitals. Work knew how wide the gap is between theory and reality, but, like others who saw a regulatory system that failed to protect patients, he felt powerless to change it.

It was 7:30 on a crisp, snowless night in January when Ken Cawthorne reported for work at Charlotte Memorial. This evening was an important personal milestone: he would officially resign his job as a pharmacist at Charlotte Memorial. Now in his early 40s, Cawthorne had never meant to stay when he first signed on at the hospital four months earlier. It was really a stepping-stone to his new love: tailoring computer systems for pharmacies. The task fit him perfectly. An exacting man lacking in so-called people skills, Cawthorne felt at home in the precise, orderly world of computer and pharmacy work.

Sloppy colleagues upset Cawthorne. Once, when a pharmacy technician typed an X in a box to designate a type of solution, days later Cawthorne would remember how perfectly that X fit inside the box; that was the kind of attention to detail he appreciated. In 1987, Cawthorne wanted to build his computer consulting business, but first he needed a backup job that wouldn't interfere with regular business hours. Charlotte Memorial was just the place; the hospital was happy to find weekend help at a time when pharmacy workers were scarce.

The shortage would get so bad that next year a nationwide survey of hospitals found pharmacy workers among the most difficult to recruit. Vacancies often went unfilled for three months or longer, forcing hospitals to tempt fate by working pharmacists overtime, by temporarily substituting other personnel for low-level pharmacy jobs, or by turning to temp agencies.

Cawthorne's preference for the graveyard shift was an added bonus for Charlotte Memorial; he was intelligent and extraordinarily well qualified, having previously directed pharmacies at two other hospitals. To accommodate Cawthorne, the hospital offered what had become a standard package in the industry: a compressed work-week at full pay. This staffing strategy had in the past helped hospitals patch holes in nursing schedules; now, it was helping cover shortages elsewhere. Cawthorne's job worked this way: show up at 7:30 P.M. Friday, work straight through until 7:30 the next morning, then repeat the process on Saturday and Sunday nights. Monday through Friday, Cawthorne worked daylight hours as a computer consultant. In exchange for 36 intensive hours over a 72-hour period, the hospital paid Cawthorne full benefits. Each side got what it wanted. Whether patients got quality care from such arrangements was another question.

Although Cawthorne regarded his hospital hours as ideal for pursuing his other career, he almost didn't take the job. The pharmacy's drug dispensing wasn't the way it ought to be, he thought. The dispensing pharmacist, for example, didn't get direct copies of physicians' drug orders. This practice, said some pharmacy experts, increased the chances of prescribing error, because a middleman was involved. "I thought over whether I'd be able to safely practice pharmacy in that environment," Cawthorne would say later. But he decided to go ahead anyway. The hospital was moving toward a better dispensing system, and besides, he thought, Charlotte Memorial had enough checks and balances to catch any serious errors. So, after delaying his decision for a day, he decided yes, it was a place he could work.

Once on board, Cawthorne's work went smoothly enough, although not without pockets of turbulence. There was the time one night when he mistakenly switched Trandate, a hypertension drug, with Trental, used in treating arterial disease. No one was harmed, but the error earned him a counseling session with his night supervisor. There was also a "personality conflict" with a fellow worker.

But Cawthorne was most bothered by the feeling of some that perhaps he didn't work fast enough. Even night shifts on weekends could be busy. The pharmacy filled drug orders not only for the mother institution but also for several affiliated medical facilities. Some nights, the pharmacy filled as many as 300 to 350 orders. The accusation of slowness bothered Cawthorne because he felt he worked as fast as safety allowed. He even asked one veteran pharmacist familiar with that hospital's ins and outs to work the night shift with him so he could see if there was a better way to do his job. "I was trying to work faster and faster and faster," he recalled. "There was pressure; whether it was put on by myself or from the outside, I felt the pressure to work faster."

It wasn't so big a problem, however, that it jeopardized his job. And so Ken Cawthorne went about his work until the Friday evening of January 22, 1988, when he handed in his resignation, effective February 7. Frustrated by his inability to build a thriving computer consulting practice, Cawthorne had decided to work full-time for a computer firm in Raleigh. A couple of weekends more and he would be through. No more Charlotte Memorial, no more graveyard shifts.

Cawthorne didn't know it, but that particular Friday was also a significant day in the life of a 33-year-old truck driver from Lenoir, North Carolina; he suffered a heart attack. And although the man survived the attack, it set in motion a chain of events that would intertwine forever the fates of Dillon Murphy and Ken Cawthorne.

The following Monday, five days before Murphy's surgery, Cawthorne left the hospital at his usual quitting time, 7:30 A.M. Having already accepted the Raleigh job, he had no scheduled consulting appointments over the next five days. Meanwhile, inside Charlotte Memorial's pharmacy, a new week was beginning and there was much to be done. One task seemed ordinary enough: converting all 1,000-cc glass bottles containing an IV nutritional fluid to 1,000-cc plastic bags. The change was precipitated by the hospital's decision to buy a new-model IV infusion pump, which worked better with plastic pouches.

On Wednesday at 4:30 P.M., the pharmacy routinely prepared a batch of this nutritional fluid, called hyper-al for short. And in accordance with new pharmacy policy, the IV mixture was placed in transparent plastic pouches and stored in the pharmacy's refrigerator.

At 7:30 P.M. Friday, Cawthorne returned to work at Charlotte Memorial. He would later say he had slept several hours before reporting in. About this time, an order arrived from Dr. Robicsek in heart surgery, asking that eight bags of cardioplegic solution be sent to the operating room for two open-heart operations the next morning.

The task of filling that order fell to 19-year-old Laura Green, who had worked full-time at the pharmacy for five months. Her job was to type patient-specific information for each bag—in this case, four bags for Murphy and four for Amick. Then she was to pull the correct product from the pharmacy refrigerator and attach patient labels to all eight bags.

Laura Green was not a pharmacist. She had no formal training in pharmacy. She was not licensed by any government agency, nor was she certified by any private group. She was not periodically tested by the hospital to evaluate her knowledge of basic pharmacy policy. Her first job evaluation—well before Amick and Murphy entered the hospital—called her a "marginal employee." Nevertheless, she remained. Her previous work experience included stints at a dry cleaner and an ice-cream store.

Green was a pharmacy technician, someone who helped licensed pharmacists do their job. She had plenty of company. In addition to 33 licensed pharmacists, Charlotte Memorial employed 34 other pharmacy technicians. Such young, untrained workers were common around the nation, as hospitals sought to cut labor costs and lighten work loads of pharmacists, who already were spread too thin.

Green, as ordered, removed eight bags of solution from a pass-through refrigerator—one door opening to the IV-mixing unit of the pharmacy, and the other to the dispensing side of the pharmacy. By 9:15 P.M., Green had attached her patient labels and had asked a pharmacist to verify that the order for cardioplegic fluid had been filled correctly. What Green did not know, however, was that she had mistakenly pulled bags of IV solution at the same time. Incredibly, both substances were kept near each other in the same refrigerator in almost identical plastic pouches.

The folly of such a practice was self-evident, yet it happened. In March 1985, Fred Hicks, Sr., checked into Vanderbilt University Medical Center for same-day cataract surgery, a minor procedure. But instead of getting his prescribed medicine, he was given oil of wintergreen, an air-freshener. Both were green liquids. Both were kept in clear glass or plastic bottles. And both were kept in the same refrigerator. Because of the mix-up, Hicks died of respiratory arrest.

At Charlotte Memorial, Laura Green had made a similar mistake, but the first open-heart operation was still 12 hours away. Ordinarily, another pharmacist—not Cawthorne—would have checked Green's work, but that person was busy, so Cawthorne stepped in.

The medication for this order had two significant features: it was an uncontrolled substance, and it was always kept in stock. Pharmacists are particularly fastidious when handling any controlled substance, because laws are very strict governing how they are to be handled. "Everyone's attention level rises, and they cross their t's and dot their i's," said David Work of the pharmacy board. But, he added, pharmacists are sometimes less careful in dealing with drugs that aren't subject to abuse.

Because the order was also a stock item, Cawthorne said, his guard may have been down. "Your thought is, Well, this is going to go and be received by someone who's going to put it on a shelf . . . presumably, there are additional checks." Against this background, Cawthorne walked over to the eight bags of solution, which had been separated by patient: four for Murphy and four for Amick. He checked the top bag for each patient, comparing the contents label with the patient-specific information. Both plastic bags, he would later say, did in fact contain cardioplegic solution. Cawthorne then committed a grave error—he assumed that so did the remaining bags.

He might have checked closer had he known one crucial fact: while he was off duty that week, the pharmacy had stopped storing IV nutritional solution in glass bottles and switched over to plastic bags, similar to those used for cardioplegic solution. The change was discussed at a Monday, January 11, meeting attended by some pharmacy department workers, but Cawthorne had not attended. He was off duty. He worked weekends. Upon arriving each day, Cawthorne was supposed to read a logbook of policy changes, then initial each entry to show he had read it. That Friday, Cawthorne had opened the book, but he saw no mention of the packaging change. In fact, he had never received any written notice of it.

Cawthorne verified that Dr. Robicsek's order had been filled correctly. Over the next 12 to 14 hours, as Murphy and Amick slept and waited for surgery, four more people would handle the bags of fluid, yet each one would fail to catch the pharmacy's error.

One such person was a second pharmacy technician, who took the plastic pouches to a dumbwaiter for transport to the operating room. At this point, fate almost intervened. After a few moments, the technician could tell that the dumbwaiter had not been unloaded on the other end, so she retrieved the bags. But 15 minutes later, around 9:30 P.M., another call came for the cardioplegic fluid. The same bags were sent again, only this time they were unloaded immediately by a nurse, who put them in the operating room refrigerator. This nurse also failed to notice from the ingredient labels on some of the bags that they contained the wrong solution. She became the fourth person to handle the pouches and not catch the error.

It was now Saturday morning. Soon, hospital workers would begin prepping patients Amick and Murphy for surgery. But there was still time. Surely, someone would catch the error.

Open-heart surgery involves more than just the person who cuts and stitches the heart. The surgical team consists of a dozen people, including the surgeon, the assistant surgeon, four nurses, and three people administering and monitoring anesthesia. All of them must work closely together. One weak link, and the whole team fails.

There is another part of the team that is less well known to the public—the perfusionist. During the operation, the surgeon places a tube in the patient's aorta and hands the other end to the perfusionist, who uses it to pump cardioplegic solution directly into the heart. Like pharmacy workers, perfusionists are in short supply in many areas of the country; many are also unlicensed and uncertified. And, like pharmacy technicians, perfusionists often get their training on the job.

It was a perfusionist who opened the operating room's refrigerator, removed the bags, and attached them to the pump used in Amick's surgery. He thus became the fifth person to handle the bags without noticing that the labels identified the contents as IV solution. Another perfusionist took the remaining bags and attached them to Murphy's pump. Nor did she notice. Nor did anyone else in either operating room. The operations proceeded as scheduled— with disastrous results.

Pharmacist Cawthorne reported back for work Saturday evening, not knowing that Murphy and Amick were barely clinging to life. Informed of his role in sending the wrong solution to the patients, he left work early, never to return.

The media first reported the deaths on Wednesday, February 3.

The hospital said little. The next day, Charlotte Memorial's public-relations staff gave its first detailed account of the tragedy in a press release. It began:

> We deeply regret the deaths of two cardiac patients this past weekend. Our first concerns were to conduct a thorough investigation, make any adjustments to hospital procedures that may have played a role and to preserve the privacy of the patients [sic] families during their time of mourning. Now that funeral services have been completed, we feel it is time to reassure our community.

The hospital pinned the entire blame for both deaths on Cawthorne. In doing so, it presented at best a misleading—if not downright inaccurate—account of what had happened. The press release continued, "A pharmacist, who has resigned, filled the request [for cardioplegic solution], but used another solution kept in the pharmacy called hyper-al instead . . . The pharmacist inadvertently mislabeled some bags of hyper-al as cardioplegia. The bags of hyper-al were sent to the operating room labeled as cardioplegia."

The hospital's "thorough investigation" did not mention that a teenage unlicensed technician, who hadn't undergone periodic testing, had actually filled the order. It didn't mention that the same teenager had labeled the bags. It didn't mention that the bags sent to the emergency room did, in fact, carry labels stating that the solution was hyper-al. It didn't mention that six people had handled the solution without catching the error, or that the pharmacy had changed its method of storing cardioplegic solution from glass to plastic bags but had not formally notified the dispensing pharmacist.

"The mistake was human error," the hospital concluded. "The fact remains, that if the solutions had been labeled correctly by the pharmacist, the unfortunate error would not have occurred." Charlotte Memorial had many subsequent opportunities to clarify its earlier comments but chose not to.

The hospital's statement also didn't explain why patients Amick and Murphy had undergone weekend surgery. Dr. Robicsek said later that he saw nothing wrong with weekend surgery and that he did it often. But Wallace Respess, Jr., a lawyer representing the Murphy family, said it was a "damn shame" that the surgery had occurred on a Saturday morning, when the hospital was staffed with weekend help. Respess said he asked the hospital's lawyer why that had happened. "I never got a response," he recalled. "That told me something, and I made both a mental note and a note in my file that that was one of the things that the jury would hear in opening statements and maybe one of the last things in closing statements." The hospital eventually reached an undisclosed settlement with both the Murphy and Amick families.

In many if not most states, Charlotte Memorial might have gotten away with its distorted effort to hang one man for the sins of an entire institution. But not in David Work's state. Backed by the findings of investigator Steve Hudson, the North Carolina Board of Pharmacy cited the pharmacy, including its boss, Wayne Rinehart, as well as Ken Cawthorne for violating state pharmacy laws. All faced the possible loss of their pharmacy licenses.

Also doing her part to challenge the hospital's account was Karen Garloch, a reporter for the *Charlotte Observer,* one of the nation's best midsized newspapers. The *Observer* knew what it was like to stand up to powerful institutions, having previously won Pulitzer Prizes for unmasking the evangelical empire of Jim and Tammy Bakker and for exposing the effects of brown lung on textile workers. Garloch took the extra step of getting other health care workers to say that the mistake at Charlotte Memorial should have been caught by other hospital personnel before it killed someone.

But while the pharmacy board and the newspaper did their jobs, there were others who stood silently by, including the state hospital licensing agency, the U.S. Health and Human Services Department, and the Joint Commission on Accreditation of Healthcare Organizations. If they did know of systematic problems in the pharmacy, they didn't force the hospital to fix them, or to warn prospective patients. HHS said its policy was to inspect hospitals when the media reported serious deficiencies, but more than a year after the deaths of Murphy and Amick, it had completed no such investigation. Ditto for the state hospital licensing agency. The Joint Commission didn't immediately investigate the deaths, either, but in September 1988 it did renew Charlotte Memorial's accreditation for three years.

Charlotte Memorial's response to Murphy and Amick's deaths wasn't atypical of the industry, or of some regulators; rarely do they view hospital-induced deaths as a systematic problem. When *The Wall Street Journal* in October 1988 reported that more than half the patients who had died at one accredited hospital had gotten sub-standard care, the Joint Commission called the finding a "string of anecdotes." When families told the New York City Council how hospital mistakes had killed their loved ones, the president of the city's Health and Hospitals Corporation dismissed their tales as "anecdotes of bad experiences"—a characterization that one angry councilman denounced as "callous" and "offensive."

The industry's reaction is even more indignant when regulators find serious breakdowns that haven't killed anyone yet. Responding mostly to complaints of poor care, federal inspectors in 1986 and 1987 found problems that threatened patient safety in 156 accredited hospitals. Many hospitals disparagingly called these technical or paper violations. Only when these deficiencies killed someone, it would seem, did they become anecdotal.

Charlotte Memorial was no doubt sincere in expressing regret over the deaths of Murphy and Amick. But seven weeks after the deaths, the hospital's president, Harry Nurkin, blasted the media for "inexplicably" continuing to focus on the incident. In his first public comment since the deaths, Nurkin opined, "Our media tend to be preoccupied with the failure of human beings to be perfect."

Nurkin could hardly blame the media or Ken Cawthorne when, three months later, his pharmacy helped to kill a third patient. This time, the pharmacy mistakenly sent to a 69-year-old woman a hydro-chloric-acid solution that was 10 times too strong. She went into cardiac arrest and died. For six weeks, the hospital kept the death a secret from the only licensing agency that seemed interested in investigating patient deaths: the North Carolina Board of Pharmacy.

Board investigator Steve Hudson heard of the incident in a phone call from a Charlotte Memorial lawyer. Looking at his handwritten notes from that conversation, Hudson said the lawyer told him that his research had found no legal requirement for the hospital to report the death, but that he was reporting it anyhow because the patient's family had threatened to go to the media. "That speaks volumes," Hudson later remarked. Once news reporters learned of the death, Charlotte Memorial explained its silence by saying that the family had "directed [the hospital] not to publicize details of the death."

With Charlotte Memorial now facing disciplinary action for three deaths, not two, it decided to attack the pharmacy board itself, claiming in state court that the board had no jurisdiction over the hospital. That responsibility, Charlotte Memorial said, belonged to the North Carolina Department of Human Resources, which had already renewed the hospital's overall operating license.

Reacting angrily to this position, the North Carolina Society of Hospital Pharmacists filed a friend-of-the-court brief on behalf of the pharmacy board. Noting that Charlotte Memorial's legal argument referred to a "single" pharmacy error, the society wrote, "There was not a 'single' error. Three people to our knowledge are dead because of problems with the Petitioner's hospital pharmacy. This pharmacy has a history . . . of failing to comply with state laws governing the practice of pharmacy." The society also bitterly attacked the appropriate state licensing agencies for failing to investigate the deaths. North Carolina state court ultimately struck down the hospital's argument.

Finally, on a humid, 95-degree day, one and a half years after the deaths of Murphy and Amick, Charlotte Memorial was called to account for its mistakes. At a disciplinary hearing in Charlotte on July 11, 1989, six pharmacy board members listened as Steve Hudson methodically presented evidence of a systematic breakdown in quality control inside the hospital pharmacy.

Facing the loss of its pharmacy license, the hospital abandoned its simple "human error" defense. Now, it spoke of instituting broad reforms, such as making pharmacy technicians undergo periodic testing, making hospital employees check medicine before passing it down the distribution chain, improving recordkeeping, and removing the pharmacy's longtime director, Wayne Rinehart.

The pharmacy board had gotten what it wanted. But just to make sure, the board suspended the hospital's license for a year—then stayed that suspension so long as Charlotte Memorial faithfully carried out its reforms.

One of the pharmacy board's biggest cases had come to an end. Some board members and staff retired to a suite at the Adams Mark Hotel to celebrate their victory. Looking back over the last year and a half, David Work said he would most of all remember how slowly Charlotte Memorial had implemented its reforms. Investigator Hudson said he was struck by how much medicine had become "a dollars-and-cents business." Later, staffers and board members would watch themselves on television, as local news shows carried lengthy accounts of what had transpired at the disciplinary hearing only hours before.

Meanwhile, back at Charlotte Memorial, hospital officials had to be feeling a sense of relief. The worst was over now, the crisis weathered. Soon, details of the tragedies would pass from public consciousness. In coming months, other hospitals would take their turn explaining medication mistakes. In 1990, two dozen open-heart patients at a Nebraska hospital would get contaminated heart solution, resulting in two deaths. In making the solution, the hospital committed 19 violations of federal drug-manufacturing standards. Less than a month later, three infants would die at Philadelphia's Albert Einstein Medical Center after receiving an incorrectly mixed intravenous solution. One study found that in one large New York State hospital, medication errors averaged 2.5 times per day. This particular hospital had a system that caught the errors in time, but other hospitals may lack such a system, researchers warned.

Outside Charlotte Memorial, hospital construction crews were winding down after a long day in the hot sun. In a while, they would finish building one of the nation's largest medical-office buildings. Then there was the $40 million hospital tower to complete, along with the parking garage and the new helipad. "Our vision is ambitious," the hospital explained, "but it is focused by the compelling urgency to ease human suffering."

Seven hundred miles north, in Washington, D.C., the vision of the hospital marketplace solving its own problems still burned bright. Medical lobbyists could soon claim success in blocking bills that would have slowed hospital construction, and in watering down government efforts to punish doctors for providing bad care to Medicare patients. The American Hospital Association would also report that hospital personnel shortages for 16 occupations were growing worse.

The White House, meanwhile, seemed to be making its own statement about what it deemed important. Six months into his term—with the quality and availability of hospital care around the nation increasingly under attack—President Bush still hadn't installed his choice to run the Health Care Financing Administration. No other agency, public or private, had more influence over hospitals. Only the Pentagon and Social Security had a larger budget. Seven more months would pass before Bush's selection, Gail Wilensky, finally took control of HCFA.

5 | The People-Pushers

IT had been night now for six hours, and a January chill was settling over the nation's capital. On Capitol Hill, legislators emotionally argued the merits of waging war in the Persian Gulf, a debate noteworthy both for its time—late Friday night—and its sincerity. It would continue into the early hours of Saturday morning.

Two miles to the north, inside the modern emergency room at Howard University Hospital, physicians were bracing for their own war to save the expected stream of gunshot victims from the surrounding neighborhood. Weekend nights were sad occasions here—a marked contrast to decades ago, when on this very site the old Washington Senators hosted baseball greats of yesteryear in what was then Griffith Stadium.

Two miles to the east, amid the leafy hills of 22nd Street, was the middle-class neighborhood that was home to 69-year-old Veleria Dempsey. The twin dormer windows of her tidy brick house emitted a soft, warm glow of yellow. From a nearby vantage point, she could see waves of twinkling lights spread out below in the distant suburbs of Prince George's County.

Mrs. Dempsey had lived there for decades, although time had brought unwelcome changes. Nearby violence, of course, was worse than ever. Now her husband, who was retiring, wasn't well. There was also the problem of her sister, Lucille Arrington. Born with a mental disability and subject to seizures, Lucille, at 70, had never held a job. Although capable of enjoying simple pleasures—the greatest coming from visits to church—Lucille still needed someone to provide shelter, to care for her. That responsibility fell on the willing shoulders of Mrs. Dempsey, herself a devout churchgoer, who could never envision turning her back on her sister.

For 25 years, Lucille had lived with Mrs. Dempsey and her husband on that hill on 22nd Street. Mrs. Dempsey read to her, took her to church, and gave her a room to herself, where she wouldn't have to climb stairs. Tonight, however, her room was empty, as it had been for many months now. Tonight, Lucille slept in a distant state, cut off from the only world she had ever known, waiting for nothing much except death.

How Lucille Arrington came to live in a Delaware nursing home—where her loyal sister had been able to visit her only once in the last seven months—was a story of dehumanization. It was about a national health system that fitted together like a railroad track changing gauge every couple of miles. It was about a system that forced hospitals to discharge patients earlier without providing adequately for them once they left.

No one wanted to send Lucille away, yet in the end, no one could afford to keep her. Not the money-losing local hospital, which sent her to Delaware. Not any local nursing homes, which couldn't make a profit on her. In the end, she was treated much like an old mule at a farm auction: displayed, inspected, and passed over, until a bidder finally stepped forward and claimed her.

What drove Lucille and her sister apart was a story that had to compete on the national agenda with other compelling causes in an era of limited budgets: turmoil in the Persian Gulf, war against drug dealers, murder on the streets of Washington. Although the story lacked the graphic impact of dead bodies or invading foreign armies, it was nevertheless imbued with a special irony: the hospital that sent Lucille away without concern for her family's wishes was the same one that had been built specifically to give shelter, food, and medical care to former slaves and other dispossessed members of society. More than 100 years ago, Howard University Hospital—then called Freedmen's Hospital—sprang from a mudhole into an institution known for welcoming the forgotten.

Today, Howard University Hospital said it, too, must occasionally forget. Either that or close for good. Neither was an option it said it wanted, but in the 1990s, it was cold reality. If it could happen at Howard, it can—and does—happen almost everywhere.

• • •

Howard University Hospital would not look out of place in a fashionable big-city suburb. Its 500-bed building is tasteful and modern. A giant medical-office building rises elegantly behind it. Howard offers technically advanced care, including open-heart surgery, and it carries the cachet of a teaching institution. On one January afternoon in 1991, there were four cars parked adjacent to the front entrance in spots marked for visiting physicians: three Mercedes-Benzes and a Jaguar. The hospital itself, a private, nonprofit enterprise, was not so prosperous. Two years ago, it lost about $16 million—and $13.8 million last year—forcing it to turn, hat in hand, to Howard University for an infusion of cash. That couldn't continue.

Howard's problems were not all of its own making. Its inner-city location and busy emergency room attracted many indigent or uninsured patients, so Howard collected only about 50 cents on every dollar it billed. Howard was also ill-equipped to profit from elderly Medicare patients—the single biggest patient source for most hospitals. Because Medicare essentially rewarded hospitals for providing fewer services, rather than more, hospitals everywhere rushed to discharge Medicare patients as quickly as possible.

When Kevin E. Lofton became Howard's administrator in late 1990, he found that his Medicare patients stayed longer than those at any comparable institution, so he set out to identify the responsible doctors and change their behavior. His predecessor had already laid off 10 percent of Howard's staff, including general housekeepers, social workers, dietitians, and such—all of whom made hospitalization more pleasant, if not safer, for patients and families alike.

But these were relatively easy answers to a financial crunch. Telling patients they weren't wanted was more difficult. One nearby hospital actually paid to keep certain patients away. When the poor showed up seeking nonemergency help, the hospital summoned a cab, then paid the driver to haul them away to a government-funded medical clinic. A cab fare, the hospital reasoned, was more easily digested than an unpaid four-figure bill that might result from hospitalization.

Recently, Howard, too, had grudgingly begun turning away indigent, nonemergency patients. Although Lofton said Howard won't abandon its historical mission, he added, "We also have to look at how to change the patient mix, change services, and attract more paying patients." In doing so, Lofton was merely following the lead of thousands of other hospitals. It was one reason hospitals in the

1980s suddenly began offering weight loss programs, sleep disorder clinics, and chemical abuse centers—a strategy all too often geared to chasing money, rather than serving a need.

"It's very difficult for members of the surrounding community to understand," said Norman Brooks, a Howard official who began working for the hospital in 1970, when it was still called Freedmen's. "People in our community who are in low to lower middle class, they say, 'You treated my grandmother at Freedmen's, and you treated my mother; why can't you treat me?' To them, this will always be Freedmen's."

Freedmen's, however, is long gone. In 1975, it moved two blocks and became Howard University Hospital—a new location, a new name. Then came Medicare's prospective payment. "After DRGs, the tough times really began," sighed Brooks, pausing at the end of a lengthy hospital tour that he gave to a visitor. "It is big business now."

By the late 1980s, Lucille Arrington's seizures had begun to worsen. Once, during a service at Israel Baptist Church, she suffered a small seizure that so upset her that she didn't want to return. To control these seizures, along with other problems, she required heavy medication, including tranquilizers. That also took its toll, and she began to drift in and out of reality. Occasionally, Lucille would require hospitalization, where oxygen was administered. One time, Mrs. Dempsey visited her sister at a local hospital (not Howard), only to find that no one had fed her. "Sometimes, after a seizure," Mrs. Dempsey explained, "it would take her a couple of days to find herself again, and she wasn't able to feed herself." Doctors said she was too weak to eat, but Mrs. Dempsey found that she did take food when it was given to her.

Even so, Mrs. Dempsey couldn't be around all the time, and Lucille eventually became dependent on tube feeding. Finally, when Mrs. Dempsey felt she could do no more, she put her sister in a nursing home several blocks from her house. It was the best possible arrangement: with her sister just a short walk away, Mrs. Dempsey could still visit every day, read to her, and hold her hand. Soon, however, Lucille suffered another major seizure, and the nursing home rushed her to Howard University Hospital.

Although her condition stabilized, Lucille now needed a ventilator to help her breathe. It did more than just make her a captive to her machine; it made her an outcast. Technology could keep her alive, but suddenly, no one wanted her. She was too sick to move back in with Mr. and Mrs. Dempsey. Even her old nursing home refused to accept her again, saying it couldn't handle a ventilator patient. Who, then, would take her? Other area nursing homes capable of caring for such a patient either were booked solid or wouldn't accept anyone without a big bank account or private insurance. Lucille had neither.

Howard University Hospital, meanwhile, knew right away it had a major problem on its hands. Under prospective payment, Medicare paid Howard only part of Lucille's $700 daily hospital costs, which kept mounting as she required respiratory therapists, nurses, housekeepers, pharmacists, and dietitians, not to mention food supplements and medication. With every click of her ventilator, with every passing day, Lucille added to Howard's growing multimillion-dollar deficit.

Had Lucille been a solitary case, Howard might have covered her expenses with profits from other patients. But fewer and fewer patients admitted to Howard were profitable. And besides, Howard had a growing number of patients like Lucille; anyone who wanted to help them couldn't, and anyone who could wouldn't.

Lucille had become an elderly version of a "boarder" baby. But while babies abandoned in hospitals got widespread media coverage, the Lucilles of the world were left mostly to suffer in private. Somehow, some way, Howard had to push them out the door, but not onto the street. This unpleasant task fell to a group of hospital workers at Howard and elsewhere whose mission has taken on vast new importance in the restructured hospitals of the 1990s. In the vernacular of hospitals, they are called discharge-planners. In reality, they often function more like the Japanese who are employed to push commuters into packed railcars so doors can close behind them. In Japan they are called "oshiya," or, simply, people-pushers.

Jacqueline Tillman, like the tour guide Norman Brooks, had worked at Howard since it was Freedmen's. As a discharge-planner, her job had grown increasingly difficult. "We are a more mobile society," she observed. "Extended families don't exist anymore, and elderly are left on their own." Couple that with nursing homes that won't accept certain patients, and last year Howard had as many as 50 elderly patients at one time (and 20 babies) with no place to go. "You have to build up an emotional immunity to do this job," Tillman said.

The stress level wasn't any lower at competing D.C. hospitals. George Washington Hospital recently discharged a patient who had stayed three years; the longest stay was five years. "The pace in a hospital is intense," said Sandra Butcher, director of social work at George Washington. "You're dealing with people who are very, very ill. If you're not very ill, you're not in the hospital these days. And you're dealing with a lot of losses: people losing their bodily functions, losing what they'd hoped their future would be."

Families can be quickly overwhelmed. "It's not in the natural course for the family to say, 'Okay, I'm going to decide between today and tomorrow to take my mother and find some place for her,' " said Lynn Lewis, director of social work for Georgetown Hospital. "Social workers don't like to push some decision that in the normal course of events would take much longer."

Moreover, social workers who do discharge-planning aren't the patient advocates they used to be—thanks in part to prospective payment. Now, they face hospital pressure to push out patients who might not be ready to go. With social workers vulnerable to staff cutbacks, it takes courage to say no. One D.C. social worker stated, "I have said to administration, When we're under pressure [to improve profits], you don't say to the surgeons, 'Make big stitches.' So you don't tell us, 'Start doing sloppy discharge-planning.' "

Pressure to discharge wasn't by any means limited to Medicare patients. Private insurers and HMOs also want their patients out quickly, said Mary Genevieve Hagan, an assistant administrator at Georgetown Hospital. In this environment, social workers can quickly burn out. Besides getting pulled in opposite directions by hospitals and families, social workers often carry excessive caseloads. On top of all that, competition for nursing home beds has turned hospital against hospital, social worker against social worker.

This everyone-for-himself attitude was epitomized by an incident that occurred in Washington late in 1990. A meeting had been convened at a D.C. nursing home so that social workers and nursing home operators might discuss their common problems. Among the 20 or so who attended was Lynn Lewis of Georgetown Hospital. "I was new to the Washington community and didn't know any of the other social workers," Lewis recalled. At one point, the discussion turned to the practice whereby each hospital made dozens of calls weekly to various nursing homes in search of beds.

Lynn Lewis raised her hand. "How about we split the phone work and share what we find with others?" she asked.

The crowd reacted as though Lewis had just dropped in from Mars. Some chuckled. "Honestly, Lynn," replied one social worker from another hospital, "if we find a bed, we're not going to tell you."

Although others thought her suggestion naive in the extreme, Lewis said she was not surprised by the reaction she got. No one had cooperated in Pittsburgh, either, where she had previously worked.

As Lucille Arrington's hospitalization stretched from weeks into months, her sister never stopped coming to visit her. Three times or so a week, Mrs. Dempsey traveled two miles to Howard University Hospital, sometimes bringing nieces or nephews. She said Lucille appreciated the visits. "I tried to care for her the way I'd like to be cared for," she told *The Wall Street Journal*'s Ken Bacon. "I'd hold her hand. I'd tell her about the day. I'd quote her favorite Scripture to her. She likes the 23rd Psalm."

Lucille was trapped. Howard didn't want to keep her, but no area nursing home would accept her, because her post-hospital care would be paid by Medicaid. Since states fund part of that program, many tried to limit their costs by keeping Medicaid reimbursement rates low or by restricting the number of nursing-home beds. Nursing homes, meanwhile, wanted to improve profit margins by picking patients who required less care, rather than more, or by finding wealthy, private-pay patients.

It was, in short, a buyer's market: if nursing homes didn't want, they didn't buy. "You basically market the patient in terms of putting up their good points and hoping that their bad points don't come out," said Howard's Jacqueline Tillman. "They [nursing homes] might say, 'We have X number of insulins, X number of decubitus [bedsores], so today we are looking for a good patient who if he had a family wouldn't even be in a nursing home," Tillman said. "If you send them a private-pay patient, you might try to skirt a heavy-care patient right behind them."

The search didn't necessarily end when a nursing home accepted a patient, Tillman said. "You can send a patient to a nursing home signed, sealed, and delivered. They will look at the patient and say, 'No way, that's not what we wanted.' [And] they will send that person back, sometimes in the same ambulance."

That people in their last years of life were marketed like junk at a garage sale didn't sit well with many social workers, but they did it nonetheless. Many even went along with the most dehumanizing side of this process, which occurred when hospitals opened their doors to nursing home representatives. These "buyers" reviewed patient medical records and trolled the halls for prospects who might yield them a profit. Hospitals justified this arrangement on the ground that the quicker they discharged patients, the more money they would have to treat other indigent patients.

Howard welcomed buyers. Each week, usually, at least one buyer visited patients. Some came from faraway states. "Nursing homes don't like surprises, and sometimes paper [medical record] and body don't always match," Tillman said. "They have learned it's better to look . . . they literally look at the patient right down to the skin."

Some places, however, like the Hospital of the University of Pennsylvania in Philadelphia, almost never admit buyers, said its social-service director, Kathy C. Forrest. But when Forrest worked in Massachusetts, she said, the practice was rampant. "Patients get psyched up, and when they are passed over they are let down," Forrest said. "Some poor old ladies would have their hair all brushed up, and the staff would make sure that Mr. Jones didn't have any crumbs that would imply he couldn't feed himself." She added, "Aside from the ethical and confidentiality issues, how dare anyone presume to look at a medical record and look over a patient who was not invited by a patient?"

It was not surprising that such buying and selling existed in Massachusetts. One day in 1989, some 1,800 patients in that state were ready to be discharged from a hospital but had no place to go. Today, federal health officials believe about 25 percent of the nation's nearly 6,000 hospitals have a "boarder elderly" problem.

Mrs. Dempsey remembered that it was a beautiful, warm day in early summer when they took her sister away. "I was at the hospital when the ambulance arrived," she recalled. "I even went up into the ambulance and gave her a hug and a goodbye. I said we would see her as soon as we could. I think she knew she was being moved but didn't know how far. We were holding hands for a long time."

After nearly a year of trying, Howard had successfully placed Lucille in a nursing home. The only problem: it was in Delaware, nearly a three-hour drive away. "I didn't have any say in this," Mrs. Dempsey said softly. "I said, 'Does it have to be so far?' but they said, 'This is the only one that will take her.' "

Mrs. Dempsey herself had tried finding a nursing home for Lucille. The homes asked whether she had money. She didn't. Once, it appeared that a bed had been found in nearby Baltimore, but that fell through when the nursing home demanded a $32,000 up-front payment to cover the first two months of care.

In the many months since the day they took her sister away, Mrs. Dempsey has visited her only once, because she can't drive and her husband is ill. But after that one visit, Mrs. Dempsey said, nurses told her they had never seen Lucille respond that way before. "She can respond to voices. I cut her hair. And as I was talking to her, she squeezed my hand."

Today, Mrs. Dempsey has only memories of when she was close enough to visit her sister. "I would tell her about everybody, and that we loved her, and I always gave her a kiss. I pray that people don't have to go through this. In reading the Scriptures, I told my sister you have to have the patience of Job."

She paused for a moment, then added, "I said, 'Just hang on and this, too, will pass.' "

The boarder elderly problem is but one small component of a health system that poorly manages the discharge of its hospital patients. Before prospective payment, hospitals kept patients until, as one social worker put it, "they ran laps in the hallways." And why not? After all, Medicare and many private insurers basically reimbursed hospitals for whatever costs they incurred. Administrators often defended long hospitalizations ("Our patients are sicker," they said), but privately they gamed the system whenever possible. Friday admissions and Monday discharges were commonplace, even though little was done for patients over the weekend.

Prospective payment, however, abruptly changed the rules of making money, and hospitals suddenly began disgorging patients by the tens of thousands. Corporations also pressure insurers to effect early discharges for their employees. Nursing homes are supposed to take many of the elderly who are discharged early, but beds aren't always available. Moreover, despite calls for reform that have echoed for decades, nursing homes don't always provide good care. Among many unresolved problems, federal investigators reported in 1990 that the abuse of residents by nursing aides often goes unreported and may be worsening. Although Congress belatedly passed a landmark law in 1987 to improve nursing-home care, Health and Human Services ineptly waited more than three years to issue the regulations needed to carry it out.

The movement toward early discharge was, in part, healthy. It cut costs while reducing patient exposure to hospital-acquired infections and medication errors. But some hospitals carried the idea too far and discharged patients who were still unstable with rapid heartbeat, chest pain, or other ailments. These patients, a Rand Corporation study revealed, died at a higher rate than those allowed to fully recover in hospitals.

One day in May 1987, some 250 people crowded into a New York City union hall to hear horror stories of patients discharged without good post-hospital care. They came in wheelchairs and crutches. They came from nursing homes and hospitals, near and far. One by one they stood, and as they told their stories some began to weep.

Virginia Wagner of Middletown, New York, whose husband had advanced heart disease, said:

My husband was told at 6 A.M. [Friday] that he had to go home that morning at 11 A.M. No home care arrangement had been made. He was too ill to come by car, so I called an ambulance. My husband was nonambulatory, very short of breath, and needed daily Lasix shots and oxygen. I am a senior citizen with no hospital training, living alone with my husband and no one to help me. It was very hard because he would not eat, couldn't walk, and had a chart of medications to take at different hours of the day and night. . . . I was up all night because my husband couldn't breathe. On Saturday, I was able to get a nurse to come from 10 A.M. to 2 P.M. at $22 an hour. While the nurse was there, my husband slept quite a bit and seemed to breathe better, but when she left he couldn't breathe. Even from outdoors you could hear him gasping for breath. My brave husband, who had suffered so long without complaining, cried, and wanted a gun to kill himself. [He died the next morning.] Every man has a right to die with dignity and this was denied to my husband.

Mary Agrillo, whose 71-year-old father suffered complications after hemorrhoid surgery, told the group:

A few days after surgery, he fell out of the hospital bed. He was badly bruised on his right side and in a lot of pain. . . . Since I visited every day after work I had expected to be notified of his discharge date. . . . I came into his room to find him in his shorts on a stripped bed, no pillow or sheets, telling me he was discharged at 11 A.M. It was then 5:30 P.M. [He was later readmitted after falling down at home.] While they were still running tests on my father, I was called at work at 10 A.M. by the hospital utilization department. I was told I had until 11 A.M. to take my father home or begin paying $500 a day privately.

Melvin Sadowsky of Queens, whose father had advanced heart disease, said:

One day I arrived at the hospital to visit my father, only to learn that either the doctor or the hospital had ordered an ambulance to send my father home. He still had oxygen and a catheter and the home care was not arranged for, and they were sending him home with 14 prescriptions for different medications. I canceled the ambulance.

Such stories prompted New York State to require that hospitals hand patients a written discharge plan. But many hospitals refused to comply, said Bonnie Ray, who oversaw a hospital hot line for patients who thought they were being discharged prematurely. "Very often, if a patient gets anything at all in writing it will be, 'Take three aspirin a day and call if there is a problem,' " Ray said. Some discharge plans are wrong, illegible, given to the wrong person, or impractical. Wealth guarantees no protection. "You can be rich and go home to die if you are discharged too soon," Ray said. "We have wonderful regulations [in New York] but very, very poor compliance." Most states don't even have the "wonderful" regulations.

Instead of strengthening discharge-planning, many cash-starved hospitals have laid off social workers. Job stress drives others out of the business. The highly regarded Montefiore Medical Center in the Bronx lost nearly half of its social work staff in a 20-month span, *Newsday* reported in May 1989. Almost two years later, a social worker at another Bronx hospital confessed that she hadn't given a written discharge plan to a patient in the previous two years.

One reason lies in the numbers. "Some hospitals carry horrendous caseloads," said Susan Haikalas, who in 1992 will become president of the Society for Hospital Social Work Directors. "It's not uncommon that people may be expected to see 80, 90, 100 people a month. In my mind, there is no way you can do this, trying to juggle that many life situations." She thought a caseload of 30 to 32 was reasonable.

Overworked discharge-planners faced hard choices. Kathy Forrest, director of social work at the Hospital of the University of Pennsylvania, said her social workers carried caseloads as high as 70. "One of the things a social work director says to a person who has such a caseload is 'We are not going to get another person [on staff], so what can we do to manage that?' "

The answer: triage. "You prioritize needs and suffering, and that's very hard to do," said one New York City social worker. Many hospitals mistakenly turned to overworked nurses to handle the overload. "They don't have the time, or resources, or expertise," Susan Haikalas said. "They have a heavy load, are going through tests, going through procedures, changing medications. They don't have the training to know what resources are out there in a community."

Haikalas said one hospital (not her own) concluded that her father, a stroke victim, was too old to get better and should go to a nursing home. Haikalas didn't believe it. She found and placed her father in a Medicare-covered geriatric rehab center. He later improved enough to return home. "Unfortunately, the person who worked with us wasn't social work–trained," she said. "Another family member wouldn't have known what to do. They wouldn't have even heard of a geriatric rehab unit."

Prospective payment, apart from prompting early discharges, also worked to keep patients out of the hospital altogether. Some hospitals, for example, asked patients to undergo complex and risky medical procedures, such as cardiac catheterization and radiation therapy, as outpatients, because those services can then be provided more cheaply. But since health officials didn't vigorously police these "freestanding" centers, congressional investigators concluded that consumers can't be assured that they are safe. "Time and time again, elderly people say, 'It was worse than I anticipated. I could barely do it,' " said Sandra Butcher, social work director at George Washington Hospital. "People are just barely hanging on in some of these situations, and they're not even admitted to the hospital."

Many hospitals thought the best discharge-planning meant

"dumping" unprofitable patients before they were admitted through the emergency room. During one three-month period, 15 hospitals made 190 requests to transfer patients to the Regional Medical Center at Memphis; about 90 percent mentioned financial status as the reason. At least they made the request; most just shipped the bodies. One in four patients sent to Regional Medical Center was medically unstable.

"We aren't talking about a patient with no money who wants a tummy tuck or a face-lift," the head of Regional's emergency services told *The Wall Street Journal.* "We are talking about heart attacks and seizures and strokes and gastrointestinal bleeding." One congressional committee concluded that 250,000 patients are dumped yearly, yet by 1991 only 140 hospitals had been named as violators, resulting in imposition of sanctions on just 19 hospitals. Even when the indigent did gain hospital admittance, according to a study of about 500,000 patients hospitalized nationwide in 1987, they were three times as likely as insured patients to die there.

Time and time again, hospital administrators have said they aren't happy when they must admit some patients while rejecting others or discharge patients into nursing homes they would never consider for their own relatives. "We do what we must to survive" is their common refrain. It is, in fairness, not the fault of hospitals that government policymakers have failed to set up a safety net for those patients lacking the knowledge, money, or just plain luck to get good medical care in a society that commits 12 percent of its GNP to health care.

Still, it's troubling to see the extreme measures that hospitals will take to compete in the DRG era. Texas's McAllen Medical Center sits just north of the Rio Grande, in the crossing path of many illegal aliens. Like other hospitals, McAllen has its own security force, but it doesn't dress them in traditional uniforms. Instead, they are outfitted in olive-colored clothes. Legal-aid lawyers say they know why: U.S. Border Patrol agents wear similar uniforms, so the sight of the hospital guards scares off poor people seeking medical care.

Over the last decade, hospitals have largely changed from social-service institutions into something less noble. "We are talking about an industry which is now a profit motive industry," said Dr. Gerard Anderson of the Johns Hopkins Center for Hospital Finance and Management. "It's a change in responsibility . . . and I think it's bad."

TWO | The New Ethics

6 | On the Threshold

IRAN released 52 American hostages. The Boys of Summer staged their first midseason strike, and "M*A*S*H" topped TV's Nielsen ratings. The year was 1981, the ideological beginning of a decade that would encompass Ronald Reagan's baffling reign as one of the nation's most popular presidents.

On a cold January evening, within days of Reagan's inauguration, the telephone rang at Richard Kusserow's rural home 30 miles from downtown Chicago. He took the call in the kitchen.

"Richard Kusserow? This is David Newhall, chief of staff for Richard Schweiker."

Kusserow had no idea what a former United States senator from Pennsylvania could want from him. As an FBI agent, Kusserow didn't get involved in politics. He knew little about Schweiker, except that he had just been picked to head the Department of Health and Human Services and, as a liberal Republican, seemed out of place among the conservatives in Reagan's cabinet.

"We are on a major search for an inspector general of HHS," Newhall said. "That's the first job Secretary Schweiker would like to fill. Would you want to come to Washington to be the IG?"

Kusserow was stunned. He wasn't a health specialist any more than he was a politician. "How did you decide to call me?" he asked.

Kusserow should have known better. At age 40, he ranked among the FBI's top experts on white-collar crime, having written an FBI manual on the subject. Well over six feet tall, with a knack for talking tough and fast, he might have just walked over from Central Casting.

Even so, he wasn't the white-bread clone that FBI management historically favored.

A former college lecturer with a master's in history, Kusserow had specialized in African studies. He had also managed to avoid the military draft, more out of stubbornness than ideology. "I didn't want anyone telling me I had to go," he explained. As soon as he beat the draft, he walked into a U.S. Marine Corps recruiting office and enlisted; he left a captain. Along the way, Kusserow attracted the attention of CIA recruiters who liked his blend of military training and African expertise. Kusserow joined the CIA but soon became disillusioned working in its covert section. He moved to the FBI in 1969.

Kusserow made his biggest mark in weaning the bureau from its old Texas Ranger approach to crime. In the past it was one agent per case, no matter how big; if an agent needed help, he would informally ask a colleague. Figuring that the FBI could combat white-collar crime more effectively through better use of its resources, Kusserow helped set up special FBI investigative squads, personally directing a number of them in Chicago.

Off the job, he enjoyed his country home on five acres with horses and a barn. But, always the investigator, Kusserow made the most of his lengthy railroad commute by picking up leads from well-lubricated commuters unwinding after a stressful day at the office. "If you couldn't make it as an FBI agent in Chicago, you can't make it anywhere," he joked.

Success bred crisis, however. One day Kusserow's supervisors asked him to leave Chicago for a promotion to FBI headquarters in Washington. Many agents privately coveted management jobs inside the coldly imposing J. Edgar Hoover Building, one of the capital's big tourist stops. But not Kusserow.

"I don't like to push paper, so I said, 'No, I'll forgo the honor,'" he recalled. "Well, you don't do that in the bureau. You either make yourself available for promotion or get out of management entirely." So Kusserow returned to the street, giving up all his squads and his pay grade. It was what one might have expected from an agent who fondly recalled his early years as a G-man, digging fugitives out of the back hills of West Virginia. Tough but thoughtful. It was precisely this mix that made Kusserow so rare—and so desirable—inside law enforcement circles.

After the call from Schweiker's office, Kusserow began to consider seriously the offer of becoming inspector general of Health and Human Services. Although he had previously rejected a move to D.C., this time he would run an entire agency, monitoring nearly $1 billion a day in federal spending, or one-third of the entire federal budget. Kusserow also appreciated the IG's independent role in keeping the executive branch honest and efficient. After Watergate, separate IG offices were created in many government departments, but Health and Human Services' remained the biggest. Even the president couldn't remove the IG without first informing Congress in writing of his reasons.

Kusserow decided to accept Schweiker's invitation, formally interviewing for the job several weeks later in Washington. The meeting went well. Schweiker would later tell congressmen that Kusserow reminded him of a junkyard dog. But while a draft-averse, white student of African culture was out of place at the FBI, so were junkyard dogs in the Reagan era. Political points in that administration were earned exposing misdeeds not of the regulated but of the regulators, whom Reagan blamed for many societal ills.

"We tried as a Government not to get on anyone's back," said a senior official with Congress's General Accounting Office. Only as the decade came to a close would the enormous cost of this policy become fully evident in the scandals that rocked the savings and loan industry and the Department of Housing and Urban Development.

Schweiker himself would soon depart Reagan's cabinet, a politically bad fit who registered barely a blip in Reagan's reign. Except for one thing: Schweiker recommended that Reagan nominate Richard Kusserow for inspector general. He was approved, and by strange political happenstance, the president had picked the toughest cop on the block to oversee the nation's biggest domestic programs—programs that benefited many of the president's biggest political supporters in the medical community. Moreover, Reagan did so at the very moment in history when Medicare began lurching toward a radical cost control plan that would give hospitals an unprecedented incentive to reduce waste, but also an unprecedented incentive to cut corners and cheat.

The medical community, to say the least, didn't expect a Reagan appointee to be snarling at its every move. "I make my living in large measure by going after the bastards out there that are in fact doing bad things in medicine," Kusserow barked. When doctors said they resented insinuations that some of them might be dishonest, Kusserow retorted, "Let me put it this way. I do not believe that physicians are any less human than other Homo sapiens bipeds."

He scolded doctors for failing to report incompetent colleagues. He rebuked other medical investigators for their "squad room" mentality, waiting for easy referrals from law enforcement agencies on crimes unrelated to professional competence. "If I'm going to go under the knife in some hospital," Kusserow said, "and I have a choice between two physicians—physician A being one who is honest but incompetent, and physician B being one who is competent but a crook—I'll take the crook if he's going to stick a knife in me."

While other Reagan regulators fought public scrutiny of their activities, Kusserow welcomed it. In a statement extraordinary for the time, he told journalists, "I'm no longer with the FBI, and no longer with the CIA, and I think that's important because nothing we do is secret." He went so far as to offer up for public inspection specific work plans. "You don't have to do a Freedom of Information Act request or anything else. Just ask for it and we'll send it to you."

Kusserow's brash style of law enforcement won him broad support in Congress and among consumer groups. Even so, powerful forces threatened to undermine his efforts. One incensed Houston lawyer, in a speech to hospital conventioneers in Washington, D.C., compared Kusserow to Lenin. The American Medical Association, meanwhile, accused the inspector general of running a bounty system that offered financial rewards to one top IG official for his success in prosecuting physicians. Kusserow, the AMA complained, didn't understand that "sensitive methods" should be used to evaluate medical care and "physician motivation."

On top of that, Reagan's budget-cutters sat like buzzards in a treetop, waiting to feast on dead enforcement and oversight programs in federal offices near and far. Besides, how much could one man, or one agency, do? At best, Kusserow was little more than a sentry. Lacking any broad, policy-making authority, he could yell and stomp, but would anyone care to listen? Or did only a precious few in the medical community know the dangers that lay ahead?

In June 1981, just as Kusserow was being sworn in as inspector general at HHS, a prophetic and profoundly disturbing article appeared in *The New England Journal of Medicine*. Hardly as provincial as the name suggests, the journal's pages, then as now, constitute the most valued plot of real estate that money can't buy in the medical profession. Scientists the world over vie for space in the journal to announce medical breakthroughs affecting millions, not to mention their own careers. Publication is the medical researcher's equivalent of winning the Academy Award.

Although the journal's raison d'être is its peer-reviewed articles of original reserach, shorter works of special interest also appear. The June 1981 article was one such piece, written by a San Francisco medical doctor, Donald W. Simborg. When he submitted his 2,000-word article for publication, Dr. Simborg never imagined the interest it would stir. Oddly, he didn't consider the article a crowning personal achievement, in part because he had done it almost as a lark, an offshoot of a hobby he had developed early in medical training at Johns Hopkins University. While fellow students there dreamed of the wealth and glory they would win as hands-on healers, Simborg could be found in the back room nerdishly programming computers. For a young doctor, this fascination with clunky, impersonal machines might have been considered strange, particularly in the early 1960s, long before computers assumed their dominant role in everyday life.

It wasn't that Simborg didn't enjoy treating patients—he would become a board-certified internist—he just wondered whether computers couldn't do more to promote the healing process. "A hospital," he noted years later, "is one of the most heterogeneous and complex organizations of any industry, with some 60 to 70 different departments or functions—each contributing in some way to taking care of the patient." The right computer system, he believed, could integrate all those functions, if only hospital managers would just stop funneling all their computer money into the business and accounting side and try using some of it on direct patient care.

With the promise of freedom to explore new computer applications, Simborg left Johns Hopkins in the late 1970s for the University of California at San Francisco. There he began exploring how hospitals might fare under a radical new cost containment proposal that had caught the fancy of budget-conscious regulators. Relying on the work of two Yale researchers, and financed in part by a $5.3 million federal grant, New Jersey had begun a pilot program that promised to restructure the hospital industry. While the current system rewarded overtreatment, the pilot program did just the opposite—it rewarded undertreatment.

Since Medicare's inception, it was thought hospitals generally shouldn't profit from a program for the elderly. Essentially, hospitals submitted their bills and they were paid, regardless of how wasteful. But with hospital costs rising an average of 19 percent a year, threatening Medicare's very solvency, the New Jersey plan seemed divinely inspired. By rejecting patchwork solutions of previous years, the program in one dramatic sweep promised to attack the disease itself, not just its symptoms.

Medicare, if it adopted the plan, would pay hospitals a predetermined amount of money, depending on the diagnosis or diagnostic-related group. Suppose Medicare paid $1,000 for a certain diagnosis but the cost of hospital care totaled $1,500; the hospital then would lose $500. But if the hospital could provide the same care for less than $1,000, it got to keep the difference. In all, there would be more than 400 diagnostic-related groupings, known as DRGs.

The timing for such a plan was perfect. With Reagan's free-marketeers hyping deregulation, what could be more philosophically appealing than a cost control program built on the profit motive? No national health insurance. No price controls. Just the gospel of profit working its magic. Inefficient hospitals could either reorganize or go out of business. In that respect, they would be no different from a poorly run dry cleaner, butcher shop, or widget factory.

Simborg, however, suspected that the program wasn't the panacea many believed it to be. For one thing, the system of grouping diagnoses had been devised for the study of disease, not reimbursement. An epidemiologist, for example, doesn't care whether a clogged artery is cleared by balloon angioplasty or open-heart surgery, yet the cost difference between the two procedures is enormous. No less a problem was the fact that payment was tied to the primary diagnosis, even though multiple ailments may be present. "There is nothing in medical school that teaches you to pick the primary diagnosis," Simborg explained. "Yet now it makes a difference in what you get paid."

Simborg and others feared that savvy hospital administrators might use computers to exploit the plan's vulnerability. If their fears proved correct, the DRG plan could prove embarrassing: its highly touted cost controls might end up producing mountains of profits for an industry already widely judged to be greedy and wasteful.

Simborg set out to test the DRG system, using actual patient records at his own hospital. He quickly discovered how easy it would be for an unprincipled hospital administrator to "game" the system. In one analysis, Simborg isolated 159 patients who in one year underwent some major surgery with a secondary diagnosis of renal disease. The average charge: $4,210. Switching the two diagnoses, however, more than doubled the charge to $9,322. In some cases, renal disease could legitimately be the primary diagnosis; in other cases, it could not.

To assess the financial impact of intentional code manipulation, Simborg wrote a computer program that automatically picked the more lucrative diagnosis, whether it was the primary or the secondary. In nearly one of every four cases, flipping the diagnoses meant a higher reimbursement. Applied across the board, this would have produced an unprecedented windfall profit for his hospital.

Simborg now had enough to write his article. On June 25, 1981, *The New England Journal of Medicine* carried his findings under the headline DRG CREEP: A NEW HOSPITAL-ACQUIRED DISEASE. Simborg wasted little time getting to the point: "This article," he wrote, "is intended to provide a case report of 'DRG Creep,' a new phenomenon that is expected to occur in epidemic proportions in the 1980s." It was a bold prediction but one he felt comfortable making.

Simborg concluded that DRG creep need not result only from unethical acts. He envisioned computer programs that would automatically flip the diagnoses when some justification could be found. Even without computers, he believed, hospital administrators would foster DRG creep by "educating" doctors to select the better-paying diagnoses when the facts of the case were sufficiently murky. "Minor diagnostic nuances and slight imprecisions of wording have little practical clinical importance, yet under DRG reimbursement they would have major financial consequences," Simborg wrote.

In professing hope that hospitals would avoid the more "virulent" forms of DRG creep, Simborg nevertheless acknowledged the capacity for evil that computers might have in a DRG system. He concluded with the following warning: "In the ensuing technologic arms race between the regulators and the regulated, it may be difficult to distinguish the disease from the cure."

Simborg's popularity soared with the article's publication. "I've published 50 to 60 articles in my life, but nothing got more press and publicity than that one," he said a decade later. Speaking invitations flooded in. Not surprisingly, many came from hospital administrators wanting to learn Simborg's secrets for manipulating the system.

Two years later, despite the alarms sounded by Simborg and others, the prospective-payment system would become reality in hospitals across America. By then, regulators had refined the DRG payment system to protect it against some of the more obvious abuses. Still, more than a few observers wondered how Congress had managed to pass so tough a cost control program on such a politically influential industry. If DRGs were really to strike at the heart of inflated medical costs, why were so many hospitals supporting the plan? It was enough to make a skeptic wonder: did they know something the rest of the public didn't?

As 1981 came to a close, one could begin to sense the imprint the year would leave on the future of the hospital industry, from Reagan's vision of deregulated medical care to the warnings of Dr. Simborg. But 1981's biggest contribution wouldn't be known for more than a year. And the importance of that contribution flowed in part from what was happening at places like Richmond Heights General Hospital in suburban Cleveland, where two executives were planning a trip to China.

A few top teaching hospitals, like nearby Cleveland Clinic, occasionally sent emissaries overseas in search of exotic potentates in need of heart surgery; to snare a foreign dignitary was a public-relations bonanza. But Richmond Heights, a modest, 220-bed osteopathic hospital, had no such grand ambitions. Operated largely by a father and his three sons, the hospital had trouble keeping beds filled in the highly competitive Cleveland market. Like many community hospitals, Richmond Heights offered help for certain medical emergencies, convenience for friends and families wishing to visit patients, and a place for doctors to admit neighbors they have known for years.

But it definitely was not an institution that would attract top Chinese rulers. No, the two Richmond Heights officials were going to China not specifically to seek patients but to experience a foreign culture and enjoy themselves. Even so, they didn't plan to pay for it. Picking up their $12,000 tab: Richmond Heights General Hospital, a nonprofit institution, which the two men helped to run. The hospital said the trip was for educational purposes.

The hospital's largess wasn't out of character. As many workers there discovered, the hospital had a festive air—at least for the fortunate few who ran it. When the hospital's founder had turned 65 years old, the hospital spent $1,500 on a party. In 1981 and 1982, it paid $4,400 for golf outings, $2,055 for Cleveland Indians box seat tickets, $9,000 for parties and liquor, $5,100 in dining bills at a single restaurant for two hospital executives and their guests, as well as thousands of dollars for car rentals and theater tickets.

The hospital's bosses weren't satisfied with just entertainment perks, either. They also promoted the private business interests of certain board members. Patients may have wondered why a savings and loan branch office, of all things, was conspicuously located inside the hospital. One likely reason: three of the hospital's board members owned stock in the S&L. And as if that weren't enough, Richmond Heights dumped nearly $1.5 million of its own funds in the S&L's low-interest passbook accounts—when some certificates of deposit were paying upward of twice the amount of that interest. So cavalier was the hospital in its business dealings that a single director on the 10-member board once authorized the hospital's purchase of nearly $400,000 in land from three other board members.

Given Richmond Heights's loose style of money management, only an advertising executive could concoct a promotional theme for the hospital that began: "We are concerned about the high cost of health care, especially in this time of economic uncertainty. We are taking bold and innovative steps to keep costs down. . . . We do care."

Richmond Heights's conduct raised ethical questions common to many hospitals of that era. Should board members of a nonprofit, tax-exempt hospital—guardians of a public trust—spend so lavishly on themselves? And who ultimately picked up the tab for China trips, liquor, and parties? In this regard, Richmond Heights was no different from many of its counterparts. The hospital tried to stick Medicare, a program already hurtling toward insolvency, by including many of those expenditures in its annual Medicare cost report. Before the advent of DRGs, cost reports determined how much Medicare money hospitals got. The higher the costs, the higher the federal reimbursement. That prompted some creative scheming. One Las Vegas hospital boosted costs for intravenous solution 800 percent, essentially by selling and reselling goods to itself.

By 1981, however, most hospitals realized the game couldn't last.

Inflation, helped along by rising hospital costs, had helped push Jimmy Carter from the White House. Clearly, government had to do something—and that something was the enactment of the prospective-payment system. The new program couldn't fully succeed, however, unless DRG rates reflected only the real cost of medical care, minus wasteful and unnecessary services. With that in mind, it was decided to set those rates using operating costs submitted to Medicare by hospitals for the year 1981. Any undetected mistakes, or intentional cost padding, in those reports could bloat DRG rates for years to come. Never before would it be more important for regulators to identify and cut out this disease.

Back in 1981, when Richmond Heights and other hospitals submitted expenses like trips to China, no one knew those cost reports would later provide the heartbeat of prospective payment. The question then became: did Medicare have the smarts to catch hospitals that tried to slip in wasteful operating costs? The answer would go a long way toward determining the success or failure of the government's ambitious plan to restructure an industry at whose mercy so many Americans eventually find themselves.

7 | Buried Secrets

DANIEL R. Garcia's world was an orderly and tasteful one, where every hair was always combed, clothing carefully matched, and work schedule precisely set. So it was with great dismay that one frosty spring day in 1984 Garcia opened a motel room door to discover that for the next several weeks he would be living a nightmare of lavender and orange. Was this the assignment he wanted so badly, he wondered? Alone, cold, away from his wife and young child, trudging home every night to a room that resembled an LSD hallucination.

Most people wouldn't be bothered by motel decor. This place was on the interstate bypass outside Baltimore, after all, not some bed-and-breakfast in Vermont. Yet Garcia's aversion to imperfection, whether in a motel room or a government program, made him an ideal choice for what would become the biggest assignment of his career.

A veteran investigator in the General Accounting Office, the research arm of Congress, Garcia had come to Baltimore to begin his agency's probe into the government's highly touted DRG program. He faced an enormously complex task. Trained auditors needed at least a year to master the complexities of Medicare regulations. Garcia was no accountant. He had never seen the tomes hospitals must file with Medicare, nor did he know the arcane, 17-step formula Medicare used to set reimbursement rates for individual hospitals.

Garcia had come to Medicare's headquarters in Baltimore to learn the basics, never a pleasant task, be it ice skating or hospital finance. But patience has its rewards. As he struggled in his new world, Garcia never dreamed that in a little more than a year he would help uncover one of the costliest financial foul-ups in GAO history. His explosive findings required that every number, every calculation, every interview be precise and accurate. Any mistake, no matter how small, could be used to discredit his conclusions, himself, even his agency, which had built a stellar, nonpartisan reputation for accuracy. With billions of dollars at stake, the GAO needed a patient investigator not prone to the sort of disorder he was meant to expose.

Daniel R. Garcia was the right man for the job.

Garcia had stumbled onto the GAO by accident. After leaving the air force in the early 1970s, he went to work teaching high school in the inner city of Fort Worth. Although he never considered himself naive, this son of a California factory worker nevertheless was unprepared for the frustrations of a school where teachers had to collect quarters from children to buy a movie projector, where lessons were taught using a world map printed in 1949, the year of Garcia's birth. Unhappy, Garcia decided to transfer to the more upscale Dallas school system. The very day he applied, however, a Dallas teacher was shot by a parent upset over a child's grade. "I told my wife, this is a perfect time to get my master's," Garcia recalled.

Later, with a master's in public administration, and his wife expecting their first child, Garcia got a call from an accountant friend suggesting he apply for the job of investigator—officially called evaluator—in the GAO's Dallas office. A long shot at best, the idea nevertheless intrigued Garcia because of a fantasy he had about working as an archaeologist, slowly stripping away the deposits of time in search of buried secrets. The GAO dug for secrets, too, but mostly in the starched white shirts of the accounting profession, from which the agency drew nearly all of its staff. Fortunately for Garcia, the GAO hired him because his background in government studies fitted with the agency's growing move away from narrow accounting issues and into broader policy examinations.

Garcia ultimately settled in the GAO's health care financing section in Dallas, directed by a matter-of-fact GAO veteran, Thomas G. Dowdal, whose short-sleeved shirts and prosaic dress made him look like a police detective running a murder investigation. Not one to suffer fools gladly, the Baltimore-based Dowdal had heard hospitals complain about how little they got from Medicare. He just didn't believe them. To gauge the fairness of Medicare's reimbursements, Dowdal had his staff sample medical tests at 16 hospitals in eight geographic regions. The GAO concluded that 6 percent were unnecessary, yet costs for these services were built into the DRG rates. Dowdal later looked at respiratory therapy, pacemaker surgeries, and intensive care units—each time finding errors, or unnecessary services, all of which bloated the new reimbursement rates.

These findings, however, barely got a rise out of Medicare officials. The mistakes didn't add up to all that much, they said. Dowdal didn't agree. He wasn't through digging, either. Dowdal's instincts told him there were plenty of secrets buried in the lengthy reports that hospitals filed with Medicare on their annual operating expenses, reports that now helped to set the base payment rates for all DRGs.

Dowdal suspected that improper costs might have slipped into those reports, permanently embedding themselves in the payment rates. This wasn't idle speculation. In 1980, the GAO had investigated how Medicare implemented a program to control home health care costs. For the program to work, Medicare had to set a reasonable cap on those payments: too low, and no one would provide the service; too high, and the program would be useless.

Medicare badly botched the job. First the government used incorrect data to set the cap, then it made a computer programming error. Even worse, it used figures that it knew full well came from unaudited cost reports.

It seemed hard to believe that Medicare would perform so poorly again, especially on a program so big and far-reaching as prospective payment. Nevertheless, Dowdal remained suspicious, and assigned Daniel R. Garcia of the GAO's Dallas office to see whether Medicare had also botched the setting of DRG rates. This time, the GAO wouldn't settle for a small sampling of hospitals that Medicare could dismiss as a statistical aberration. It wanted proof. If Medicare had messed up this time, the GAO didn't want to leave any escape routes.

And who better to lead the charge than a man with the initials DRG?

• • •

Garcia's investigation began without much dramatic action. There were no whispered, late-night confessions, no shortcuts around the piles of mind-numbing numbers, no Deep Throats, no caches of hidden documents neatly summarizing Medicare screwups. For the first nine months, beginning March 1984, two-thirds of the GAO's time went toward trying to understand Medicare's terminology and various data bases.

Investigators, meanwhile, were required to sit down with green GAO legal pads and write in longhand the who, what, when, and why of each key interview, and conclusions. Why review this hospital's records and not another one's? Why interview this particular government official? Each report had to be signed, then reviewed and countersigned by the project leader, Daniel Garcia, before becoming part of the permanent record. The GAO wanted no mistakes.

The simple act of retrieving a hospital file could take days, as the GAO's Ken Brake discovered. Because of a recent reorganization inside Medicare, several files couldn't be found, including one on New York City's Bellevue Hospital. Brake learned that Medicare had hired Blue Cross to audit Bellevue. Simple enough—except that on a trip to New York, Brake learned that Blue Cross had subcontracted that job. Another interview established that the audit file had been sent back to Medicare headquarters in Baltimore. But on returning to his home base in Baltimore, Brake checked in with Medicare, only to discover that the file had been shipped back to New York. Further inquiries proved fruitless, and Brake, deciding he had wasted enough time, dropped Bellevue from his sample.

To assess how well Medicare had extracted cost data used to set DRGs, Garcia's investigators examined cost reports from 100 hospitals, retracing the complex formula Medicare used to gather data, code it, and compute final reimbursement rates.

Medicare's sloppiness appeared everywhere. On his green legal pad, carefully skipping every other line for readability, the GAO's Cleo Zapata wrote: "We found that HCFA [the Health Care Financing Administration] made coding and computational errors while extracting the data in 51 of 100 cases reviewed." That was more than half. Although only 8 percent of those errors involved significant sums of money, Medicare's cavalier handling of such important numbers sent an important message: the government's figures were not to be trusted. Virtually every number would have to be double-checked, every calculation redone.

The final tally of Medicare's bumbling startled even the GAO. An investigation that promised to be long and arduous had just gotten longer.

As the investigation progressed, Garcia increasingly came to rely on Ken Brake, a genial Kansas native who each year left his home in Baltimore to help out on the family farm during harvest season. Although 15 years older and one civil-service grade above Garcia, Brake's gentle humor and secure personality made him an unthreatening and ideal partner, willing to accept Garcia's ideas, never feeling the need to pull rank. Their work on this project fused their different backgrounds and personalities into a solid, long-term friendship.

It was Brake who helped Garcia during his difficult first days in Baltimore. Together they had patiently surveyed the changing landscape of hospital care, probing for weak links in the government's defense against the hustlers who had begun to gather in menacing numbers. "I remember seeing full-page newspaper advertisements from a Texas hospital offering to send a chauffeur-driven Rolls-Royce to pick up patients," Garcia recalled. "That told me there was plenty of money to be made." And plenty of temptations. For a while, Garcia and Brake considered investigating companies hawking computer software that promised to maximize a hospital's return on DRGs. A shortage of leads, however, put an end to that idea.

Finally, an accidental discovery persuaded Garcia to focus his inquiry solely on the hospital cost reports. That breakthrough came when Garcia and Brake obtained Medicare computer tape No. 032747, which contained the names of 5,630 hospitals that had filed 1981 cost reports. Brake happened to notice that the tape also included a small checklist indicating which hospitals had been audited and which hadn't. Since Medicare had used 1981 cost reports to set DRG payment rates, Brake naturally expected that all had been audited to prevent improper claims from slipping in. The checklist, however, suggested otherwise. Stunned, he walked into Tom Dowdal's office.

"You'll never believe what we found," Brake said anxiously. "Only 80 or so hospitals out of more than 5,000 were audited."

"That can't be," replied Dowdal, ever the skeptic. "You must have made some mistake."

Brake didn't think so, but he wasn't about to disagree. Not yet, anyhow. Not before he and Garcia had a chance to do a little more detective work.

First, they had to learn whether hospitals were, in fact, making improper claims in their cost reports. Otherwise, the audits—and their discovery—would be mostly meaningless. As a beginning, Garcia and Brake pulled three audited hospital reports and compared them against the original, unaudited ones. When the comparisons proved inconclusive, they began pulling more, dozens more, not only from 1981 but from subsequent years as well, since the reports continued to determine a part of each hospital's Medicare payment during the three-year transitional period between the old system and the new preset DRG rates of prospective payment. Finally, the numbers began to paint a clearer picture. Yes, hospitals were packing their federal cost reports with improper—even unconscionable—items, such as liquor and Mercedes rentals, although the extent of those claims wasn't known.

California hospitals were particularly bad. One Los Angeles hospital stuck Medicare with plane fare to London for a hospital executive's spouse, as well as $2,381 for Los Angeles Kings season hockey tickets, $1,186 for Kings play-off tickets, $232 for a 10K race, and $10,741 for a city referendum. A senior Medicare official speculated that the regional peculiarity might stem from California's high proportion of for-profit hospitals. "They seem more creative and less inhibited," the GAO was told.

The GAO also noticed that the same improper claims often appeared in cost reports year after year, suggesting they weren't innocent mistakes. "[Auditors] go back every year and say, 'You can't put that in there,' and the next year it would be there again," said Don Hass, one of Garcia's investigators.

Some claims—the nickel-and-dime stuff—appeared to have been inserted to distract auditors, to keep them from finding even bigger items. That view was bolstered when Garcia and a fellow investigator decided to witness personally a hospital audit in progress. Together they drove to a town just outside of Dallas where two auditors, under contract to Medicare, were reviewing the books of a midsized hospital. At a meeting inside the hospital conference room, the two auditors got quickly to the point.

"If I didn't have to spend so much time making adjustments to recurring nonallowable items, I could spend more time reviewing the minutes of board meetings," complained Gordon Dyer, one of the auditors. Those records, he explained, provide valuable hints on where unallowable expenses might be found.

The other auditor, Rosalind Hicks, was equally direct. "If I had more time, I'd increase my emphasis on looking at bad debts," she said. Hicks had seen enough evidence, for example, to conclude that hospitals frequently collected twice on the same "bad debt." First, they wrote off the debt, entitling them to recover a portion from Medicare. Later, when patients paid their bills, they failed to inform Medicare.

Both auditors also accused hospitals of using stalling tactics to disrupt their reviews. Although hospitals receive two months' notice of a pending audit, auditors often arrived only to find necessary records missing. A perfect example: the very hospital they were now in. "Two weeks ago, I called the controller to confirm the records request I had made six weeks earlier," Dyer said. Nevertheless, they found the general ledger of business transactions incomplete—November and December were totally missing. Hicks wondered whether the hospital had done this intentionally. "Since many parties occur during November and December, the hospital may not want us to uncover expenses for such things as liquor," she said.

Their appetite whetted, GAO investigators visited the Dallas office of the HHS inspector general, where they learned another hospital trick: how to hide income that should be used to offset expenses. "I had one hospital that received income from the sale of silver recovered from x-ray film processing," said Fred Mosely, who headed the office. The hospital hid that revenue, he explained, by giving it to a volunteer candy stripers' group, which then "donated" the money back to the hospital. Since Medicare doesn't consider donations revenue, the hospital claimed higher expenses and ultimately got more Medicare money.

Clearly, only shrewd auditors could catch hospitals at such games. But how shrewd were they? Garcia decided the best way to find out would be to avoid the generals' tent in favor of the enlisted men's. With that in mind, he boarded a plane for Los Angeles, where he planned to start at the bottom.

In Los Angeles, Garcia rented a car and headed northwest into the San Fernando Valley and movie country. He felt upbeat. A stiff breeze had cleaned the valley of smog, revealing a pristine landscape that reminded Garcia of how exquisite it had been to grow up in the 1950s in southern California.

Just outside Los Angeles, he stopped at a stylish new office build-ing tastefully terraced and adorned with plants and benches—the home of Blue Cross of California. Garcia had come to attend an intensive two-week training session for accountants assigned to audit hospitals. With Medicare's passage, Congress thought it could save money using private insurance companies, rather than govern-ment workers, to help administer the program. This decision also served to buy off the insurance industry, which bitterly opposed government intrusion into its domain.

How well this arrangement worked no one really knew. Garcia's first impression, however, wasn't favorable. To his surprise, most accountants in the class either were fresh out of college or had recently been dismissed from major accounting firms for failing to measure up. During breaks and at lunch, Garcia discovered that many students weren't lacking for career plans, either. "They viewed Blue Cross as only a stopping-off point," he recalled. "The plan was to get to know as much as possible about what the insurers looked for in the hospital cost reports, then get a job in the hospital industry, where they could use that information."

Garcia would later confirm that unfavorable first impression. "Many hospital accountants know how to get around the regula-tions because [hospitals] hire people who have worked for the fed-eral government," one auditor told him. In addition, insurers in Wyoming, Colorado, Florida, and Iowa had many of their top audi-tors hired away by hospitals.

Garcia emerged from the training session more suspicious than ever. He subsequently learned that Medicare's financing agency, for example, had never expected Congress to pass DRG legislation so quickly in April 1983. With only months remaining before the first hospitals entered the DRG program, Medicare ordered a rush audit of hospitals from coast to coast. Auditors, however, were ill-equipped to carry out that order. Compounding the problem, Medi-care issued confusing audit guidelines, then failed to monitor the audits properly.

To assess the damage from that frenzied period, Garcia and his staff visited Medicare auditors around the country. One stop was San Francisco. "We hired subcontractors to handle the extra work load," a Blue Cross official there said. Unfortunately for U.S. taxpayers, the subcontractors used Medicare as a training ground for inex-perienced junior staffers. Some lied about their Medicare experience.

Others stayed for only a week or two, disrupting the audits. "We had to redo much of their work," one Blue Cross official complained. Blue Cross of California ended up firing two of its subcontractors; more than a dozen more were fired around the country.

In-house auditors weren't necessarily any better. Because of previous federal budget cuts, insurers found their Medicare auditing ranks depleted. When Medicare called for a rush audit, the companies had no choice but to restock with inexperienced employees, even though 12 months' experience was necessary to become fully versed in Medicare's complex regulations. The result was predictable: one Houston hospital got away with overstating kidney acquisition costs by $300,000 because of an inexperienced audit manager. The inflated claim remained in the hospital's reimbursement rate, the GAO was told.

The grimmest assessment came from Blue Cross officials in the Los Angeles area, who flatly admitted that the government had been taken in those hasty 1983 audits. If accountants "had been given a longer lead time, our audits could have generated more savings," said Joe Tuma of Blue Cross. He said the audits were inferior to ones conducted later.

According to the GAO, Tuma voiced many of the same complaints as other insurers, with one significant addition. "The auditors hired by the subcontractors were snooping around, trying to find things to use against Blue Cross," he said angrily.

Why? Because they planned to seek employment in hospitals, Tuma answered. "It was a sad experience," said one Blue Cross auditor.

Even sadder was the government's poor record in punishing hospitals that were caught trying to cheat Medicare. Fear—law enforcement's best tool—had never found its way into the hearts of hospital administrators. "I'm sure some of them put in some questionable entries," said Charles Booth, director of policy reimbursement at the Health Care Financing Administration. But, Booth added, if his agency had tried, for example, to punish one major Texas hospital that in 1983 submitted $10 million in improper costs, "I'd have every congressman in Texas in here—and a few other people, starting with the governor, I suppose."

The GAO also wondered whether Medicare officials weren't getting too cozy with the hospitals they were supposed to be regulating. Garcia and his staff were suspicious enough to investigate one incident in which Medicare, several years earlier, had suddenly changed how it computed inpatient hospital reimbursement under a pre-DRG program. To learn why the change had been made, GAO investigators visited Medicare headquarters in Baltimore, where they got a surprising civics lesson on whom Medicare views as its prime customers. Taxpayers? Elderly beneficiaries? Apparently not. One reason for changing methodology was to create a situation where any errors would tend to favor the hospitals, explained HCFA's Paul Olenick. "HCFA could then easily defend itself if the hospitals complained about rates being too low," he said.

This bureaucratically timid attitude carried over to DRGs as well. Capital costs, for example, were supposed to have been excluded from DRG rates, since hospitals were already collecting some Medicare money for buildings and equipment. Medicare, however, failed to exclude those costs, meaning that hospitals, in effect, got paid twice. "HCFA believed that by allowing these costs in the rates, reimbursement would benefit the hospitals and they would accept prospective payment with less resistance," Olenick told investigators.

Keep the hospitals happy . . . a strange song for hospital regulators to be singing. And HCFA wasn't the only empathic regulator. The biggest responsibility for ferreting out fraud rested with the insurance companies hired to audit hospitals. They were supposed to refer cases of dishonesty to the inspector general of Health and Human Services, who then decided whether to pass it to the local U.S. attorney for possible prosecution. That rarely happened.

Carl Gruninger, of the inspector general's Dallas office, had long worried about why his office got so few referrals. "I even tried scare tactics, telling the auditors that if my office discovers unreported fraud cases, they may be implicated," Gruninger said. That tactic proved unsuccessful, however; he could only recall a handful of referrals to the Dallas IG in the last five years.

Although Garcia did not know it, Richard Kusserow, the HHS inspector general in Washington, was about to launch an investigation that would later yield the worst example of an auditing breakdown. Ironically, the probe began with a tip from a most unlikely whistle-blower: the American Medical Association. The AMA's tolerance for unsavory moneymaking schemes among its members is legendary, yet even it couldn't stomach a plan conceived by the Paracelsus Healthcare Corporation to increase Medicare profits at some of its 26 U.S. hospitals. The plan called for participating hospitals to split profits from DRGs with their physicians, thus giving doctors a financial incentive to provide less care.

The AMA believed that the plan—later discontinued—smacked of a payoff, but Kusserow concluded that weak antikickback laws precluded any prosecution on those grounds. Nevertheless, Kusserow's investigation did uncover discrepancies in Paracelsus's cost reports to Medicare. Paracelsus, it turned out, had submitted expenses for golf tournaments in Monterey and Lake Tahoe, spousal travel, country club dues and expenses, gifts to physicians, limousines and charter jets, political contributions, and foreign acquisitions. So damning was the evidence that Paracelsus agreed to plead guilty to mail fraud and paid $4.45 million in reimbursements, fines, and interest.

The conviction offered no reason to cheer, however. Paracelsus's thievery most likely would have gone undiscovered if not for the publicity given to its incentive plan. If Medicare's auditors couldn't catch such blatant cheating, what could they catch?

Insurance auditors, understandably, weren't anxious to shoulder all the blame. "U.S. attorneys don't want to prosecute," a senior Blue Cross official said. "Hospitals avoid prosecutions by saying they didn't know the regulations or blaming it on new and inexperienced bookkeepers." The official even hinted the frustration might be getting to the inspector general. "When we did have a clear case of abuse, the inspector general's response was simply to make the adjustment, without penalty to the hospital."

Yes, the GAO investigators concluded, there was plenty of blame to go around. Government records weren't always reliable enough to build the paper trail needed for prosecution. And even when they were, the complexities of health care financing caused the eyes of all but the most earnest of U.S. attorneys to glaze over. Mix in the fact that the cheating often involved relatively small amounts of money at politically influential institutions, and it was no wonder that expense padding became nothing more than a cat-and-mouse game between hospitals and auditors.

The only losers, of course, were the nation's elderly, who, along with other taxpayers, would sooner or later have to pay for it all. By decade's end, Paracelsus would stand as the government's sole successful prosecution of a hospital for Medicare expense fraud in the 1980s.

After months of expeditions and interviews all across the country, Daniel Garcia figured the time had come to learn, once and for all, whether Medicare had used the unaudited and inflated cost reports to set the DRG rates. It wasn't as simple as picking up the phone, however. "The learning curve was tremendous," he recalled. "You will go into an interview and realize this isn't who I need to talk to, either because the person is too high in the agency to know what is actually happening in the field, or too low to know where the real problems are. Then when you do find the right people, they turn out to be unavailable. We literally interviewed one person while she walked between meetings."

It was the summer of 1984 when Garcia finally found the Medicare official he wanted to interview: Rose Connerton, a compact bundle of energy. No matter whom they talked to about Medicare reimbursement rates, all echoed the same refrain: "See Rose. She knows." At times, GAO investigators joked that if anything were to happen to Connerton, the entire cost containment program might collapse in a pile of rubble. Indeed, her input was so valued that, according to Medicare folklore, her dependent staff once felt compelled to contact her using a ship-to-shore radio while she vacationed on the open sea.

With Connerton finally cornered, Garcia popped the question: had Medicare actually used unaudited 1981 hospital cost reports to set the DRGs? Privately, Garcia never fully believed it, despite the GAO's earlier discovery of the computer tape checklist. But what he heard from Connerton gave him the jolt of his career. Medicare had indeed used those unaudited reports, and except for a few isolated cases, Medicare officials hadn't bothered to remove any improper costs.

"I was just dumbfounded," Garcia said. "We were all so low-keyed, and when we heard that, it was suddenly as though the clouds had parted and the sun came out. We turned and looked at each other, realizing the implications." Garcia had experienced the rush that every investigator lives for. He had found the mother lode. Suddenly, other promising leads seemed unimportant. His investigation, once so uncertain, now had a clear end in view. All he had to do was find a way to calculate what this grotesque oversight— assuming it was an oversight—was costing American taxpayers.

After months of tedious work, the fun was about to begin.

The GAO lacked the staff to analyze the 1981 cost reports from more than 5,000 hospitals, so investigators picked a sample of 418. By comparing the dollar differences between the unaudited and the audited reports from those hospitals, the GAO could project the total overpayment for the universe of hospitals. With so much left to be done, Garcia felt fortunate that his investigation wasn't scheduled for completion until July 1985, nearly a year away. Everything was coming together so perfectly.

Then he got a phone call. It was October, and Garcia was in Encino, California, interviewing a Medicare auditor, when he learned that Thomas Dowdal, head of the GAO's health care financing section, and one of his bosses, was on the line.

"Dan, I've got some news for you," Dowdal said. "We've just got a congressional on this DRG investigation."

Garcia thought he must be joking. In GAO circles, "a congressional" meant that a member of Congress had requested a GAO study. These studies took priority and had a deadline. Garcia's investigation, on the other hand, had resulted from the GAO's own initiative and thus had no deadline. Garcia worried that he might have to cut short the biggest investigation of his life because of some congressman.

"What kind of time frame are we talking about?" he asked.

"Hearings are scheduled for March. Can we make it?"

Garcia, the ultimate planner and organizer, now faced a deadline four months earlier than he had planned.

"No way. That would be impossible," he replied with irritation. But after more reflection, Garcia and Dowdal agreed to discuss the request again after Garcia returned to Texas.

Garcia immediately caught a flight to Dallas, where he met the GAO's Ken Brake, who had flown down from his office in Baltimore. Together they reviewed what had to be done: investigate the cost reports of 418 hospitals audited by 40 insurance companies spread out across three dozen states. It was a daunting task, but yes, both concluded, they could meet the deadline if they split up the country, blitzing every hospital on their list. That could be done only with more people. So they agreed to go back to their respective supervisors and request the impossible: more staff.

To their surprise, they got it.

Ironically, Garcia faced many of the same problems insurance firms encountered when Medicare ordered its rush audit of hospitals. Like the insurers, Garcia got more bodies to help meet his deadline, but they, too, lacked experience; a few recruits had never as much as seen a hospital cost report. Fearful of mistakes, Garcia brought his entire team of 15 or so down to his Dallas war room for a week-long training session.

Garcia's original game plan called for the GAO to obtain copies of cost reports from each of the 418 hospitals, plus audit workpapers used by Medicare's fiscal intermediaries. Key numbers would be extracted and run through a computer program, making it possible to estimate the size of Medicare's debacle. Problems with the documents quickly developed, however. Some photostats were unintelligible. Some weren't the right documents. Additional requests had to be made. It was all too time-consuming and unreliable, so Garcia changed strategy. He decided that he and his staff would go personally to each insurance auditor for the 418 hospitals—some 40 in all—and work only from original documents to reduce the possibility of error. He split his squad into two-person teams.

"I had this big map of the United States showing where the fiscal intermediaries were," Garcia recalled. "Because time was of the essence, we literally plotted out the country, figuring who would go to where from where, arranging flights and times. We didn't want to be crisscrossing each other."

For this assignment, Garcia's staff temporarily jettisoned its legal pads in favor of professionally printed books designed specifically for collecting data. As soon as one team member finished extracting cost figures from documents, the other would repeat the process, double-checking the data. Then, at the end of each day, team members sent their completed books by overnight mail to data key-

punchers who stood ready in San Antonio, Texas. Fearful that someone in San Antonio might make a keypunch error, Garcia arranged
to have the work rechecked once it got to Dallas. "I had seen the
mistakes Medicare made, and I didn't want us to repeat them,"
Garcia said.

After blurry weeks of airports and motels, the last of the numbers
had been gathered and sent for processing; Garcia returned to Dallas, where he nervously watched his computer terminal. Soon, the
mainframe computer in San Antonio would begin spitting out on his
screen the final tally of Medicare overpayments. That one number,
more than anything else, would define the past year of Daniel
Garcia's life. A big figure would most likely bring media attention
and recognition inside the mammoth GAO bureaucracy, where
thousands of people labored in obscurity.

Suddenly, Garcia's terminal came to life. "I remember watching
data being printed in column after column, data from each hospital,
printing out line by line," Garcia said. "It was like watching a ticker
tape or a horse race. At that time, we had no idea what the bottom
line would be, millions or billions. The data was so massive, no way
could we imagine what we had."

Finally, his screen flashed the numbers he was waiting for: nearly
$1 billion in Medicare overpayments for fiscal year 1986, and a
projected $8 billion in overpayments over the next five years.

At 10:05 A.M. on May 14, 1985, Congressman Fortney H. (Pete) Stark
banged his gavel in Room B-318 of the Cannon House Office Building in Washington, D.C. It was Stark who, as chairman of the House
Ways and Means subcommittee on health, had asked that Garcia's
investigation be put on the fast track. "We are here today to try to
learn what has happened in the months since Medicare began using
the prospective-payment system," Stark announced.

No person on the Hill made the medical establishment more
wild-eyed than Stark, a Democrat from California who had made a
fortune in banking before he turned 40. No ordinary dollar-counter,
Stark had startled conservative neighbors when, during the Vietnam
War, he erected an eight-foot-high neon peace symbol atop his
bank. Although first viewing Stark as little more than a maverick
when he was elected to Congress in 1972, the AMA began taking him
more seriously as he proved adept at building consensus through

his wit and attention to detail. During the 1980s, Stark repeatedly savaged greedy doctors and hospitals for selling out their principles for a few extra dollars. The AMA responded by spending heavily to unseat their tormentor. Although more liberal than his district, Stark proved equal to the challenge. By 1984, the only candidate Republicans had been able to field against him was an 80-year-old who had legally changed his name to J. T. Eager Beaver. Mr. Beaver garnered only 26 percent of the vote.

Stark's hearing, which had been delayed for several months, brought out the hospital industry in force. A proposal by Reagan budget-cutters to freeze—not cut back—the DRG rates drew a sharp attack from Jack W. Owen, executive vice president of the American Hospital Association. He accused Medicare of playing unfair. "The association believes that [the freeze] should result from legislative, rather than regulatory, action," he pleaded, leaving unsaid the fact that his group's campaign donations could be used to influence individual legislators. "The AHA recognizes that hospitals will have to contribute their share to the solution of the deficit problem. However, hospitals . . . should not be required to bear more than their fair share."

The wailings of the industry grew louder later during the Stark hearing. "Quality of care may suffer," warned Donald R. Oder, representing the Illinois Hospital Association. "DRGs don't adequately account for the cost of care."

The hospital industry also brought out its most effective lobbyist: Michael D. Bromberg, who headed a trade group representing for-profit hospitals. "We have kept our part of the contract," Bromberg lectured. "[B]ut if Congress unilaterally changes it or changes the rules of the game by freezing payments, then we can hardly be expected to continue to endorse the system."

Garcia attended the hearing and listened to these pleadings with increasing amazement. What are they saying? Do they really think they can get away with it? Garcia would not personally have the honor of dropping his bomb on all this nonsense. That job belonged to Michael Zimmerman, a higher-ranking GAO official.

As Garcia sat nearby, Zimmerman began his testimony with a striking tale of profiteering that went unchecked due to bureaucratic errors, miscalculations, and general stupidity. If this situation were left uncorrected, America's hospitals could pocket $8 billion in Medicare overpayments over the next five years, Zimmerman said.

Moreover, he pointed out, Medicare already knew that DRG rates were badly inflated, having eventually audited the raw 1981 hospital cost reports. Medicare just hadn't seen fit to make any adjustments. "We believe . . . an adjustment would be appropriate," Zimmerman said, in perhaps the biggest understatement of the day. He even offered the GAO's help in making things right. "As a longer-term strategy, however, we believe HCFA should recompute the base rate using more current data reflecting hospitals' operating experiences."

All reasonable suggestions—except that Medicare would have none of it. "Don't misunderstand me, I think $940 million [in over-payments for one year] is more than a slight error, but we did our best under the circumstances," HCFA's Charles Booth told the *Dallas Morning News*. In explaining its use of error-ridden data, Medicare said the law required only that the most recent cost data be used—and said nothing about accuracy. That lame excuse was akin to a student saying he got a poor grade on a test because the teacher never said that answers need to be correct.

Privately, of course, Medicare recognized that DRGs were bloated. But cut them? No way. A freeze would be better, Medicare officials argued, so as not to appear "punitive of the hospital industry."

These, then, were the people who in the 1980s were at the helm of the nation's second largest domestic program, the ones responsible for steering the hospital industry toward a new age of efficiency and responsibility, all without compromising patient safety.

Stark's hearing, despite the GAO's explosive disclosure, went largely unnoticed. The next day, *The New York Times* carried not a word; *The Washington Post,* just eight paragraphs on an inside page. The media began to grasp the story's significance only about two weeks later, when the wire services picked up an article in the *Dallas Morning News* that blasted Texas hospitals for trying to cheat Medicare. The article, quoting Garcia, made the point that Pentagon overcharges, the scandal of the moment, paled when compared to Medicare's overpayments.

Hospitals took umbrage at the comparison and launched a fierce counterattack. Suddenly, Garcia—the messenger of bad tidings—found himself summoned before GAO bosses to defend his public comments. Although he satisfied his superiors, and ultimately received one of the GAO's highest honors, a Meritorious Service

Award, the entire experience left him chagrined. Feeling burned out, Garcia took a six-week vacation, then applied for—and got—a GAO post in the Far East, about as far away from American hospitals as he could get. He spent the next several years traveling throughout Asia, leaving others to fight the battle of DRGs.

Back in the States, Inspector General Richard Kusserow eventually rode into the fray, demanding again and again that Medicare rebase the DRGs—all to no avail. Federal health officials countered that they dealt with the overpayments by simply holding down subsequent annual adjustments to the DRGs. That, however, failed to account for millions of dollars in overpayments already made.

Then, on June 14, 1990—five years after Garcia issued his findings—Congress once again heard testimony that Medicare would overpay up to $1.5 billion in 1991, this time because federal health officials had decided to reduce even further their anemic auditing and oversight procedures. A clearly frustrated Pete Stark said he feared "that for every $600 toilet seat the Pentagon bought, Medicare has bought a $600 bedpan."

The line prompted more than a few snickers. But to the taxpayers and the millions of elderly Americans on fixed incomes, witticisms were scant compensation for the increasing financial burden placed upon them by the nation's floundering health care system. Moreover, the overpayment scandal raised an ominous thought. If federal health officials had botched the setting of DRG rates, how good could they possibly be at ensuring that hospitals didn't manipulate those rates—as Dr. Donald Simborg had predicted they might, years ago in *The New England Journal of Medicine?* The temptation was clearly there.

8 | Keys to the Kingdom

ONE good thing about living in Columbia, Maryland, Patricia Brooks discovered, was that the man across the street cooked a fine southern-style barbecue. It was the kind of talent that can make a neighbor mighty popular.

And so it was with Don Nicholson, the barbecue man. Like many residents of Columbia, a planned community between Washington and Baltimore, both Brooks and Nicholson worked for the federal government. Beyond that, they had little in common: she, a medical-records specialist with an explosive laugh who liked to look for the good in people; he, a slightly overweight investigator who was trained to look for the bad. But because of barbecue and proximity, Brooks got to know Nicholson, and one day early in 1983 they casually began discussing their work.

"Congress has just passed this big initiative to control hospital costs," said Nicholson, an assistant inspector general under Richard Kusserow in HHS. "It's called prospective payment, and I'm going to help oversee it."

What a coincidence, Brooks thought. "My profession is pretty excited about the new law, too," she said.

Some years back, as a disabilities examiner for Social Security in North Carolina, Brooks had visited hospitals and found that world intriguing. Later, during a visit to her future mother-in-law's house, she noticed letters offering jobs in medical records. Figuring this field had a good future, she enrolled in a one-year medical-records program taught at the Public Health Service. In exchange for free tuition,

Brooks owed the government one year of work, and that led to her current job with the federal prison system.

"There are going to be a lot of problems with the new system," Brooks warned. And Nicholson listened intently as she explained its many pitfalls, most of which related to the use of complex medical codes.

"Oh, you mean codes are involved?" Brooks recalled Nicholson asking. "I didn't know that."

Nicholson's reaction was common, even in government. While many knew there would be nearly 500 diagnostic groupings in the new Medicare payment system, few people understood the arcane procedure for picking the DRG. Upon a patient's discharge, hospital personnel must consult a bulky, three-volume reference, *International Classification of Diseases*. From there, they select the appropriate five-digit code for one of 10,171 diseases and a four-digit code for 1,086 diagnostic and therapeutic procedures. These codes are then fed into a computer program called Grouper, which determines the DRG. Another computer program, called Pricer, makes adjustments for local economic conditions, such as the cost of labor, before selecting a final Medicare payment.

One problem, Brooks explained, was that the disease classification books were outdated. Besides, she said, the references were designed not for reimbursement but for the study of disease.

Don Nicholson was taken aback. The IG's staff didn't have any medical-records people on staff. How could the IG oversee such an important program if its staff didn't even begin to understand it?

"Would you consider coming to work for us?" Nicholson asked.

"Yes, I would," Brooks said. Her employer, the Public Health Service, permitted assignments to certain outside agencies.

Through this accidental social contact, the inspector general of HHS came to acquire his first medical-records expert. Although Nicholson would eventually leave government to market his barbecue skills, Brooks went on to become one of the nation's foremost experts on medical coding, eventually launching one of the longest investigations in IG history.

Her new assignment began one spring morning in 1983. She remembered it well. It was April Fools' Day.

Brooks's job took her to Baltimore's far west side and a street called Security Boulevard, a bureaucratic beehive with a distinctive suburban flavor. Each day, thousands of government workers funnel into the massive headquarters of the Social Security Administration and the many offices of the nearby Health Care Financing Administration. On this street, anonymous analysts in the financing agency made key decisions affecting the health of the nation, from how much to reimburse doctors (and patients) to the regulation of medical labs, nursing homes, and hospitals.

The inspector general of HHS, wanting to be near the action, leased local office space from HCFA. It wasn't prime footage, but the IG, a natural adversary, wasn't very popular, either. With DRGs a mere six months away, Brooks hardly noticed that her cramped office left no room for even a bookshelf. Her first task: find out what HCFA—which administered Medicare—was doing to plug the gaping holes in the medical codes that were being used to determine Medicare reimbursements.

Very little, it turned out.

"HCFA was getting ready to implement this whole system, and they did not have a single coding expert," Brooks said. "To show you how pathetic it was, the person in charge of coding when prospective payment started was a pharmacist." Making matters worse, the code books were already four years old, and Medicare had no system in place to update them, even though technology was rapidly changing the face of medicine.

Not surprisingly, when Medicare rolled out its newly christened cost containment program six months later on October 1, 1983, leaks began springing everywhere—millions of dollars in leaks that benefited hospitals eager to exploit government bungling. Suddenly, for example, hospitals across the country began to perceive the financial wonders of performing surgical debridement, the removal of foreign material or dead tissue from near a burn or wound. Adding the code of this relatively costly procedure to the other procedural codes produced a higher-paying DRG. And because this particular code was imprecise, hospitals inserted surgical debridement at every absurd opportunity. "People discovered that if you debride a nail, trim a nail, you can get two, three times the amount of the [proper] DRG payment," Brooks said.

Strokes surfaced as another area of abuse. Brooks found that hospitals were coding a stroke when patients had only suffered a far less serious transient ischemic attack, which mimics a stroke but usually lasts minutes and never more than a few hours. That generated Medicare overpayments of $31.5 million.

But hospitals struck their greatest treasure not in the head but in the heart. Coronary bypass, a common major surgery, produced a high-paying DRG because it requires a highly coordinated team of up to 12 people, the cutting open of a patient's chest, a heart-lung machine, and delicate stitching, for a total cost of $20,000 or more. A much less expensive procedure is coronary angioplasty, in which a balloon catheter is inserted into a blood vessel, then expanded as a means of opening clogged vessels. Angioplasty requires fewer people, no cutting of the chest, and less recovery time. It promised huge cost savings—except that official code books didn't recognize the procedure. As a result, hospitals got reimbursed for angioplasty as though they had done coronary bypass surgery at more than twice the cost.

"The hospitals loved it," Brooks said. Some even joked about it. The final two-year tab for this single procedure: $100 million in overpayments. Still, with no formal procedure to change the code book, Medicare took more than two years to fix the problem. Even dead people got into the act. Heart attack victims deposited DOA in emergency rooms were nevertheless coded as being alive. "We had to explain that you can't admit somebody who's dead," Brooks said. Nearly 200 changes had to be made when the code books were finally updated in 1986.

The importance of coding may have caught government regulators napping but not most hospitals. The ability to spot profitable DRGs and so coax the most dollars out of the new prospective-payment system quickly caused a fundamental reordering of the hospital hierarchy. Before DRGs, medical-records personnel ranked barely above floor polishers. They had to chase down doctors who, believing paperwork to be beneath their calling, contemptuously refused to complete patient records in a timely manner.

DRGs changed all that. Gold could be mined from medical records by those who knew how. "Suddenly those folks who were down next to the boiler room in the subbasement of the hospital are on the top floor with the hospital administrations," said Inspector General Kusserow. "In many cases we're finding that the success or failure of the hospital could rest on the medical-record staff."

To milk the most from Medicare, medical-records specialists turned to computers, just as Dr. Simborg had foreseen in his article in *The New England Journal of Medicine.* By the very first day of prospective payment, some hospitals had already pinpointed which doctors would make them money because they specialized in high-paying DRGs, and which doctors would lose them money. The latter could then be pressured to change their practice style or leave.

As the inspector general overseeing the prospective-payment system, Richard Kusserow took a personal interest in such computer programs. One day, he asked Pat Brooks for a demonstration. Already deeply suspicious of DRGs, Kusserow grew angrier by the minute as he saw these programs suggest better-paying DRGs "with dollar signs literally popping out of the computer screen."

They aren't going to get away with it, Kusserow vowed. But how to stop them? Exposing a problem could take months, even years. The IG often released investigative findings through public reports, a lengthy process that underscored the IG's independence, provided tangible proof of the IG's accomplishments, and increased public pressure to correct the problem. This time, however, Kusserow didn't want to wait. The highest-ranking officials of Health and Human Services had to know of this immediately, he decided.

With Brooks and her computer programs in tow, Kusserow walked over to HHS headquarters on Independence Avenue several blocks from Capitol Hill. Wanting to make the biggest splash possible, he had asked Brooks to wear her U.S. Navy–styled uniform from the Public Health Service. Officers of the service had the option of wearing their uniforms when assigned to another agency, but the tradition had begun to wane. Although Brooks almost never wore hers, she went along with the suggestion.

Kusserow and Brooks marched into the office of John J. O'Shaughnessy, an assistant secretary of HHS. Although the Health Care Financing Administration, headed by Carolyne K. Davis, ran Medicare's DRG program, Health and Human Services ran HCFA and thus bore ultimate responsibility for any screwups.

"We've got something to show you," Kusserow announced. And show they did.

Brooks recalled what happened when she plugged in her software. "I had this little dog-and-pony show where I would sit down and pick a DRG. Now I'd say, 'If I list the diagnosis like this, versus this, here's how much more money I could get. And look what happens when I sequence the code this way.'"

Moments after the demonstration ended, Brooks said, an agitated O'Shaughnessy picked up the phone. "I'm calling Carolyne Davis right now," he said angrily. "I'm going to tell her she has to do something. They're doing nothing in HCFA on coding. We need to put some people on this."

He needn't have bothered. Carolyne Davis was already on Kusserow's list for a demonstration.

When Kusserow and Brooks arrived in Davis's office, they found the former nurse who had risen to HCFA's top post, wearing a lime-green suit and surrounded by a cluster of senior staffers, all anxious and clearly embarrassed by the imminent prospect of being shown up.

"You are very vulnerable with your coding," Kusserow declared, sounding very much like an ex–FBI agent. "You need to put more effort here. Show 'em, Pat."

Looking authoritative in her uniform, Brooks ran through her routine. "Now, here's debridement," she said. "There are no coding rules here. It's just begging to be stolen from."

Every so often, Davis, sitting in front of a computer screen, could be heard sighing, "Oh my, oh my."

Kusserow, the hard-driving investigator, loved confrontations like this. Brooks, however, felt uncomfortable. Everywhere she went, bureaucrats hated to see her coming. "Any time the IG [staff] comes in, their job is to embarrass you," Brooks said.

In the end, Patricia Brooks never adjusted to Kusserow's style. After several years with the IG, she joined the same agency that she had investigated: the Health Care Financing Administration. Why waste time probing someone else's performance when she could do the job herself? she reasoned. It turned out to be a big job, even for Pat Brooks. She would spend the rest of the 1980s trying mightily to stay one step ahead of the hospitals and their computers. She didn't always succeed. Range-riding hospital consultants always seemed to find a new twist on how to make extra money for no extra work.

Some consultants came from major accounting firms, others were merely students in the art of medical coding. "The latest problem we have is gallbladder surgery," Brooks said one day in the summer of 1990, sitting in her Security Boulevard office. From telephone tips, she ascertained that several consultants in the Midwest had begun teaching hospitals how to cheat by coding not only gallbladder removal but also, separately, a bile duct procedure, which is actually part of any standard gallbladder removal. By adding the extra code, hospitals got a higher-paying DRG.

For the most part, however, Brooks didn't blame the hospitals, which she saw as merely taking advantage of a flawed system. If they did enter erroneous codes, she believed, it was more likely out of ignorance than deceit. In truth, she lacked the heart of an investigator, not wanting to embarrass, extending the benefit of the doubt whenever possible.

The IG, for his part, was not one to agonize over the bruised feelings of hospitals or Medicare administrators. "There are a lot of people advocating for the provider of services, great lobbying forces that educate Congress, quote, unquote," Kusserow said once. "[But] there are very few, in my judgment, all too few, that advocate for the interest of the beneficiary. . . . That is part of our mission."

If hospitals chose not to play fair, Kusserow would do something about it. And he didn't care whom he offended.

Kusserow's concern over the vulnerability of DRGs took root early. Before Congress bought into the new system, Medicare's New York office had looked into a pilot DRG program in New Jersey and found that 10 percent of the claims it examined had a wrong DRG, with each "mistake" resulting in higher payments to the hospital. Another review group, analyzing a second set of claims, found 15 percent of them inaccurate. Those findings prompted Medicare to warn of "the potential for hospitals to manipulate diagnosis reporting." If Congress was to adopt DRGs nationally, the agency warned, it had better devise a mechanism to catch abusers.

The Reagan administration, in the name of cutting government bureaucracy, didn't do that, however. Upset with that decision, Kusserow joined with the General Accounting Office in successfully pressuring Congress to create peer review organizations, known as PROs, to find cheaters and substandard medical care. But even that didn't go far enough, Kusserow believed. He wanted accountability within the hospital itself, someone to point a finger at, should financial chicanery be discovered. In Kusserow's mind, that had to be the person who, in his words, "held the keys to the kingdom."

Before DRGs, that designation belonged to the financial officer who filed annual reports on operating costs with Medicare, since those reports determined Medicare reimbursement levels. Now, for the first time, individual medical records took precedence, and whoever controlled them had a hand on Medicare's money spigot. Yes, Kusserow thought, who better to hold accountable than the attending physician, the one who established the principal and secondary diagnoses, who listed procedures and worked with the medical-records staff? He reasoned that any attempt by administrators to game the system could be blocked by requiring doctors to sign a statement attesting under penalty of law that the stated diagnoses were accurate.

When Kusserow proposed that kind of accountability, the physician community reacted angrily to the suggestion that they could be pressured into unethical acts. "I was told by doctors that was the most insulting thing they had ever heard," he recalled. "The AMA was shocked that I could even think of such a thing. They reminded me of the Hippocratic oath. I just said, 'These regs aren't going through without it.' I just wouldn't give on that point."

Sure enough, soon after DRGs began, interns, residents, and staff physicians began calling Kusserow, complaining of pressure to alter their diagnoses or treatment plans. "Some doctors say it is suggested that if they do not cooperate, they could lose staff privileges," Kusserow said. The IG's staff felt compelled to call on some of those hospitals to remind them that code gaming was a crime.

To win doctors over to their way of thinking, hospitals had more than the stick; they also had the carrot—namely, money. Free office space, income guarantees, and joint business ventures went a long way toward making doctors think of their interests as being one and the same as the hospitals'. In the competitive 1980s, administrators needed doctor loyalty more than ever. Besides being the linchpins of DRGs, physicians were counted on to steer patients into the empty beds that were such a source of distress to administrators.

Thus, Kusserow realized, physician attestation wasn't the final solution to preserving a doctor's independence. But at least it was a start.

One of Kusserow's most difficult, and most important, investigations was conceived one night early in 1983 in a well-known Chicago rib house named Carson's. Kusserow and his top staff had just finished a long day's work in the Windy City and were looking forward to well-deserved relaxation, drinks, and a hearty meal. Seated with Kusserow at Carson's were Don Nicholson, one of his lieutenants; Larry Simmons, a deputy in charge of audits; and one other supervisor.

As the evening progressed, the men expressed their increasing concern over the government's preparation for DRGs. What safeguards would be necessary to protect taxpayers? they wondered. And how would they assess the effectiveness of those safeguards once the program began? At one point in the evening, according to Larry Simmons, the idea arose for some type of national survey. The only way to learn if hospitals were cheating on DRGs, the investigators reasoned, would be to go into the hospitals and examine actual patient records.

It wouldn't be easy: what with Reagan slashing government budgets everywhere, this project would be expensive and time-consuming and require additional expertise. Nevertheless, Kusserow went for it. So began his longest and farthest-reaching investigation of the 1980s.

To find the minds capable of running such a project, the IG took Pat Brooks's suggestion and reached again into the Public Health Service, plucking a batch of commissioned officers that included a statistician, a programmer, a coding expert, a doctor, and a nurse. Even with the added expertise, the investigation proceeded fitfully. Just designing the study consumed a good part of 1984. When a few hospitals suggested they might not cooperate, Kusserow angrily fired off subpoenas. They eventually backed down, and by late summer 1985, more than 7,000 medical records from 239 hospitals had flooded into the IG's Baltimore office, occupying nearly an entire room.

A meager budget, however, continued to try everyone's patience. To help analyze the records, the IG hired a Boston-area firm, but staffers in Baltimore lacked the money for regular visits to Boston, according to Brooks. Jokes about passing the hat for the next trip to Beantown became common. When the time came to transport the records from Baltimore to Boston, the IG had no one to turn to but his statistician, Mark Krushat, who rented a truck, then personally hauled the records up the Eastern Seaboard, a grueling drive of nearly nine hours.

Months passed. Patricia Brooks left the IG to help oversee coding at HCFA. Meanwhile, the investigation evolved beyond just coding and into a massive analysis of the quality of hospital care under DRGs. But the IG persevered because the study promised some important answers. Why, for instance, had the complexity of illnesses steadily increased each year? Because hospitals were manipulating codes to get higher-paying DRGs? Also, did prospective payment's emphasis on recordkeeping force hospitals to reduce recordkeeping errors, which previous studies had found in 17 to 76 percent of cases examined?

Finally, nearly five years after the Chicago rib dinner, *The New England Journal of Medicine,* on February 11, 1988, published the IG's findings on coding accuracy. They were distressing. One in five DRGs inaccurately reflected the diagnosis and the treatment actually provided. But that wasn't the worst of it. Previous studies had found errors to be random, as likely to harm hospitals financially as to favor them. Now, the errors distinctly favored the hospital. For example, hospitals used DRG 129, the designation for cardiac arrest, incorrectly more than half the time, with 83 percent of those errors favoring hospitals. Across the board, overpayments outpaced underpayments two to one. The total damage: $308 million in hospital Medicare overpayments for one year alone.

The study stopped just short of accusing hospitals of cheating. "It was not within the scope of . . . this study to determine a hospital's 'motive,' " the IG wrote in one of many separate reports on the study. Nevertheless, the conclusion was inescapable. "A hospital that influences the coding process in an improper manner . . . engages in a practice known as 'DRG Creep,' " the IG wrote, echoing the term used by Dr. Simborg in his article seven years before. And yes, "creep" did occur, researchers concluded.

The study also pinpointed where in the hospital the errors occurred. About half, researchers found, resulted from physicians designating the wrong diagnosis or listing the wrong procedures. In some cases, a medical-records staffer should have informed the physician—but didn't—that the diagnosis had no support in the medical record. That failure suggested that coders were poorly trained, afraid or unwilling to confront the physician, or under pressure to complete the coding.

Another 27 percent of the errors resulted from someone listing the secondary diagnosis as the principal diagnosis—exactly what Dr. Simborg had warned of. "My guess is that someone in the billing office is running the data through the Grouper and fiddling with it," said one key member of Kusserow's research team. The remaining errors involved the use of wrong codes to describe the diagnosis, and other assorted mistakes.

• • •

The hospital industry's reaction to a report that didn't name names was predictable. "I am surprised the error rate was as low as 20 percent," said Jack W. Owen, executive vice president of the American Hospital Association. People were still learning the DRG system, hospitals explained, even though it had been around for a full year before the study began. "[T]he spanking administered to hospitals in a recent study by the Department of Health and Human Services inspector general appears unjustified," concluded an editorial in *Modern Healthcare*, a weekly magazine covering the hospital industry. "We believe in the integrity and honesty of those in health care who must cope with coding."

Ironically, the thoroughness of the study provided hospitals with their best defense. Suppose what the IG said was true, they argued; still, it happened three years ago, and the bugs have since been worked out of the system. Without another study, Kusserow could not counter that statement.

Unfortunately, Kusserow's study wasn't designed to identify hospitals that criminally gamed the system. At no time in the 1980s was either a hospital or doctor prosecuted for DRG creep. But the IG's staff could do only so much. Whether he wanted to admit it or not, Kusserow just didn't have the resources for thoroughly policing 144,000 employees, 1,600 sites, 250 programs, and 1,000 mainframe computerized systems. "We issue 6,000 reports a year," Kusserow said in 1988. Apart from Medicare, he had oversight responsibility for Social Security, Old Age Survivors Insurance, Black Lung Program, Office of Refugee Resettlement, Administration on Aging, Head Start Program, Foster Care, Centers for Disease Control, and the National Institutes of Health, among other programs and organizations.

In short, not only was the prospective-payment system loaded with lucrative temptations for the cheaters, there was also very little likelihood that they would be caught. The rare exceptions were those hospitals whose cheating was so flagrant that it could not possibly be ignored.

9 | Sacred Heart

AT 7:45 A.M., Janet Covington walked past a statue of Christ just outside Sacred Heart Hospital in Hanford, California. It was June 8, 1987, and she was about to begin her first day as a permanent employee of this small-town hospital at 1025 North Douty Street.

Although Covington had enjoyed two previous jobs at big urban hospitals, she now looked forward to the warmth and camaraderie of Sacred Heart, a place that would allow her to get close to the healing process. Her move wasn't without risk, however. Smaller hospitals, particularly those committed to serving the poor, were more prone to financial instability. Covington knew that. What she didn't know was that Sacred Heart's saintly facade masked perhaps the worst financial scandal to hit a hospital since DRGs began. In trying to expose it, Covington would suffer great personal anguish and very nearly ruin her professional career.

What happened inside Sacred Heart went beyond one institution's finances; it revealed the hollowness of the government's heralded war against rising medical costs. If regulators could neither prevent nor discover DRG coding abuses as gross as these, how many other Sacred Hearts might there be?

Midway between San Francisco and Los Angeles, right next to the Overland Stockyards, is the city of Hanford, a quaint little settlement with a big water bill, live Shakespeare, and a history that dates back to a horse thief called the Teacher (local Indians were his most famous students) and an auditor (after whom the town was named). The city, conceived and planned by the railroad, labors to make itself green and comfortable in what otherwise would be desert sand. "Old money" is said to reside here, perhaps explaining why the two big charity fundraisers in 1989 and 1990 featured Bob Hope and Red Skelton.

Among the oldest local fixtures in Hanford is Sacred Heart Hospital, established in 1914 by six nuns from the Dominican Sisters of Kenosha, Wisconsin. Legend has it that one Sister saved the hospital when she walked miles with a cow to the home of a wealthy landowner. "Take it," she said. "It's all we have and there's no reason to keep it anymore." Embarrassed, the man made a large donation to keep the doors of healing open.

From their quarters behind Sacred Heart, the Sisters ruled with compassion over this four-story, 88-bed hospital located several blocks from the main downtown square. Their control began to wane, however, as hospitals became more financially complex in the post-Medicare era. Following the industry lead, the Sisters put Sacred Heart's future in the hands of someone whose expertise was money, not healing.

That worked for a time, but by 1986 the hospital was again foundering. The administrator would soon depart, just as the Sisters began to experience their own problems. "Sister Angela is now at St. Agnes in Fresno with a very poor prognosis," department heads were told at one meeting. Another sister "continues to have bouts of depression. Sister Sebastian remains confused following surgery." Several weeks earlier, Sister Immaculata, a former administrator, had died following a stroke.

There were other problems. "The organizational structure . . . is totally inoperable," a management company concluded after studying the hospital. "Lack of direction has resulted in acquisition of properties, the planned use of which is either ill-conceived or wholly unknown." The hospital didn't even have a quality-assurance coordinator.

Then, as if by divine intervention, Sacred Heart's luck turned. The hospital had heard about a woman doing fine work at the much larger Fresno Community Hospital, a 50-minute drive away. Her name: Janet Covington. An outgoing woman, Covington had fine credentials, among them a master's in nursing, administrative experience, and a fistful of glowing reference letters.

Covington worked in the area of quality assurance, a hugely important job inside any hospital. It was with great pride, then, that Fresno Community had listened to inspectors from a national accrediting agency praise its quality-assurance program as "the finest" in California. Not only had the inspectors credited Covington, they had asked to use her methodologies to teach others in the industry. "She is truly a trendsetter," observed Connie Siffring, Fresno Community's assistant administrator.

Not wanting to hoard its riches, Fresno began lending its experts, including Covington, to smaller, outlying hospitals. In return, Fresno hoped someday to get patient referrals. The plan, however, worked too well. Covington did such a good job of consulting that nearby Sacred Heart Hospital asked her to move there permanently. She accepted.

Covington's limited duties as a consultant at Sacred Heart had given her only a vague sense of how the hospital operated. She knew next to nothing, for example, about its business side. Once she became a permanent employee, however, she set out to talk to as many employees as possible. Only then did the hospital's disorganization become fully apparent. No problem, she thought—people would listen to her suggestions, as they had in the past. Eager to make her mark, Covington began moving aggressively to implement changes. In retrospect, perhaps too aggressively. Employees who might have become invaluable allies bristled at this new woman telling them how to do their jobs.

Before long, Covington had more on her mind than a few bruised egos. Her ear had been picking up whispers of something far more disturbing. What it all meant, she didn't yet know, but she began collecting information like pieces of a jigsaw puzzle. At night, in the quiet of her home some 25 miles outside Hanford, she laid each new fact on the table, hoping that a picture would emerge.

On these nights, Covington often sought counsel from her husband, Stanley Sidicane, who knew what it was to wrestle with shadows. Years earlier, before he met Janet, Stanley had made the acquaintance of men with a dangerous dream: they wanted to remake the Teamsters Union leadership. That brought them face-to-face with one James Hoffa. Short in stature, Stanley was brought into battle for his lawyerly skills rather than his biceps, although he

did many times witness the Teamsters' version of democracy—
fistfights—including one in which combatants struggled over a
pistol as it wildly discharged bullets into the ceiling. At such moments, Stanley had the good sense to seek refuge in a closet or
whatever safe haven he could find.

Yet Stanley, in his own way, packed more wallop than a thug's
right cross. He had waged his guerrilla warfare in the courts, firing
off motions, trying to outmaneuver Hoffa's camouflaged tentacles of
power that reached almost everywhere, including the courts. Years
later, Stanley would wonder whether the people he had fought to
install in the Teamsters were any better than those they had sought
to replace, but at least he had tried. That alone required courage.

At Stanley's urging, Janet Covington pursued the mystery that was
unfolding at Sacred Heart. Although she didn't yet know the full
plot, she suspected early on that the protagonist was the hospital's
hero: Wallace Flemming, the administrator who had arrived in 1977
to save the hospital from financial ruin. Known around the hospital
simply as Wally, he had departed Sacred Heart for good on April 1,
about two months before Covington took over.

In one of his last official acts, Flemming had signed a typed,
one-sentence statement:

Dear Sister:
I hereby submit my resignation as Administrator of Sacred Heart
Hospital effective April 1, 1987.

Sincerely,
Wallace Flemming

Such a curt resignation seemed odd for a man who had been CEO
for a decade. Adding to the intrigue was another letter, of the same
date, addressed to Flemming and written by one of the Sisters. In it,
Sacred Heart promised Flemming up to $98,000 in severance, as long
as he agreed not to disclose hospital secrets, or even the terms of his
settlement. The hospital said Flemming's severance agreement was
standard.

Covington knew the hospital had problems with Flemming; she
just didn't know how deep they went. His demise, she learned,
began in early 1987 after Sacred Heart hired an outside firm, Catholic
Health Corporation, to help oversee the hospital. Although sharing
Sacred Heart's religious orientation, Catholic Health was an inde-

pendent company, managing under contract more than 30 hospitals. It was Catholic Health, Covington said, that told her during her job interview at Sacred Heart that it had found links between Flemming and "some discrepancies" involving Medicare billings.

"What are you talking about?" she asked.

"Evidently, he had a resequencing computer . . . in his office," she was told. According to Covington, a Catholic Health official explained that the hospital plugged patient data into a computer and then, using special software, switched the principal and secondary diagnoses of a case to see if this produced a higher-paying DRG. In and of itself, that wasn't improper. The program, after analyzing patient data, might suggest that the hospital double-check the diagnostic sequencing. Or it might ask whether the hospital forgot to include a medical procedure usually associated with a particular illness. A problem arose only when hospitals used the program to maximize reimbursements by falsely portraying a patient's diagnosis and treatment. How long Flemming had this computer was unclear.

As Covington recalled her interview, she was told that problems existed on only 30 or so records. "It's all out in the open, and all cleaned up, and nothing to worry about," Catholic Health said.

Fine, Covington thought. Better to know than not to know. Now she could focus all her energies on managing the dozen departments under her control. There was so much to be done.

Yet try as she might to build for the future, Janet Covington couldn't help being consumed by the past. The harder she struggled to set her own agenda, the deeper she became entangled in Wally Flemming's web. Everyone, it seemed, had a story to tell about the former administrator. Some employees feared Flemming, while others found him shy and disarming. "He only had to dig his toe in the ground and put a straw in his teeth and he would win you over," said one former employee. Everyone agreed he was very much in control. Conservative and circumspect, he parceled out power like pearls. And he didn't take kindly to anyone challenging his authority.

Covington learned of one unpleasant incident some years back involving Flemming's former secretary, Mona Andres, who had gone to the Sisters with an accusation of her boss's financial improprieties, mostly on his expense accounts. As a reward, she was fired. That day, crying and emotionally shattered, Andres angrily confronted one of the Sisters. "I don't believe in God anymore," she blurted out.

Later, in 1982, Andres filed a lawsuit, accusing the hospital of dismissing her because she refused to keep silent about what she had found. Andres said the hospital paid her a sum of money—the amount of which she declined to disclose—to settle her claim out of court. Subsequently, the hospital declined to comment and Flemming couldn't be reached.

Flemming's victory over Andres sent a chilling message to everyone: challenge me at your own peril. He had helped build the hospital's bottom line, and now it was the hospital's turn to stand behind him. It wouldn't be the last time, either.

In January 1986—two years after DRGs began, and with Flemming still firmly in charge at Sacred Heart—Medicare watchdogs put the hospital on intensive review after a spot check turned up 29 questionable DRG entries. A facility assessment survey, commissioned by Catholic Health after Flemming had left Sacred Heart, attributed the special review "to the fact that the previous CEO was changing some of the DRG codes and 29 of the DRG codings were called into question." Though Medicare ultimately took no action— it uncovered no more serious problems—the intensive review did raise questions about the hospital's billing procedures, particularly given Flemming's strange edict that all Medicare records must pass his personal review.

One person who criticized Sacred Heart's coding practices was Margaret Meyer, a part-time medical-records supervisor for several area hospitals, including Sacred Heart. She implored Flemming to change his ways. In a memo dated August 14, 1986, Meyer warned the administrator, "This hospital has more DRG errors than all my other five acute hospitals combined. I'm very concerned about it."

"I'm not," Flemming flippantly replied. He further mocked Meyer's serious concerns by drawing a frowning "happy face" on her memo.

Meyer, angry and frustrated, had written the memo to protest Flemming's coding instructions for two Medicare patients. After pointing out that one of his decisions went "against all coding guidelines," Meyer pleaded:

Please believe me. If I went to you for tax advice and you told me I could not deduct something as a business expense, I would believe you. There are coding guidelines just as there are principles of accounting. I studied coding for one year in school and I have had fifteen years of experience in coding since then. It is a very elementary principle of coding that the disease must be coded first, and then the organism which caused the disease. I am sorry that the payment is lower, but all hospitals are in the same situation.

Flemming himself had no formal training in medical-record coding, according to two coding specialists at the hospital. Several years later, Meyer would say that as far as she knew, Flemming had never acted illegally, but she noted, "I was repeatedly concerned that he shouldn't have input because he didn't have any background for it," she said.

If Flemming didn't worry about Margaret Meyer, his coding decisions would have had to pass one final safeguard that HHS Inspector General Kusserow had demanded for the protection of American taxpayers. Federal law required attending physicians to sign and date the following statement: "I certify that the narrative descriptions of the principal and secondary diagnoses and the major procedures performed are accurate and complete to the best of my knowledge." On paper, such assurances looked good. In reality, Sacred Heart showed them to be virtually worthless.

Janet Covington had never before encountered an administrator who participated in the DRG billing process. "I was shocked," she recalled. Her suspicions peaked after she talked to others at the hospital, who sketched out Sacred Heart's strange paper trail.

Upon a patient's discharge, practically all hospitals prepared a summary of the medical record, accompanied by a blank physician attestation to its accuracy. Once the appropriate signature was obtained, the patient data went to the billing department, which filed for reimbursement from Medicare. Sacred Heart, however, improvised a new system. Instead of preparing a single summary, hospital coders sometimes prepared multiple summaries, each one different, for the same patient. One summary might list a principal diagnosis and secondary diagnosis, while another might flip the two, or maybe try out a third primary diagnosis.

Covington said one coder later admitted that she had filed as many as six summaries for a single patient. Another coder would later say that no more than two forms were prepared per patient, and that was done only because coders couldn't decide on the correct diagnosis. The multiple forms were then delivered to Wally Flemming's office. Sometimes, different summaries were first sent to Mary Quilty, the quality-assurance coordinator, who checked the one she .thought worked best. "I would take it to Mr. Flemming," Quilty said later. "He would look at it, and I can see him yet taking the other[s] . . . wadding them up and throwing them in the trash." Another records supervisor added, "There was an unwritten policy that Mr. Flemming initialed all attestations before they went to the billing department."

The DRG system wasn't supposed to work that way. If coders had questions about a patient's record, they were supposed to ask the attending physician or further research the medical record—not prepare a multiple-choice test for someone outside the medical-records department. "Your end product should be one form," said Margret Amatayakul of the American Medical Record Association.

Sacred Heart's doctors could have easily put an end to the alleged manipulations. But month after month, year after year, they signed hundreds of statements attesting to the accuracy of diagnoses that were, in fact, incorrect. "They are too busy to read it," said one former HHS investigator. "That's the fallacy of the system. You have doctors who don't review these documents and just sign them."

In May 1987—years after the alleged coding abuse first began at Sacred Heart—a few doctors finally questioned Catholic Health about whether someone had been changing their diagnoses. If the hospital fully investigated the questions, it didn't report its findings to Medicare officials. By then, Flemming was long gone.

Meanwhile, Covington, stunned by what she had been hearing, began checking medical records for coding accuracy. When too busy during the day, she stayed after work. Coding irregularities were everywhere, she discovered. That's when it hit her: oh, my God, this has been going on ever since DRGs began.

And that wasn't all. Covington also discovered what she believed to be another, totally separate financial scandal. Medicare, it turned out, had grossly miscalculated upward the hospital's reimbursement rate. That meant Medicare had overpaid patient bills already bloated through the hospital's own miscodings. Moreover, Sacred Heart knew of Medicare's mistake but had not moved aggressively to correct it, according to Covington.

Blue Cross of California, which processed Sacred Heart's Medicare billings, would later say the hospital took three years "to bring it to our attention in writing." Even then the hospital didn't clearly specify the problem, said Michael Chee, a spokesman for Blue Cross. Subsequently, the hospital would deny Covington's account and say that it had tried repeatedly, without success, to get Blue Cross to correct the problem.

Whatever the case, Covington wanted to report her disturbing discoveries to her superiors as soon as possible. That opportunity came early in July 1987, when three officials from Catholic Health Corporation arrived in Hanford for a visit. Covington had been interim CEO for less than a month.

"I need to talk to you about this DRG stuff," she said anxiously.

The reply surprised her.

"We are not having this meeting to talk about that," Covington said she was told.

Later, Kaye Mickelson, senior vice president for Catholic Health's western region, privately suggested that Covington continue to gather information. "We'll take care of it," Mickelson assured her.

On July 8, 1987, Janet Covington spelled out her findings in a confidential letter sent to Mickelson at her office in Spokane, Washington. "It appears that instead of 30 fraudulent DRGs, there are hundreds of charts reflecting fraudulent DRGs covering the period of about January 1984 to December 1986," she wrote. Covington reported that multiple attestation forms had been prepared on the same patient, and that on average each fraudulent DRG brought the hospital an extra $1,000. "[T]he amount of overpayments to the hospital for fraudulent DRG claims could well be millions of dollars," she wrote.

Covington also reported that Medicare's fiscal intermediary, Blue Cross, had mistakenly classified Sacred Heart as an urban hospital, rather than a rural one, and thus had been reimbursing the hospital at an inflated rate. (Urban hospitals are paid more because their costs are higher.) "I believe that [Blue Cross] should be properly notified of the overpayments as soon as possible. They have already overpaid us over two million dollars now," Covington wrote.

Her letter ended, "Please advise me as soon as possible regarding how you wish to proceed in investigating and reporting the fraud."

If everything wasn't out in the open before, it certainly was now. Covington felt relieved. She had done her job. Now, it was someone else's responsibility. Later, Catholic Health Corporation would deny that it had ever received the letter.

Days and weeks passed as Covington waited for the hospital to act on her findings. She applied to be permanent CEO at Sacred Heart, but despite her credentials and success at unearthing hospital secrets, she didn't even make the final cut. And once the new CEO took over, Covington was told she would have to move into an office over the boiler room. Meanwhile, she continued to dig. And the more she dug, the more her relationship with hospital management seemed to deteriorate.

Dispirited and emotionally frazzled, Covington resigned in early October. At first she just wanted to run away from it all, but her conscience and her husband, Stanley, wouldn't let her. She decided to fight, filing a suit in state court that accused the hospital of a laundry list of bad deeds, many of which she said had figured in her departure. Sacred Heart, denying that it had acted improperly, defended itself vigorously against Covington. "They questioned me in deposition for parts of a dozen days," she said. "The file of my deposition alone is nearly two feet thick."

Janet Covington had proven to be but a minor irritation to the hospital. She became a genuine threat, however, on November 5, 1987, the day she and her husband filed a lawsuit under protective seal in U.S. District Court in Fresno, alleging that Sacred Heart had defrauded the Medicare program. Known informally as a "whistle-blower" suit, it entitled her to a percentage of what the government collected in penalties and back payments on false claims. More important, the U.S. Justice Department was now required to review her charges and, if warranted, litigate the case on behalf of Covington and her husband.

A whistle-blower lawsuit was a last line of defense. There seemed to be no alternative. In this case, Sacred Heart should have aggressively rooted out the Medicare abuses and alerted authorities. Medicare's peer-review organization should have identified the faulty hospital coding and stopped it. Medicare's fiscal intermediary, Blue Cross, should have spotted its own reimbursement mistakes. And the Department of Health and Human Services should have made sure all of those units protected taxpayers and Medicare beneficiaries by doing their jobs properly. In the final analysis, they all failed.

Until her whistle-blower lawsuit, Covington had been shoulder-
ing the entire fight alone. That changed, however, with a phone call
she received one morning early in 1988 at her home in Selma,
California, proclaimed by local billboards to be "The Raisin Capital
of the World."

"Janet Covington? I'm Special Agent Wybaillie with the inspector
general's office of Health and Human Services. Can I come over and
talk to you?"

Covington agreed, and they talked. And talked. And talked. To
Janet Covington, Edmond Wybaillie was the sound of the cavalry
charging to her rescue at her most desperate moment. To the others
he spoke to, he was . . . well, on the strange side.

Mary Quilty, the former quality-assurance coordinator at Sacred
Heart, was in bed recovering from a stroke when Wybaillie paid a
visit to her home. "My daughter came out and said that there is an
inspector general from Social Security," Quilty recalled. "I quickly
got up, barefooted, and put on my robe. I had applied for disability,
and I thought how nice of them to come to the house. Well, I was
very cooperative. I had him sit down. . . . He had me repeat at least
three times exactly what I did with and for Mr. Flemming for the
DRGs, and after about two hours he said—I don't actually remember the question—'You mean to say that Mr. Flemming never . . .
cheated the government?' I said, 'No, he did not.' He said, 'I can put
you in jail for lying.' Well, I saw red. I got up on my cane and chased
him out of the house. 'Get out.' "

Wybaillie, blue-eyed and wiry, moved about as if perpetually
connected to a subway's third rail. Not easily confused with the local
parish priest, he had the investigative soul of a man born to ruffle
feathers. A former IRS criminal investigator, Wybaillie had learned
his trade working organized-crime cases in mob-infiltrated Manhattan. He knew that the best way to get the unvarnished truth was
often by surprise. "At the IRS, we were taught to do the unan-
nounced interview," he explained—before the lawyers arrived and
the facts got massaged.

Working in the IG's San Francisco office, Wybaillie had taken a
call one day from the U.S. Attorney's Office asking him to look at
Covington's allegations. The Sacred Heart saga quickly consumed
him. "A true criminal investigator eats, sleeps, and drinks a case—
every moment thinking, How can I break it?" Wybaillie said. "You
put yourself out. You don't look at the clock. You drive late at
night."

Soon, many people around Hanford began hearing a knock on their door and finding Wybaillie outside. As reports of these encounters filtered back, an air of tension filled Sacred Heart. Any lingering doubts about the seriousness of the matter, however, vanished the day Wybaillie showed up at the hospital with his own copying machine. Your patient records, please, he said.

The tide of battle had turned. And Janet Covington allowed herself to hope that maybe, just maybe, she might triumph after all.

Because everyone Wybaillie spoke to denied wrongdoing at Sacred Heart, Covington had to convince him that, whatever people might say, the proof of abuse would be in the records. Before leaving Sacred Heart, she had managed to isolate 80 or so suspicious cases. Wybaillie, armed with a subpoena, seized those records and brought them to Covington's house, where they compared billing records with patients' actual diagnoses and treatment. "All of them turned out bad," Covington recalled.

Wybaillie sent the dirty records to Kusserow's headquarters on the East Coast. Once his experts had a chance to review them, Wybaillie reported back with their response. "They are really hot. They are really excited," he said. "It's just like you said—every record spoke for itself."

Wybaillie still needed a systematic way to find and prove coding manipulation. Covington volunteered that she knew just how that might be done. She described what, in essence, was a key that would unlock the hospital's secrets. Find that, she said, and the hospital's deceit could be proven. Covington wanted Wybaillie to obtain a master list of patient diagnoses that the hospital used, for planning purposes, to track the type of care it provided. Sacred Heart sent patient data to an outside firm, the McAuto Abstracting Service, which compiled it and then sent the hospital periodic summaries. Get those summaries, Covington told Wybaillie, and we can compare what the hospital billed Medicare against its own internal records.

Good strategy, Wybaillie thought. He confronted Sacred Heart's new CEO, Michael Arishita, with his demand for the McAuto reports. Much to his surprise, he was told that the summaries didn't exist. (Margaret Meyer would later offer a different account and say she mistakenly gave Wybaillie the wrong records.)

Covington was outraged. "They do exist. And I can tell you where to find them."

Wybaillie returned to the hospital. Following Covington's instructions, he went to the basement. There they were. "He called me screaming with laughter," Covington recalled. "He said, 'I can't believe it. I can't believe it. They were right where you said they would be.'"

Wybaillie brought the McAuto reports to Covington's house, and they quickly discovered, she said, that discrepancies did exist. Even so, according to Covington, the government delayed hiring independent record analysts, which would have been necessary to confirm that fraud had occurred inside the hospital. Tired of waiting, Covington and her husband threatened HHS in writing to spend up to $50,000 of their own money to hire the analysts.

HHS finally relented, and Wybaillie arranged to bring in a record consultant from Blue Cross in Los Angeles. The Blue Cross analyst and Wybaillie set up shop in Covington's home. Wybaillie would seize the records they wanted, and the consultant and Covington would examine them. Late in February 1988, the consultant reported finding "multiple instances of incorrect coding in all 3 years, '84, '85, '86."

That confirmation gave the IG a green light to proceed to a full-scale review of the hospital's Medicare records from 1984 to 1987. Again, many months were to pass before the American Medical Record Association, under contract to the IG, began examining nearly 20 percent of the hospital's Medicare billings under Wally Flemming. On January 9, 1989, the association finished its first batch of 152 records.

"Documentation is poor," it concluded. "Coding quality is poor." It also noted discrepancies between the physician-attested diagnoses and patient discharge summaries, with the "mistakes" heavily favoring the hospital rather than the government. Moreover, 90 of the 152 records had errors in selecting, sequencing, and/or coding principal diagnoses, and 123 had errors in selecting and coding the secondary diagnoses. To be sure, some of the errors were due to inexperienced coders. Nevertheless, the kinds of errors made federal investigators suspect that something funny was going on. The IG's top men in Baltimore and Washington spoke excitedly about Sacred Heart possibly being the hospital industry's biggest scandal ever—certainly unrivaled by anything since the DRG system began.

Nearly lost in the rush was another serious, and unexpected, finding. The records, the reviewers said, suggested unnecessary hospitalizations—something the Blue Cross analyst had also noticed.

Sacred Heart later dismissed the suggestion as unfounded, pointing out that ultimately the government never pursued the issue.

Then, just as the Sacred Heart investigation seemed to be gaining speed, the government inexplicably downshifted into low gear. "The United States is aware that this review is proceeding at a slow pace," the Justice Department admitted in court papers. Covington, after doing so much to help the government build its case, now felt betrayed. "I quit logging hours after I reached 500," she said. "The supervisor at HHS in San Francisco [said] they were understaffed and had a large caseload, so that was why they could not give my case adequate attention."

Many more months passed. Finally, on August 4, 1989, the Justice Department revealed its final, stunning conclusions: "Over seventy percent (72.8%) of the records reviewed evidence errors in selecting, sequencing, and/or coding principal diagnosis. Nearly ninety percent (88%) exhibit errors in selecting and coding secondary diagnosis, and over forty percent (44.4%) evidence inflated payments from Medicare to Sacred Heart."

The Justice Department added, "The review clearly demonstrates that blatant and systematic abuses occurred to the Medicare reimbursement system at Sacred Heart." All told, the government accused the hospital of filing an estimated $1.4 million in false Medicare claims. Federal lawyers didn't even bother to mention that record reviewers again questioned the necessity of admissions. Sacred Heart later denied its error rates were that high, and blamed overpayments on inexperienced coders making innocent mistakes.

Covington was pleased but not overjoyed. The government's final report merely confirmed what she already suspected. Moreover, no one had yet been called to account for the abuses that occurred at Sacred Heart. With each passing day, that appeared increasingly unlikely. The previous year, Covington had lost her main ally, Ed Wybaillie, who quit the IG altogether after a long and bitter dispute with his superiors over an unrelated work matter. Janet's husband, Stanley, wrote a letter to Inspector General Kusserow, begging him to return Wybaillie to the case. No one knew the case as well as Wybaillie, Stanley argued; lose him and you lose valuable momentum. Kusserow rejected the appeal, saying his office had plenty of competent agents.

In truth, it had taken a wired Wybaillie to charge up a Justice

Department that never demonstrated much passion for pursuing fraud cases against hospitals. Wybaillie believed Sacred Heart had committed fraud. So did the Justice Department's own lawyers. "An initial summary of the investigation has . . . concluded that fraudulent upcoding of DRG codes occurred," the Justice Department said in court papers filed in March 1988.

With Wybaillie still on the case, the U.S. attorney had even gone so far as to issue grand-jury subpoenas. But the criminal division would quietly close its probe without ever calling key witnesses. Subsequently, the Justice Department declined to discuss the case. Not only had Wybaillie departed while the investigation dragged on, but so had the assistant U.S. attorney running the criminal probe, as well as the Justice Department attorney litigating Covington's whistle-blower lawsuit. That meant new people, new assignments, new personal agendas.

In this environment, the federal government exhibited little concern that Sacred Heart for almost four years had continued to accept overpayments, stemming from a government error, on virtually every single Medicare bill. Then, when the error was finally discovered, Medicare allowed Sacred Heart to keep interest earned on the $2.3 million in overpayments. Medicare didn't even require that the overpayments be repaid; it merely withheld portions of future reimbursements. Moreover, Medicare's administrator in California subsequently discovered five other hospitals that were being reimbursed incorrectly. Apparently, none of them had to repay interest on any overpayments, either.

Meanwhile, nearly three years after Janet Covington had filed her whistle-blower suit, the Justice Department had neither taken her case to trial nor settled it. A year earlier, Covington said, the IG's office told her that "something big" would break after Christmas in 1989, but by late 1990, nothing had happened.

Covington's struggle wasn't without cost, which she described in a letter to federal lawyers. "Because of my investigation assistance and my unwillingness to cover up the facts of the fraud, I suffered . . . emotional distress, defamation of my professional and personal character, loss of friends and support of colleagues, the inability to be rehired into an executive health care position, and general 'blackballing' within my profession." She returned to work in a Veterans Administration hospital because "no one in the private sector would hire a 'whistle-blower.' " Wallace Flemming did better. He became

CEO at John C. Fremont Hospital in Mariposa, California. Flemming, who would eventually leave that job, could not be reached for comment. Sacred Heart said Flemming had denied any wrongdoing.

Today, Edmond Wybaillie works in a small IG office in another federal agency, a few blocks from Health and Human Services. He has deep respect for Kusserow's big-picture approach to policing health care, particularly his pursuit of systemic reform. But Wybaillie also believes Kusserow lacks sufficient numbers of seasoned criminal investigators to handle individual cases. And he won't easily forgive the government's failure to probe Sacred Heart aggressively. "You are talking about a precedent-setting case, the best case to come along in HHS history," he said. "This case was a starmaker."

In 1984, HHS Secretary Margaret Heckler offered a stern warning to those people with DRG larceny on their minds. "The hospital industry is on notice," she said. "I intend to curtail DRG creep. We cannot allow manipulation."

Despite this tough talk, however, HHS never assigned a high priority to rooting out DRG creep. Peer-review organizations were supposed to uncover coding abuses, among other things, but HHS did a poor job of supervising them. Instead of uncovering fraud, two of the nation's biggest PROs, in California and Florida, were themselves implicated in alleged schemes to defraud the federal government by claiming to have reviewed hospital records when they hadn't. Both PROs were exposed through whistle-blower lawsuits, not by HHS.

Even worse was PRO incompetence. When the nation's leading medical-record coders were asked at a 1988 conference if PROs contribute to the improvement of coding accuracy, "the resounding response was NO." In fact, the participants concluded, PROs contribute to "coding inaccuracy" because they hire poorly trained coding personnel.

HHS also failed to oversee its independent auditors, the fiscal intermediaries, who are supposed to make sure hospitals don't cheat Medicare. "The government says, 'We are going to do self-policing,' " said Ed Wybaillie. "They say, 'We'll cut the intermediary's budget.' But what they fail to see is their return on money is two to one."

Privately insured patients were subject to the same abuse as Medicare patients. When Blue Cross and Blue Shield of South Carolina audited 1,500 hospital bills from 30 hospitals, it found more than $1 million in overcharges. Many hospitals employed the services of unethical consultants, who goosed up hospital billings by inserting charges for undocumented services that most likely were never rendered. "In the past three years, I have had to beat off the [consulting] firms with a stick," said Scott Miller, a senior vice president at Florida Hospital in Orlando.

Over the years, hospitals have often complained that they were the true victims of DRGs. Even with bloated DRG rates, hospitals said, prospective payment didn't treat them fairly. But when Inspector General Kusserow investigated their claims, he reached an embarrassing conclusion: the first two years of the most celebrated cost controls in history produced some of the biggest hospital profits in history. Teaching hospitals led the way, with an 18.28 percent profit the first year. One Ohio hospital realized $24 million on $88 million in Medicare revenue.

"Those windfall years really provided the industry with an opportunity to make the transition to the future," Kusserow said one summer day in 1990. "Instead, they hired the MBAs, and the Madison Avenue types, who they thought would increase revenue. And who did they get rid of? They got rid of the low-paying jobs, the nurse's aides who actually were involved in the delivery of services. In the first few years, the census of employees dropped. And when this windfall [began] to dry up, the industry belatedly began to realize something wasn't working the way they wanted it to. Now, they have to make this transition to the future without the benefit of that windfall."

Janet Covington, meanwhile, would have to wait until January 10, 1991, before the Justice Department finally settled her whistleblower lawsuit. In announcing that the government had recovered $3.25 million from Sacred Heart and Catholic Health Corporation, the Justice Department said Medicare fraud cases were among its "highest priorities."

[The] survival of the system depends upon cost containment and vigilance. Our successful recovery in this matter demonstrates the Department's continuing commitment to investigate and litigate against those who would divert Medicare's limited resources away from their intended purposes and into their own pockets.

As part of the settlement, Janet Covington and her husband will receive $650,000.

10 | Candy from Strangers

AN hour's drive out of Vicksburg, Mississippi, across the dull flood-plains of western Louisiana, sits the city of Monroe and its network of earthen levees. Every few years, the local newspaper dutifully reports that the latest flood damage, no matter how troublesome, wasn't nearly as bad as the Big One of 1927. Back then, according to local folklore, one could float all the way from Monroe to the distant Mississippi River.

Monroe's 60,000 residents may share the perils of lowland living with much of Louisiana, but the region differs from the Cajun-influenced parishes to the south in being part of the Mississippi of staid Protestantism and good old boys. Monroe is also the only significant urban center in Louisiana's northeastern quadrant. But while the city sat atop one of the nation's biggest underground gas reserves, the local economy collapsed when the bottom suddenly dropped out of the oil business. By 1990 the downtown area, never pretty, featured a spacious pigeon roost inside one of the city's tallest but abandoned buildings, along with a thriving colony of bail bondsmen—lightbulbs flashing 24-hour service—who found their sustenance in Monroe's hard times.

Such a city would seem, then, an unlikely stage for one of the more intriguing medical dramas of the 1980s. It was not about the heroic saving of a life, or some tragic medical miscalculation, but a more complex story of greed, betrayal, fortunes won and fortunes lost. It was, above all, a stark portrayal of how the practice of medicine changed in a decade when doctors faced more competition, more indigent patients, and more public and private cost controls.

Lavish life-styles could still be attained by practicing medicine—and quickly, too—but that often meant bending rules in ways that could make a doctor or his colleagues squirm. Some opportunities sprang from technological innovations that permitted doctors to run sophisticated tests in their own offices, rather than in hospitals. That meant greater profits but also brought new temptations to overtest. Many succumbed. Why should they be denied their just rewards? they reasoned. Their predecessors had gotten theirs.

Hospitals were rocked by similar forces. Administrators who couldn't fill empty beds faced termination. New revenue streams had to be developed to pay off old construction debts. Careers were on the line. And so it happened that in the 1980s candy stripers, goodwill, and aging Catholic nuns gave way to what one health care analyst called the switchblade style of hospital management.

Such were the forces that burst over Monroe's sedate medical community like a lanced boil, poisoning friendships, turning hospital against hospital, doctor against doctor, brother against brother. Modern medicine's new conflicts crystallized in Monroe over what amounted to the buying and selling of hospital patients, a bizarre kind of auction where doctors referred their patients to the hospitals that offered them the greatest financial rewards. Similar practices existed elsewhere, to be sure, but rarely did they resonate so richly as in this threadbare Louisiana town.

The reason why had much to do with the fact that at least a few Monroe doctors hadn't forgotten a simple childhood lesson, as true in medicine as in life: never take candy from strangers.

Monroe's winds of war began to stir one day in 1984 when Dr. LeRoy Joyner, a supremely confident man-about-town, climbed aboard an airplane bound for Nashville, Tennessee. In a few short hours, he would begin laying the groundwork for a multimillion-dollar deal the likes of which Monroe's medical community had never seen. Tall, dark, and available, Dr. Joyner had a taste for fine clothes, expensive cars, and nightlife. Some doctors didn't feel comfortable with Joyner's cocksure demeanor, but they admired and respected his medical talents.

A Monroe native, Joyner had gone away to medical school, then returned to a city that had virtually no medical specialists. Unsure of how to set up and run a specialty clinic, Joyner and a colleague sought help from an Atlanta firm that counsels doctors on exactly such matters. They listened well and established their clinic in Monroe. Soon the Atlanta consultants were saying they had never seen a clinic grow so fast, pulling in annually $1 million in new receipts.

Dr. Joyner's sudden success drew a lot of attention around town. And no one looked on with more interest than Pat Gandy, a good old boy from nearby Shreveport, Louisiana. As administrator of the new North Monroe Community Hospital just outside town, Gandy worked for what was then the world's largest hospital company— the Nashville-based Hospital Corporation of America. By 1984, HCA would own or manage more than 400 hospitals in this country and around the world. HCA counted on Pat Gandy to know the people of Monroe, what they liked, and what they didn't.

Even the most savvy administrator would have had trouble making North Monroe profitable. Unlike existing hospitals acquired from someone else, North Monroe was built from scratch by HCA, which bought the land, hired the architect, and financed the construction. Besides, Monroe already had three hospitals, led by venerable St. Francis Medical Center in the heart of downtown. Founded by six Franciscan Sisters from Calais, France, the hospital had opened in 1913 as a sanitarium; by the 1980s, it had an open-heart unit and 400-plus beds.

HCA banked on North Monroe benefiting from expected commercial growth north of town, but that was the future. Gandy had to worry about today. When North Monroe opened in 1983 amid newspaper advertisements and speeches from local politicos, federal health officials were busy implementing cost controls that would empty tens of thousands of hospital beds around the nation. Pat Gandy, cowboy boots and all, was a duck-hunter's dream target. Here was this newly minted, three-story, 100-bed hospital, plenty of parking, elegantly designed, equipment just waiting to be broken in, yet it had one major problem: no business. "We peaked at, you know, 10, 12, 14 patients, and we were not growing," Gandy said. "It became obvious to me I had to do something."

Gandy needed patients. And he needed them now. His job depended on it. But soliciting patients wasn't like selling washers. You didn't usually get them by offering discounts or running full-page ads in the local paper. Gandy knew that he first had to win over Monroe's doctors. Sell them on the hospital and their patients will follow. Most patients still trusted doctors to pick the right hospital for their needs. The better physicians, aware of wide differences in quality among hospitals (even within the same hospital), tried to match specific ailments with specific caregivers. One hospital might be great at hip replacements but lousy at heart surgery, and so forth.

Unfortunately, many doctors also picked hospitals just because they were nearby, making patient visits easy; less time on the road, more money in the pocket. It was one reason why a poor open-heart unit with a death rate 10 times higher than other such units could still get patients. Doctors didn't send people to such places maliciously, knowing they might be harmed; many simply lacked the time to investigate qualitative differences, and so admissions often turned on amenities such as good hospital parking. A certain cynical attitude could also infect some doctors who, after years of practice, reasoned that since every hospital makes some mistakes, why bother to pick and choose? If your number is up, it's up.

Pat Gandy saw Dr. LeRoy Joyner as nothing less than a patient-manufacturing machine. Until now, Joyner and his fellow specialists had been sending customers to St. Francis. Gandy tried to change that by aggressively courting Joyner. Would he please send some patients his way? Would he consider joining the staff?

Dr. Joyner regarded Gandy as a pest. No, he didn't want to go to North Monroe, he said. St. Francis was only steps from his front door; North Monroe was seven miles. "Finally," Dr. Joyner recalled, "after becoming weary of Pat Gandy's pursuits, [I] just leveled with him and told him that economically our interest was downtown, our loan and our property was downtown by St. Francis, and that I basically felt that HCA was a nuisance."

Faced with that response, Gandy figured he had no choice but to go for broke, to play the game as it was played elsewhere. St. Francis wasn't going to drive him back to Shreveport. He recalled the admonishments of HCA's founder: "Pat, you need some doctors out here. We need to get some of these doctors around St. Francis." Administrator Gandy, belatedly, was about to enter the 1980s, switchblade firmly in hand.

Gandy approached Joyner again, this time with more than words.

According to Joyner, Gandy suggested that HCA "buy our building, buy all of our property, retire the entire debt, and we could still own the building." And that wasn't all. "They would build us an entire new building complex as large as we wanted and allow us to buy as much property at the new hospital as we wanted."

The offer stunned Joyner. Was this for real? His clinic owed nearly $2 million on its building. Two million dollars—and we still keep the building? Plus an HCA loan of up to $2 million to build a new clinic. It was like winning a lottery. Joyner's colleagues were excited. Eagerly, he explained the offer to his old Atlanta consultants, who approved. Joyner's clinic, the consultants said, could get much more from HCA than from stodgy St. Francis.

Gandy's offer addressed a twofold goal: more patients for North Monroe, and fewer for St. Francis. Moreover, HCA could block another doctors' group, which might send St. Francis profitable patients, from moving into Joyner's vacated building. "We wanted to put [in] some attorneys," Gandy said.

Gandy's offer was quickly followed by a phone call from HCA headquarters in Nashville. Could Joyner come to Nashville to seal the deal? Yes, Joyner said, assembling a negotiating team that included him, another doctor from his clinic, a lawyer, and his Atlanta consultant. Pat Gandy was one thing, a local boy not unlike Joyner himself, but this was the biggest hospital company in the world, summoning him to the mount. As Joyner climbed aboard the plane to Nashville, he was both excited and apprehensive. His consultant warned him to be on guard, that HCA would begin deal-making immediately. Don't be fooled by pleasantries, he was told. There was a purpose for everything.

Sure enough, Joyner found upon his arrival that HCA behaved as advertised. "They said, 'We're not going to do much this afternoon,' " Joyner recalled. " 'Welcome to Nashville. We just want to sit around and chat and meet everybody.' So they took us to this fabulous office building, and we appeared to be the only group there." The hosts made certain the afternoon included a stop at the corporate boardroom. Around the table they went: "The chairman of Eastern Airlines sits here, the president of this company sits here." HCA knew how to hook a fish.

Even the elderly cofounder of HCA, Thomas Frist, Sr., just happened to drop by. At one point, an HCA official left to take a phone call. "Boy, this is incredible," he said upon his return to the room.

The call, he explained, had been from doctors just like Joyner's group who seven years ago were unsure about joining the HCA team. "Now they were just calling to say that they needed so many more million dollars to build a big MRI [magnetic-resonance imaging] center."

And yet another coincidence: the same doctors' group had also worried about leaving the big Catholic hospital in town. "We told them that anytime we've gone into competition in a town where there was a dominant Catholic-run hospital, within eight to ten years we were the dominant hospital. That's happened every time." The HCA official had a captive audience. "Their [Catholic hospitals'] skills are 25 years behind the times. We're on the cutting edge in terms of management. . . . We bury them."

Joyner called his first afternoon in Nashville "totally overwhelming." There would be plenty of time tomorrow to work out details. But the deal, for all practical purposes, had already been made.

Once the agreement was signed, Joyner and Gandy stayed in almost daily contact. North Monroe had been averaging only 20-some patients, far too few to make money. HCA in Nashville estimated North Monroe's break-even point at 45 patients. "They felt that our group had grown rapidly and that we could solve this hospital's problem, bingo, with one move," Joyner said. And at first, HCA's projection seemed uncannily accurate. Within a week of the agreement's signing, North Monroe's census shot up into the 40s, as Joyner's clinic began referring patients. Joyner's clinic hadn't suddenly discovered that North Monroe was a better hospital. Its doctors were sending patients there for their own financial reasons.

Although HCA had assured the doctors that they wouldn't be pressured or told how to practice medicine, it was perhaps naive to have believed it. Several weeks after the initial surge in admissions, the census dropped back into the 20s due to the natural ebb and flow of hospitalizations. Then, one weekend, it dropped all the way down to 12, and Gandy panicked. The following Monday morning, Joyner and his colleagues arrived at work to find a surprise on their desks—a note from Pat Gandy. "Admit patients to North Monroe. Help me," it said. The strong implication: hospitalize patients whether they need it or not.

To those wiser heads who had warned Joyner of taking money

from HCA, the note was a prophecy come true. "Nothing is free—you're making a big mistake," Monroe's older physicians had said. "You'll soon be owned by a big corporation that doesn't really care what happens to you."

Joyner immediately sought out Gandy. "I told him it [the note] was not well received at all, and that we would have to use some other method. The guys were really incensed." The response surprised Gandy. He hadn't meant to come down so heavy, he explained, but sooner or later the hospital would have to meet its bottom line.

Joyner's clinic also had to contend with rising community anger over its planned move to North Monroe. Some doctors began deriding Joyner's group by calling it the Buckaroo Clinic or the Billionaire Boys' Club. St. Francis wasn't pleased, either; it responded by removing Joyner and some colleagues as medical directors of labs inside the hospital. On the surface, St. Francis tried to act unruffled by rumors that HCA was out trying to buy doctors. "This is the Bible Belt—we believe that it's not just the doctor that cures people," said one St. Francis official. But now, St. Francis found itself spending more and more time anticipating HCA's next line of attack.

Joyner took most of the heat for his clinic's move. "I was the only one in the clinic from this area," he said, "and I was viewed as the bad guy." With Joyner's partners getting more worried by the day, HCA stepped in again—this time, with a $60,000 lump payment to be divided up among the partners. "It was to infuse some spinal substance, more or less, into people who were losing their courage," said Joyner.

Construction of the new clinic hadn't even been completed, and already problems were worse than expected. Maybe the old docs were right. Even so, the time for turning back had long since passed.

Gandy's reign over North Monroe was about over. "Pat Gandy pissed off the doctors, pissed off the townsfolk, and pissed off the doctors' wives," said Cheryl Keller, North Monroe's director of marketing, who arrived about a year after the hospital opened. "We had all these fine employees and we had to close floors." The hospital had also made the mistake of coming on too strong with a hard-sell initial advertising campaign—"blow and show," as Keller described it. The locals resented this out-of-state company barging into town without so much as saying excuse me. "Pat Gandy was a southern boy, but he did all the wrong things."

Gandy eventually left North Monroe in 1984, and HCA wasn't going to make another mistake. This time it selected Arlen Reynolds, who had helped to run a number of hospitals for the Saudi Arabian government. Reynolds told people he was a troubleshooter who had honed his skills in a foreign land "where contracts were always broken and nothing was ever as it seemed." The line could have come straight out of *Chinatown,* with Jack Nicholson as a private detective talking about life in an alien culture where black is white and white is black. If Reynolds had sought to evoke a mysterious background, he had succeeded.

Yet Reynolds hardly looked the part of a dashing sophisticate: he was short, pudgy, and balding, and wore glasses. And he played this other role to the hilt. Dr. Joyner said that upon meeting him, Reynolds had confided that "by appearing clumsy and inept . . . the enemy camp, basically St. Francis, would allow him in their midst and he would, quote, 'have them all by the gonads' before they realized his potential. And his aim and intent was to bury St. Francis Hospital." Arlen Reynolds wasn't referring (anatomically, at least) to the Sisters who ran St. Francis, but he made his point. He played hard, and he played to win.

One of Reynolds's first calls at North Monroe was to Cheryl Keller. "I need a marketing director," he told her. "But I do not want you to be known as a marketing director, because 'marketing' is a bad word." Reynolds's approach to the community would be low-key— joining boards of charities and the like. "He took money from direct advertising and gave donations," Keller said. "Our goal was to position us as good corporate citizens."

Behind the scenes, however, HCA and Reynolds were busy plotting their attack on St. Francis. One particularly devious plan—it was unclear exactly who thought it up, although it apparently wasn't Reynolds—was to locate a poor-people's clinic in Joyner's old building. Poor black patients without insurance could be sent to St. Francis, while those with good insurance could be skimmed off and sent to North Monroe.

"The concept was to turn St. Francis into an indigent-black hospital," Joyner recalled. "Number one, they [poor blacks] weren't profitable; number two, they weren't desirable to the patients who were profitable. And we would have patients objecting to coming to St.

Francis because it was full of poor black people." Reynolds didn't object to the idea, Joyner said, and actually "signed the lease with me sitting and watching him do it." Reynolds later denied any knowledge of a plan to make St. Francis an indigent hospital.

Reynolds did, however, acknowledge pursuing other plans aimed at harming St. Francis. If Joyner's specialty clinic could be swayed by big money, why not other doctors? Reynolds began attending meetings of Joyner's specialty clinic. "He wanted the clinic to become multifaceted and . . . recruit doctors that would practice just at HCA," Joyner said. "He assured us that there would be incentives." An HCA official in Nashville even raised the possibility, Joyner said, of giving him $100,000 in HCA stock if he would act as a recruiting consultant.

So Joyner stood ready to help, even though the stock deal never materialized. When one St. Francis doctor expressed interest in moving to North Monroe, Joyner said Reynolds authorized him to offer the doctor $60,000. "He wanted it disguised in such a way that you couldn't recognize it as coming from HCA," Joyner said. "He did not want there to be direct evidence in Monroe that they were spending money to move physicians to HCA." The doctor ultimately declined to move. Reynolds later denied ever using Joyner to recruit anyone.

Undaunted, Reynolds moved aggressively to lure away a women's clinic near St. Francis, offering it the same lucrative deal given to Joyner's clinic. Dr. James Wolff of the women's clinic recalled that HCA told him, "We'll take care of your building downtown. At the end of the time, if you've been, I guess, a faithful servant out here or whatever, you'll have your building back." Dr. Wolff declined the offer, but it deeply divided his clinic.

One day, three of Wolff's colleagues called an emergency meeting of the clinic's owners, at which they announced they were leaving for North Monroe. "We were shocked by it all and started asking around," Wolff said. They found that HCA had been trying to buy doctors like cattle at a Fort Worth auction. "There's a lot of people who work hard in this community that don't know what's going on all the time, and I guess we were one of them."

Two of the three deserters eventually changed their minds and stayed, but one, Dr. Ralph Armstrong, went ahead and left. Dr. Wolff's office was right next to Armstrong's. "We discussed it," Wolff recalled. "He stated that they [HCA] had consolidated a bunch of his debts and [given] him a very favorable interest rate. . . . They were going to pay off some of his wife's debts at the rug shop she had, and he had, I think, a store complex next to the old surgery center that needed some refinancing or whatever and they straightened that out for him." David Glover, who would later become North Monroe's administrator, said he believed that the hospital had paid Armstrong a lump sum of either $60,000 or $80,000 to cover his rent for three years. Reynolds said he thought the payment was more in the neighborhood of $190,000. Both estimates fell well short. Armstrong later acknowledged that HCA gave him about $240,000 to make the move. But, he explained, North Monroe was also more sensitive to the needs of his patients.

With Monroe's medical community now abuzz with reports of easy money, Joyner's clinic hungered for another feeding at HCA's trough. Some clinic physicians had begun grumbling about steep payments on their newly constructed, HCA-financed clinic. Joyner sought to defuse their concern by going back to Nashville, where he got HCA's agreement to suspend the payments for a year. That suspension would be reevaluated annually, depending on the hospital's occupancy rate, Joyner said HCA told him. The ploy gave HCA greater leverage over the clinic's doctors.

More and more, Joyner began to wonder about the wisdom of his actions. Sure, HCA expected his patients. "Everybody gets their pay-back," he realized. But never had he grasped what a slippery slope he was on until perhaps the crowning moment of his professional career. *CHEST,* the leading clinical journal for pulmonary medicine, was about to publish an article by Dr. Joyner on his experimental work at St. Francis (before he moved to North Monroe) using a laser to treat lung cancer. An editorial comment from the famed Mayo Clinic accompanied the article.

Somehow, HCA learned of the article's impending publication, and Joyner said Reynolds confronted him about it. "We want credit for this," he said. Joyner was more than surprised—he was shocked. "Arlen," he told Reynolds, "St. Francis bought the laser, they never got reimbursed. They took all the risk of being sued. And the work was done totally at St. Francis. I cannot do that."

The discussion ended, but Reynolds wasn't swayed. He put in a call to HCA in Nashville, then summoned Joyner back to his office. Joyner had never seen Reynolds mad before. "You are the most underhanded, backstabbing person I've ever dealt with," Reynolds sputtered. His face reddened, and he had trouble getting his words out. "I've laid everything on the line for Nashville," he said. "They assume they're getting credit for this publication. I've gotten money for this laser suite [a new unit to be set up in North Monroe] and we've bought you all this new equipment and you have to change this."

For the first time, the full consequence of Dr. Joyner's financial links to HCA hit home. These guys own me, he thought. My word, what have I gotten involved with? Joyner eventually caved in and called *CHEST* requesting the change, but he was too late. The article was published crediting St. Francis.

If Joyner was worried, it didn't last long. Now a celebrity within his specialty, he flew to medical conferences around the world to appear as a featured speaker. But while he basked in international acclaim, he left his home base untended. "Arlen is going to get rid of you," a woman he had been dating at North Monroe kept telling him. But Joyner was too busy to be concerned, until one day his partners in the clinic voted him out. "They said, 'You're getting a divorce, you're causing a lot of trouble, everybody in town hates you.'" When he got the news, Joyner remembered that Reynolds had been at the meeting. The administrator would also deliver his own punishment: North Monroe no longer wanted Dr. Joyner on its governing board of directors.

Joyner's final feather had been plucked. Seduced by the prospect of a quick financial killing, he had abandoned a lucrative practice at St. Francis that he had worked so hard to build. In the process, he had painfully discovered an old truth. "There's no free meal ticket is what I learned," Joyner said. "And the big boys play rough." Soon he would return to St. Francis and start all over again.

Apparently, Joyner's new insights were lost on his colleagues. With Joyner gone, HCA prepared to serve up its sweetest deal yet. Some remaining doctors began grumbling that North Monroe hadn't installed sophisticated equipment and services as promised, thus costing the specialists income. Although not bound by any written contract, North Monroe made amends by promising nearly $1 million to be split among eight or so doctors in $30,000 monthly payments. The floodgates had been opened—why stop now?

HCA had in a few short years certainly accomplished one thing: a new competitive spirit had arrived in Monroe. And wasn't that what federal policymakers wanted, hospitals battling over doctors like vultures over a road kill? But what did all this mean to those patients who still believed that doctors selected their hospital on the basis of quality, as opposed to financial self-interest? And what were hospitals doing spending millions to buy off doctors at a time when medical costs were so high that countless people could no longer afford the care they needed?

Dr. Henry Jones, a Monroe physician, worried about these questions as he watched Monroe's medical community respond convulsively to its new environment. He saw the changes, and he didn't like them. About that he was sure. But he was far less certain as to what he should do about it.

To know Henry Jones was to understand a certain photograph hanging on his office wall. Four decades old, it showed a grinning, stocky man standing with one foot inside the cockpit of a two-seat Ercoupe airplane and the other on the wing. The man carried a black doctor's bag. The picture—missing only an aviator's scarf flapping in the breeze—seemed pure Hollywood, larger than life, such as young boys dream of while drifting into sleep.

The pilot in that photograph was Henry's father (also named Henry), who had repeatedly risked his life flying into back bayou country, landing on tiny gravel roads to help poor patients who couldn't be reached quickly any other way. Before he died, he built three hospitals around the state. The picture made Henry Jr. think of talks he had had with his father, first as a medical student, then later as a practicing physician. "How should a doctor balance his professionalism with his business interests?" young Henry wanted to know. The answer was always the same: "I consider myself a physician first and a businessman somewhere down on my list of priorities."

One memory of his father was particularly vivid. Once when Henry Jr. was seven years old or so, he pulled his red wagon to one of his father's hospital construction sites. As he carefully loaded discarded pieces of wood, a construction worker stopped him. "Who are you?" he asked.

"I'm Henry Jones's son," young Henry replied.

"Well, he's a mighty good doctor. I trust him more than anyone else in this town."

Henry Jones, Jr., recalled those long-ago days with great fondness. It was why he had decided to become a doctor. And it was one reason why, he said, he decided to speak out about what was happening to his profession in Monroe in the 1980s.

In retrospect, Dr. Jones seemed an unlikely challenger to HCA. He had been, in fact, one of the leading supporters of HCA's move into North Monroe. He had served on a steering committee that helped write the hospital's original bylaws; he had opened the first doctors' office next to the new hospital (keeping his original office by St. Francis) and become the hospital's first chief of staff.

Although Jones had a good practice around St. Francis, he and other physicians came to regard it as insensitive to their concerns. More competition, he thought, could only help matters. Dr. Jones was also at a point in his life—in his mid-40s—when many people are through fighting big battles. After years of paying off debts and building a practice, doctors usually aren't overeager to jeopardize their newly acquired comforts. Moreover, Jones was already expecting a big change in his personal life. After rearing three sons and watching them leave home, he and his wife were about to adopt a daughter.

At first, all seemed well at North Monroe. "Pat Gandy was an open, likable guy," Jones would say later. But then Gandy cut his infamous deal with Joyner's clinic. "As it got to be widely known," Jones said, "I got angry and a lot of other doctors got angry." Jones, after all, hadn't been paid any money to move out to North Monroe. Still, he was willing to forgive and forget. "Let's just cut this crap out—this was my position when I was elected chief of staff."

Gandy was soon gone, however, and replaced by Arlen Reynolds. Meanwhile, the deals continued. "I tried to work within the system," Jones said. "I first went to the hospital administrator, voicing my objections. Then I went to the new hospital administrator." Jones didn't think doctors ought to sell themselves to the highest bidder. To him, doctors were purchasing agents for their patients, ordering blood tests and X rays, hiring consultants when necessary, recommending hospitals. They shouldn't accept money for referrals any more than, say, a purchasing agent for Sears should accept money from suppliers trying to place their merchandise in Sears stores.

When hospitals pay doctors money, Jones believed, they "are in a position to manipulate that doctor's practice, suggesting more tests, [influencing] when patients should be released and who should be admitted. Once physicians are seduced into accepting subsidies, low-interest or no-interest mortgages, free office space, free computer and business consultation, as well as outright cash payments, then it is easy to convince them that what the hospital administrator wishes them to do is what they would have done anyway. It is easy then for the doctor to convince himself that he is acting in the best interest of his patient."

Hospitals may legitimately pay independent doctors, some medical ethicists say, only when they are in isolated rural areas and need to lure new doctors into the community. But that wasn't the case in Monroe, which had plenty of physicians. Here, one hospital was simply using money to steal doctors from a competitor.

Jones knew that in speaking publicly against HCA's payouts, he would alienate those doctors who benefited from HCA's largess, as well as those who hoped to do the same one day. But as a family practitioner, he was less likely to be hurt by angry doctors than a specialist who depends almost exclusively on other doctors for patient referrals.

Dr. Jones also knew that he would be tackling a political powerhouse. Although based out of state, HCA had carefully cultivated its political roots in Louisiana, a state with a rich history of politicians sharing a blanket with hospital executives. Former governor Edwin Edwards was twice indicted in the 1980s—but never convicted—for involvement in an alleged payoff scheme affecting hospitals. After Edwards left the governor's office, but before his reelection four years later, he and other politicos obtained state permission, called a certificate of need, to build several new hospitals. In essence, they traded those certificates to big, for-profit hospital chains—including HCA—in exchange for stock in those chains. Edwards didn't deny profiting by the exchange, he just denied using his position as governor to do so. HCA's North Monroe Hospital had no links to Edwards, but it did hire the law firm of a prominent state senator from the Monroe area, and it put the wife of a state representative on its board of directors.

Jones still hoped, however, to avoid bloodshed. "I always prided myself as being able to get along with everyone," he said. But Jones's beliefs would never fit Arlen Reynolds's management style. Reynolds, his detractors said, liked the loyalty that came when a doctor's finances were entwined with his hospital.

So when North Monroe saw a chance to freeze out a radiology group based at nearby Glenwood Hospital, it offered an exclusive contract to another radiologist. The angry Glenwood radiologists, one of whom had helped North Monroe get state permission to buy a new CAT (computerized axial tomography) scan, confronted Reynolds. "Arlen was severely lashed," said one doctor who was present at the meeting. Reynolds later said he was not behind the decision. He also said doctors were concerned about the quality of work done by the old radiologists.

But Jones, who was also at the meeting, wasn't satisfied this time. "I promised you," he said, "there would be no deals and everybody would have a fair shot out here. That's not happening. I can't follow through with my promise; therefore, I'm resigning [as chief of staff]."

Jones couldn't have fully anticipated what would follow. He didn't plan to stop practicing at North Monroe; he simply wanted off the HCA team. But Jones now felt like an enemy soldier inside the hospital's barbed-wire perimeter. The next day, LeRoy Joyner said a livid Reynolds told him that Henry Jones would be dealt with. "He didn't know exactly when or how, but that he would wait for an opportunity," Joyner said.

Dr. Jones soon began noticing subtle changes in his practice. For example, he no longer seemed to get patient referrals from North Monroe's emergency room. Patients who didn't specify a doctor in the ER were assigned one off a rotating list of physicians who practiced at North Monroe. To test his suspicion that he was being blackballed, Jones sent in a patient with instructions to ask for him. According to Jones, the patient nevertheless was assigned to another doctor. Reynolds said he never blackballed Jones.

Then Jones found that HCA wouldn't sell him more land around the hospital. In July 1986, HCA returned an $84,000 check that Jones had sent as payment on a lot next to his office. Accompanying the returned check was a letter from HCA's Nashville headquarters. "It became apparent to us," the letter stated, "that there were physicians who had shown promise of greater support of the Hospital and we concluded to sell the property to those physicians."

And who was showing that necessary degree of support? As it happened, it was another doctor named Jones—Gary Jones. Like Henry, he was a family practitioner. But unlike Henry, he had no qualms about accepting financial help from HCA. He was, in HCA's view, a far more suitable candidate to buy its land. Even better, Gary was Henry's brother. What better way to attack Henry's credibility than through his own flesh and blood?—one Jones fighting another, in full view of Monroe's medical community.

• • •

Almost 15 years younger than his brother Henry, Gary Jones professionally came of age in the 1980s. Like other doctors of his era, he recognized the importance of business acumen as well as medical competence. Having grown up near Monroe, Gary wanted to return there after graduating from Louisiana State Medical School in Shreveport. Moreover, he wanted to practice at North Monroe, which, like him, was young and ambitious. That posed a delicate problem, however: his brother already had a family practice there. Henry Jones offered a solution: he wanted to expand, so why didn't Gary and his friend Dr. Kerry Anders join his North Monroe family practice? Gary and Kerry accepted, although Gary said that several family members warned him that working with Henry would be difficult.

In the beginning, Henry said, he and Gary used to laugh derisively about how physicians taking money from HCA ought to be singing "Sixteen Tons" because one day they would owe their souls to the company store. Gary may have been laughing, but he wasn't happy in Henry's shadow. Apart from some intraoffice squabbles, he thought Henry seemed to be coming unglued, changing his mind from day to day on business decisions. At one point, Gary said, Henry tried to pressure him and Dr. Anders into buying Henry's building at an inflated price. Their refusal to buy angered Henry even more.

Eventually, the bond between Henry and Gary—however tenuous it may have been anyway—began to rip apart, with HCA standing by fanning the flames of their feud. While still working with Henry, his two young colleagues began talking to North Monroe about buying the lot next to Henry's clinic to build a new office for a competing family practice. This happened to be the lot that Henry also wanted.

Then one day a doctor running a nearby laboratory dropped by to tell Henry some shocking information. A woman connected to HCA, he said, had called his lab trying to get the names of patients from Henry's clinic who had had lab tests run on them. "He said that he realized that was my property and [asked] what did I want to do," Henry recalled. "I said, 'I don't want you to give it to them.' "

According to Henry's office manager at the time, Dr. Anders asked how he could get the clinic's patient list. She felt uneasy about providing that information, but she did so anyway.

Henry Jones wasn't the only doctor then who suddenly found someone poking into private records—the very heart of a physician's practice. After Dr. James Wolff of the women's clinic had rejected HCA's financial inducements, Wolff said his office manager "made us aware that sometime between the hours of, I think, 2 A.M. and 4 A.M., somebody tampered with our record computer some way." About that time several doctors at Wolff's clinic announced they were leaving for North Monroe. Wolff didn't know who had done the tampering, or for what reason.

At Henry Jones's clinic, a final showdown occurred on July 17, 1986. Aware that his two colleagues were talking to clinic employees about joining them in a new practice, Henry summoned them into his office. "Turn in your list of patients, and turn in your beeper, turn in your keys to the office," he ordered. "You are finish[ed]."

HCA couldn't have been happier, judging by how it opened its bank vault to Henry Jones's new adversaries. North Monroe immediately took the highly unusual move of allowing Drs. Gary Jones and Kerry Anders, two private practitioners, to use the hospital's emergency room temporarily as a place to see private patients. The hospital didn't charge the doctors rent. It also helped the two doctors advertise their split from Henry's clinic.

HCA was just warming up. Within two weeks of Kerry and Gary's firing, North Monroe had leased space across the street, put in a trailer, equipped it with medical gear, and opened it as a temporary office for the two doctors. North Monroe also agreed to guarantee Gary $6,000 a month in net income for the first year, provide rent-free office space for up to a year, cover half his marketing costs, lend him money interest-free to buy new office equipment, and arrange the construction of his new, permanent office right next to his brother.

Gary Jones may have thought of himself as an independent doctor, but HCA had its hooks in him. His financial agreement with HCA went so far as to require him to maintain regular office hours five days a week, 48 weeks a year, while keeping on active status at the hospital. Should Gary fail to keep up his end of the deal, "this indebtedness shall be due in full," the contract read. "Any amounts not paid when due shall bear interest at the highest rate permitted by law." Gary Jones denied that his medical judgments were influenced by HCA's financial assistance.

Henry Jones's troubles were just beginning. One day near dusk, he said, a car nearly ran over him in the hospital parking lot. He says he reported the incident to police. There were also threatening phone calls. "One day people like you, a hale fellow well met, then the next day you are to be avoided," Henry said. "You go in to make rounds, and people look down and whisper."

He often encountered ridicule. "What's the matter with you, Henry?" doctors would ask. "You didn't get a kickback. Is that your problem?" Gary, his own brother, went so far as to say that Henry was disingenuous in invoking ethical concerns to attack his critics. "It is convenient for him now that he has done a lot of [harmful] things to people . . . to blame it all on something that people will understand," Gary said.

Henry lashed out at his enemies with a series of lawsuits alleging unfair trade practices by doctors who accepted HCA money—including his brother—and by HCA. Jones ultimately dropped all his lawsuits against the doctors, saying he realized his fight was with HCA, not them.

He also wrote letters to anyone who would listen, and paid the local daily newspaper to insert a questionnaire that sought to measure patients' dissatisfaction with hospital care. With his income dropping, he closed one office, then another, before moving into a smaller, cramped office near St. Francis. His medical practice had once included six doctors and 35 employees; by November 1989 he had just one part-time doctor and a small handful of employees.

Jones protested HCA's business methods to the Louisiana State Medical Society and the Louisiana State Board of Medical Examiners, but neither agreed to investigate. The Ouachita (Parish) Medical Society said it would look into it, but first it called Jones's patient questionnaire "an injustice . . . to your fellow physicians" and referred the matter to the state's medical-ethics committee. If not for Henry, no one would have made a public issue of HCA's payments, said Fred McGaha, Jones's lawyer. "Then, as a reward, he gets reprimanded."

But even in his lowest moments, there were doctors and medical professionals who admired Henry's battle. "I appreciate your efforts to be on the front line," one Monroe physician wrote to him. And another: "You have my moral support and best wishes."

Even Henry's brother Gary, who had become chief of staff at North Monroe, got angry when the news reached him that his hospital had confessed in a legal deposition to paying one doctor $8,000 a month for a medical directorship that required very little extra work each month. Other testimony given in connection with Henry's lawsuit produced a flood of similar allegations, quickly becoming the talk of the town. HCA had given one doctor an income guarantee of $12,500 a month, another $10,000 a month, and so on.

As the list grew longer with each witness, Steve Ronstrum, chief operating officer at St. Francis, now knew for the first time exactly what his hospital was up against. It made him look back in sadness on the undelivered promises of the 1980s. "We were happy. Reagan was coming into office. All of us wanted the yoke of regulation taken off," Ronstrum said, sitting in his hospital office one overcast November day in 1989. "What I've learned is the need to go back to basics. Health care is not a commodity—we are putting our lives in the hands of other people. It's a sacred relationship.

"There is no resource where patients can go to find out the difference in quality between hospitals. And I know about quality. I lost a son to cancer two years ago. I took him around the country, and he died right here at St. Francis. So I've been on both sides of the bed. When our gallbladder goes awry, we don't have time to go to a library and get a book about it. Trust is so important, and it is trust that we have lost in the 1980s."

Ironically, Ronstrum contends, there wasn't any need for North Monroe to be built in the first place. He reached into a drawer and pulled out the latest occupancy rates of Monroe's four hospitals— each was at least one-third empty. So much money spent fighting each other, he sighed, in an area so economically barren.

Dr. Henry Jones realizes he may not win his suit against North Monroe, a battle that so far has cost him tens of thousands of dollars. The law is vague and subject to broad interpretation. But while Jones may be unpopular now, he took solace in the case of a Hungarian-born doctor, Ignaz Philipp Semmelweis, who in the mid–19th century in Vienna earned his colleagues' scorn by making the radical suggestion that washing hands before performing surgery reduces infection. "He was right, wasn't he?" Henry says with a wry smile.

Jones's redemption may be a while in coming, however. By the 1990s, patient-selling in its many forms had become deeply rooted in communities across America. Even more important, law enforcement was virtually powerless to stop it.

11 | Caveat Emptor

IT'S no wonder the Nagra body recorder is the tool of choice for spies, criminal investigators, and assorted rogues. The tiny, Swiss-made device offers high-quality stereo and fidelity, but at $5,000 is only for the truly sneaky.

Like Richard Kane. In his eight years as a criminal investigator with the Health and Human Services Department, Kane had successfully wired 15 to 20 people with the Nagra. Hiding it on the human body was usually easy. About the size of a small checkbook, the Nagra can be taped to the small of the back or to the leg near the groin. Two microphone-tipped wires running out of each end of the recorder can then be strung around the torso, or draped over both shoulders and taped to the breastbone.

One humid July day in 1985, agent Kane and his Nagra were summoned to a Houston suburb to help investigate a local hospital administrator. Kane's job: outfit a doctor named Jerry McShane with a Nagra so he could catch the administrator making self-incriminating statements. This posed a particular problem, however. Dr. McShane was fat. Once the recorder had been taped to his body, the microphone wires had to traverse great mounds of flesh before they could be positioned correctly. Then, the microphones had to be attached in such a way as not to be jostled by flabby skin or clothing.

McShane wasn't happy with what was happening, either. He had never expected to be standing in his own office with some stranger taping wires to his body. He was no spy; he was a doctor, and a successful one at that. Still in his 30s, McShane earned $400,000 a year, spun around town in a Jaguar, and co-owned a rock-and-roll club, a weight reduction center, a horse-breeding company, and a thriving doctors' clinic. Patience, however, wasn't among McShane's virtues. He wanted more, and if that meant breaking a few rules, so be it. That attitude eventually helped him make the acquaintance of Kane and his colleagues. The doctor now had this choice: carry out his undercover assignment or risk losing his cushy life-style.

Kane, after a struggle, finally attached and tested the Nagra, pronouncing it ready for use. He taped the recording switch in the "on" position. Now, it was all up to Dr. McShane.

The doctor dressed carefully so as not to undo Kane's handiwork. He then set out alone from his Deer Park office for a 13-minute drive to Pasadena General Hospital right outside Houston. Gregarious by nature, McShane was worried about acting natural, about finding a way to ask the best open-ended questions, as the federal agents had coached him to do. Every word he uttered was being recorded. He was flat-out scared.

Upon arriving at Pasadena General, McShane parked his car and entered the hospital, greeting people he recognized. He walked directly to the office of the hospital administrator, Russell Furth, the prime target of this federal investigation. After a brief wait, McShane entered Furth's office and began his performance.

To the disappointment of investigators, however, it fell well short of Academy Award caliber. McShane talked too much, was imprecise, told lies, and interrupted Furth at key moments. Nevertheless, his secretly recorded conversations with Furth on this day and one other would send tremors through the hospital industry. In a move unprecedented at the time, the federal government used the recordings to indict Furth for putting out a bounty on patients he needed to fill his hospital.

Until now, local U.S. attorneys had declined to prosecute similar cases even when evidence pointed to criminality. They viewed the federal statute barring patient-buying as vague. Not only was the crime easy to camouflage, but many in government still believed the medical world ought to police its own in matters of ethics. Prosecutors also realized that bigger game could be hunted in less risky areas. To fire on a well-connected hospital and miss was far more perilous to one's career than unsuccessfully targeting some low-life crack abuser. Timid prosecutors, however, frustrated criminal investigators at HHS, who labored to uncover payoff schemes only to see their cases die for lack of interest.

Then came Furth. The stakes were high, indeed. A successful prosecution might embolden other prosecutors to take on similar cases. It might encourage HHS investigators to keep pursuing patient-buying schemes. More important, a successful prosecution might force hospitals and doctors to reconsider the merits of joining the thriving underground trafficking in patient bodies.

At 9:30 A.M. on March 11, 1986, the unsettling saga of Russell Furth began to unfold in a crowded federal courtroom in Houston. More than just the eyes of Texas were about to see a legal system woefully out of step with modern medicine.

Linda Lattimore, chief of the U.S. attorney's criminal-fraud section in Houston, knew from the beginning that she faced an uphill battle to send Furth to prison. Although Lattimore said she had never lost a trial as a federal prosecutor, she had to face facts: the secret McShane tapes weren't top-quality—they had to be sent to a special lab to filter out extraneous noise—and the doctor had failed to get clear-cut self-incriminating statements from Furth. Moreover, her two star witnesses, Dr. McShane and his partner, Dr. Michael Spinks, had shown themselves to be greedy, unprincipled physicians willing to trade patients for money—Furth's alleged crime.

The courtroom setting wasn't shaped to her strengths, either. The trial, held in a large ceremonial courtroom, required that Lattimore use a microphone. Scrappy but not physically imposing, she lacked the booming voice that played well in such a forum. She also faced formidable legal opposition. "It was like a lawyers' convention," she recalled. A two-brother legal team represented Furth, the only defendant, while Furth's hospital, Pasadena General, and its parent company, American Healthcare Management, also had legal representation. Indicative of the trial's importance, American Healthcare hired the prominent and politically connected firm of Fulbright & Jaworski. It, in turn, summoned a top gun from its Washington, D.C., office, Richard Beckler, the former acting chief of the Justice Department's criminal-fraud section, who would later represent John Poindexter of Iran-contra fame.

Lattimore, in tackling the Furth case, had no idea how pervasive patient-buying had become in Houston or around the country. Houston's anything-goes attitude, so obvious in its lack of urban planning, also plagued the city's medical community. Overconstruction of hospital beds had created rabid competition for a limited supply of patients. One nonprofit hospital tried to lure business by spending $2.3 million on doctors for unspecified purposes while building a hunting lodge on an island in the Gulf of Mexico for friends of the hospital.

Houston physician Donald S. Winston said kickbacks were so common around town that one hospital chain mistakenly sent him a $50,000 check intended for another physician. A bank officer had delivered the check. "I grabbed it out of her hand, locked her in the waiting room, copied both sides, then returned it," Dr. Winston told *The Wall Street Journal.*

Russell Furth wasn't even the first Pasadena General official to be accused of buying physicians. Before Dr. McShane stopped admitting patients to Pasadena General, he said, the hospital (under a previous owner) had suddenly begun delivering mysterious cash payments to him. "Once a month," McShane recounted, "this check would come, and if you tried to find out much about this check, you couldn't get much information." When McShane asked the hospital administrator why he was getting money, he was told, "Well, for supporting our hospital, for helping us out."

The freewheeling ways of Houston's hospital industry were costly. Patients there paid 20 percent more than the national average.

The events of the case now coming to trial took place just outside Houston in the city of Pasadena, not a locale young would-be doctors dream of as they struggle to survive the rigors of medical school. Dubbed Stinkadina because of its gasoline refineries and petrochemical plants, the city grew from 2,000 residents just before World War II to 125,000 in the 1980s, sparked by the deepening of the Houston Ship Channel and the oil boom. Along with its environmental warts, Pasadena's industry produced a steady flow of worker injuries, fattening the pocketbooks of many a doctor and hospital. Four hospitals served the area, but according to trial testimony Pasadena General offered fewer services and was getting run down. Many patients and doctors found it less than desirable.

American Healthcare Management, a publicly traded hospital corporation based in Dallas, bought Pasadena General in 1983, believing it could save the hospital by cozying up to doctors. Russell Furth said his bosses preferred spending money on doctors, rather than bricks and mortar, "because buildings lose value, but it's physicians who admit patients."

Dr. McShane and his partner, Dr. Spinks, had all but stopped admitting patients to Pasadena General several years earlier. The loss of any regular admitter frightened hospital administrators, since a physician on average produced $400,000 annually in inpatient revenue. The weakest administrators allowed their institutions to be held hostage by bullying doctors. "I can admit to any hospital that I want to for any reason I want to," Dr. Spinks boasted. "I don't have to justify that to anybody. I can admit [or not admit] because I don't like the color of the carpet or I don't like my parking spot there."

Pasadena General believed its survival depended on recapturing big admitters like McShane and Spinks. Enter Russell Furth, a hard-working, ambitious man in his late 30s. Although he began his career in nonprofit hospitals, he quickly learned the importance of the bottom line when he moved to American Healthcare Management. Soon, he won a promotion to supervisor of a string of American Healthcare hospitals. Then, one day, the corporation called Furth in to tell him he was being transferred to Pasadena to turn that hospital around. Furth felt blindsided. "Stinkadina" was not his idea of a good career move. In a fit of anger, he typed out a résumé, but he never sent it anywhere, deciding instead to tough it out.

Upon arriving in Pasadena, he carried out his first orders: a visit with McShane and Spinks. Furth didn't come empty-handed. He presented the two doctors with a lucrative business proposition that worked this way: the hospital would buy a CAT (computerized axial tomography) scan for anywhere from $600,000 to $1 million. If the scan made money, the doctors got the profits. If it lost money, the hospital took the loss. In other words, the doctors risked nothing. But to make money they would seriously have to consider sending patients to Pasadena General.

The CAT joint venture was nothing more than an ethically tainted gift to win physician loyalty. Although joint ventures aren't as crass as passing envelopes of cash, they achieve the same result: hospital administrators get patients for their empty beds. And once that happens, as doctors know, the more tests they order, the more money they earn.

McShane and Spinks loved the CAT scan idea, so Furth plucked from his dessert cart another treat. The hospital has an advisory committee of doctors, he explained, each of whom gets $1,000 a month. Almost no work is required, except for a monthly meeting lasting usually an hour. Even the most piggish doctors could smile at the thought of earning $1,000 an hour. But just to ensure that doctors didn't collect this money while sending patients to other hospitals, Pasadena General stipulated that only doctors admitting 12 to 15 patients a month qualified for a seat on the committee. Again, the committee served the same purpose as a joint venture: hook doctors using money.

That, too, was fine with McShane and Spinks. But wasn't there more the hospital could offer? The discussion eventually turned to direct patient-buying, although accounts differed as to who first broached the subject. The hospital would pay both doctors $70 for each patient admitted. Then, to conceal the true nature of the payments, the hospital would call them consulting fees—one patient equaling one hour of "consulting" at $70 an hour.

All parties agreed, and the deal was struck. On March 21, 1985, McShane and Spinks admitted their first patients to Pasadena General. That night, Furth and his newly recruited doctors climbed into McShane's Jaguar and cruised to a private club for a celebration dinner of sorts. The doctors were happily aboard, their first checks had been cut, and Furth's first assignment had been successfully completed. It was only fitting that Furth should pick up the restaurant tab.

At his trial, Furth testified that he had never bought patients before and that the payoff scheme troubled him. Nevertheless, he said, he went along with the payments because his boss at American Healthcare had approved them in advance—a charge the company denied. "That's no problem," Furth quoted his superior as saying. "In the state of Texas . . . it's not illegal for a hospital to pay for admissions for non-Medicare, non-Medicaid patients."

Incredibly, the statement was correct. Hospitals in most states can legally buy patients like chattel so long as their bills aren't paid with federal funds from Medicare and Medicaid. On this point the government's entire criminal case would turn because no one, not even Furth, denied that he bought patients from McShane and Spinks. The jury would have to decide only whether Furth had bought any federally covered patients—and the rest be damned.

Not long after McShane and Spinks accepted Furth's largess, other doctors in the area began hearing rumors about who cut what deal with Pasadena General. As the rumors intensified, McShane and Spinks grew more nervous because in Texas, while hospitals can't be prosecuted for buying patients, doctors can be prosecuted for selling them. Finally, McShane and Spinks saw a lawyer who helped them gain immunity from prosecution in exchange for testimony. Once McShane had secretly taped Furth, Linda Lattimore moved to indict the administrator for allegedly violating a federal statute that makes it a crime to offer or pay "remuneration (including any kickback, bribe, or rebate) directly or indirectly, overtly or covertly, in cash or in kind to any person" for the purpose of obtaining the referral of a Medicare patient.

Although McShane's tapes mentioned Medicare patients, they weren't conclusive. They did, however, include many embarrassing moments for Furth—moments Lattimore hoped to drive home to the jury. At one point, Furth told McShane of his boss's impending visit. "Next week the president of our company is in; will be here on Wednesday," he told McShane. "I know you can't predict what may be happening next week, but if you have some admissions around Tuesday evening . . ." On the stand, Furth had to admit that he wanted occupancy high so that his boss would be "in a very, very good mood."

Furth's chief lawyer, Randy Schaffer, had plenty to work with as well. Like any good defense attorney, he wanted to make the government's chief accuser, Dr. McShane, appear unlikable and unbelievable. He contrasted Furth's modest life-style with the gluttony of Dr. McShane and his partner—McShane and Spinks drove a Jaguar and a Porsche, Furth a modest Chevy. The doctors earned $800,000 annually, Furth $54,800.

On the witness stand, Furth said that one night he, McShane, and Spinks decided to meet over dinner to discuss the joint venture. The doctors suggested a restaurant called Tony's. Still new in town, Furth hadn't heard of the restaurant and thought it was "a little pizza Italian place." As Furth's lawyer skillfully led the way with questions, Furth told of his shock at finding the restaurant parking lot filled only with Mercedes-Benzes and Rolls-Royces. He said he parked his "hospital Chevy . . . where the servants were." The night's tab: $329. The doctors allowed Furth to pay for it.

Schaffer had his most fun, however, slicing apart McShane, whose excess weight alone made him an unattractive witness. McShane said under oath that he would admit only to those lies which Schaffer caught him in.

SCHAFFER: "Would you tell a lie if it was necessary to save your medical license?"
McSHANE: "I guess I would."

Schaffer also argued that Furth wouldn't buy Medicare patients, because with government reimbursement rates so low, they weren't profitable. (Other hospitals found Medicare immensely profitable.) His most dramatic appeal to the jury, however, cast Furth as a loyal corporate employee who did what he was told and who didn't personally profit from his dealings with McShane and Spinks.

"I likened it," Schaffer said later, "to these universities that get their football coaches to offer incentives to football players to come and play, and when the shit hits the fan, the university backs away and says he was on his own." Then he added a chilling thought: "They couldn't single my guy out of all the people in the country and make him a felon, because that's the way the industry operated." Furth himself left no doubt about the prevalence of patient-buying when in one recorded conversation he told McShane, "Say something should happen to me, you also want to know that the next person coming in is going to be doing the same damn thing I'm doing."

Lattimore tried her best to salvage the case. "Could you assure yourself that patients who were in those hospitals needed to be there if the doctors receive referral fees on admission?" she asked the jury. But in the end, it didn't really matter. The first-ever federal prosecution of a hospital administrator for buying patients had crashed and burned. The federal jury took less than two hours to acquit Russell Furth.

The trial had delivered a clear message: patient-buying schemes may be unethical, they may exude the worst of odors, but they aren't necessarily illegal. To stay out of federal prison, hospital administrators had only to avoid buying patients whose bills were paid with federal funds, leaving hundreds of thousands of potential victims.

In this atmosphere of the late 1980s, Minneapolis's Methodist Hospital didn't worry about hiding its $2.5 million kickback to the area's largest physician group; it brazenly spelled out the payoff in a written contract. The buyers and sellers of these patients avoided federal felony charges by contractually excluding Medicare and Medicaid patients. Everyone else was fair game.

Ironically, Methodist cited competition, the Reagan-era solution to rising health costs, as its reason for paying wasteful kickbacks. "We were vulnerable," said a spokesman for Methodist, explaining that the hospital had major capital investments to protect. And protect them it did. For $2.5 million, Methodist didn't want just any warm bodies—it wanted bodies that rang up good numbers on the cash register. The contract entitled the hospital to 90 percent of every patient needing CAT scans, radiation therapy, home care, inpatient rehabilitation, and certain outpatient surgical procedures.

But while Methodist selfishly protected its financial interests, there was no one to protect the most vulnerable group of all: patients. Men, women, and children who suddenly found themselves undergoing expensive tests at Methodist never knew that their doctors—to whom they entrusted their lives—had made booty on sending them there. The Hennepin County Medical Society called the deal unethical, but as a private group it has no legal authority to punish anyone. The Minnesota Board of Medical Examiners, which licensed physicians, did have such power, but it refused to say if it had even investigated the contract. State prosecutors, meanwhile, had no legal grounds to pursue a criminal case against the hospital because patient-buying was just as legal in Minnesota as it was in Texas.

Although 36 states do prohibit doctors from getting or giving payments for patient referrals, the vast majority don't bother to monitor compliance with those laws, and thus have no way of knowing when payoffs are made. Only two states say their offices have enough resources to search out violators.

Hospitals too squeamish to pay an outright commission for patients admitted will often buy them indirectly through joint ventures. The principle, however, remains the same: fill beds not on the basis of high quality or low cost but on physician self-interest. Hospital officials by the thousands began flocking to seminars with such bluntly worded game show titles as "Making a Deal with Doctors." In the world of hospital administration the words "kickback" and "bribe" gave way to the euphemisms of "physician bonding" and "physician practice enhancement."

A May 1989 seminar in San Francisco implied that if your hospital didn't make these deals, your competitors would. With CEO turnover rates in some regions approaching 30 percent, administrators responded well to such pitches. "CEOs are told the first thing you do in the morning is figure out how to get rid of your competition so that your hospital will have a better [fiscal] record," said George Harding IV, an Ohio hospital administrator.

Without effective antikickback laws, administrators had to either pay up or risk more empty beds and lose their jobs. "Joint ventures," the San Francisco seminar noted, "are now remaking the health-care landscape. . . . This trend will continue as competition for patients intensifies." By 1990, nearly half of the nation's hospitals had business partnerships with their medical staff.

Minneapolis lawyer Terence M. Fruth witnessed firsthand the lengths to which a desperate hospital chain—in this case, Republic Health Corporation—will go to attract patients. Hoping to assure investors that the company had a plan to stay solvent, Republic invited bondholders to a January 1988 meeting in New York at the Waldorf-Astoria Hotel. Co-sponsored by the notorious junk-bond king, Drexel Burnham Lambert, the meeting made Fruth feel queasy almost from the beginning. Although Fruth represented a small Minneapolis bondholder, most attendees were high-rolling junk-bond investors—"a real cast of characters," he recalled.

Growing more uncomfortable by the minute, Fruth listened to Republic push business deals with doctors as a way to fill beds and increase revenues. Republic produced data showing that hospitals with surgical joint ventures—in which doctors shared in the profits—did more cutting than those with no joint ventures. Fruth finally decided he had seen enough. "I raised my hand," he recalled. "I said, 'Wait a minute, this is clearly, in my view, a breach of medical ethics.' " Fruth felt like the student who just told the teacher that his classmates had been cheating. "Somebody said—I don't remember who—'Maybe in Minneapolis there are those concerns, but I can tell you that in Texas and Florida there are different notions of what is proper.' I just said, 'Okay, I'm not going to argue with that one.' "

In truth, Texas and Florida were no different from any other state; administrators everywhere could be found baiting traps for doctors. Lewisburg Community Hospital in Lewisburg, Tennessee, was so hot for a joint venture that it installed an investing doctor as chief of radiology services, and as radiation safety officer. But according to the American College of Radiology, the doctor rarely visited the hospital and wasn't even a member of the hospital's regular medical staff. Critics called the arrangement potentially unsafe, a charge Lewisburg denied.

Doctors showed their enthusiasm for joint ventures by altering their practices. In 1988, Dr. Fred Dumenigo couldn't recall ever, in 20 years of practice, admitting a patient to Miami's Victoria Hospital. But by November 1989, after the hospital's owner, Columbia Hospital Corporation, allowed him to invest in its hospital, Dumenigo boasted that he was sending 60 percent of his patients there.

Many hospitals tried a different tactic; they simply bought physician practices outright. By the late 1980s, about one in five hospitals nationwide had, essentially, locked in patient referrals by putting doctors on their payrolls. Again, patients didn't always know that their "independent" doctors had lost their independence. "If you have locked in that supply of patients, then you have assured your future and you have significantly damaged your competing hospital," explained Barry Moore, of Hamilton/KSA, a medical-consulting firm.

Administrators defended buying doctors as harmless, but that would be true only if all hospitals were equally good. And they are not. For example, one Philadelphia hospital, accused by the Justice Department of paying doctors to get patients, was also accused of employing unlicensed physicians.

Arnold Relman, former editor of *The New England Journal of Medicine*, thought even joint ventures were dangerous. "Physicians are human like everyone else," Dr. Relman said. "When you're sick, by golly, what you most of all need is a reliable, honest, competent doctor who's concerned about you, and whose judgment you can trust. I'd hate to see 'caveat emptor' written above the doors of hospitals." Unless such deals are outlawed, he added, "doctors will continue to drift toward the opinion that medicine is just a business and patients are theirs to be bought and sold."

Most legislators paid scant attention to Relman's concern. Congressman Fortney (Pete) Stark led a charge on Capitol Hill to rein in the more abusive patient-buying schemes, but when his original bill left committee in 1989, the toughest provisions governing hospitals had been seriously weakened. HHS didn't help matters when it took nearly three years to write guidelines, requested by Congress in 1987, that sought to clarify what constituted an illegal kickback.

In this legal and ethical vacuum, Bronson Methodist Hospital in Kalamazoo, Michigan, could pay kickbacks to get HMO (health maintenance organization) patients and then charge them $1,200 a day, as against $600 to $650 at a neighboring hospital, according to a 1989 lawsuit filed by a unit of Blue Cross and Blue Shield of Michigan. Is it any wonder, then, that Kalamazoo's hospital care was among the costliest in the state? Or that doctors around the country who own testing equipment tend to order more unnecessary tests?

The top prize for creative bonding, however, would surely go to Leyden Community Hospital in suburban Chicago. Its vice president of surgical services distributed a memo to "ALL STAFF PHYSICIANS AND SURGEONS" outlining a plan to boost surgical volume over the slow-cutting weeks following Thanksgiving. The memo stated in part:

> Any physician who performs ten (10) major surgery cases between November 23, 1989 and January 31, 1990, will be entitled to receive by March 31, 1990 their choice of one of the following "Promotional Incentives":
> A) An In-Office fax machine; or
> B) Portable Cellular Telephone.

The memo had been marked "approved for implementation," but after the *Chicago Tribune* reported its contents, Leyden Community Hospital denied that final approval had been given, and said the plan was dead.

Stories of DRG creep, Medicare cost-padding, and hospitals bribing doctors for patients were not big news in the 1980s and early 1990s—not with so many other hospital problems competing for public attention. The sound bites of this era were crowded emergency rooms, nurse shortages, and rising medical costs, all easily quantified, if not easily explained. Not that stories of financial chicanery weren't important. By adding costs to a medical system already burdened by inflation, they aggravated other, more visible problems.

The federal government revolutionized hospitals through DRGs, but in an era of deregulation it lacked the will to prevent the financial abuses riding the back of that revolution. The Reagan administration couldn't tell the difference between cutting unnecessary paperwork and cutting government's oversight for its own liabilities. Consequently, budget cuts "fell disproportionately on enforcement, oversight, management, and accounting functions," said one official of the General Accounting Office.

Even so, there were people in federal government, like Richard Kusserow, the HHS inspector general, who emerged as dedicated defenders of taxpayers and hospital patients. Frustrated at his inability to ferret out patient-buying schemes, Kusserow once encouraged doctors to snitch on their corrupt colleagues by calling a special nationwide hot line. The medical community was appalled at such a suggestion.

On September 25, 1990, the American Medical Association called on President George Bush to demand Kusserow's resignation. The AMA, and later the American Hospital Association, said Kusserow was unfairly harassing the medical establishment and could no longer be trusted. Kusserow remained on the job. He wasn't perfect; on rare occasions, his bluster blurred his judgment. He once challenged a television reporter on camera to prove him wrong on a particular point. Amid much embarrassment, Kusserow later had to admit his error. Still, his many admirers in Congress and elsewhere thought a little anger wasn't out of line when directed at a health care system that had shown so much disdain for disciplining itself.

In October 1990, Congress passed a budget that required elderly Americans to pay one-third more in Medicare deductibles in 1991 and nearly two-thirds more in premiums by 1995. Were they getting their money's worth?

At the end of the 1980s, the Conference Board, a business research group, commissioned a survey of 7,000 families to learn how they ranked the value of 50 products and services. Money paid for used cars, in lawyers' fees, and in bank service charges was not well spent, according to the list. All of them, however, finished higher than hospital charges. Those placed dead last.

THREE | Absent Watchdogs

12 | A Gathering of Felons

ITS image sears the memory of those who lived through it. Neighbors bought firearms. No number of dead-bolt locks seemed enough. Children didn't leave home without adult escorts. The worst part, however, was that it never seemed to end. Twenty-four hours a day, this open-air drug bazaar imprisoned an entire neighborhood.

The time: late 1970s. The place: Elyria, Ohio. Crack cocaine hadn't yet gripped America by the throat. The worst drug pushers were still confined mostly to inner-city streets, hidden from mainstream America. That was what made the drug trade here so implausible. This was rural Ohio, down the road from soybean fields and dairy farms, hardly the usual gathering place for addicts, felons, and fugitives from justice. Yet this was their stage, and what an act they put on for the neighbors—stealing, beating, shooting, urinating, fornicating, snorting cocaine, jamming hypodermic needles into their veins.

The drug trade here was no secret. As business went on month after month, year after year, people began to journey to this spot from all points on the compass, and from as far as Alabama, California, Colorado, Florida, Georgia, Maryland, Michigan, New Jersey, New York, Pennsylvania, and West Virginia. Sometimes 75 cars at a time waited in line for drugs like Dilaudid, a powerful narcotic. An area prosecutor would later call this "a nuisance the equal of which has never been recorded in the history of the courts in the state of Ohio."

At the center of this strange spectacle was not some hardened, back-alley drug pusher. It was a physician, fully licensed by the state of Ohio to treat the sick and dying. His name: Dr. Leonard F. Faymore. This was the good doctor who attracted all that traffic. Not only did Dr. Faymore criminally dispense the worst kind of addictive drugs, but he did it with a flair—right down to his pharmacist, herself a heroin addict with needle tracks on her arm and a pistol at her side. One day, high on cocaine and barbiturates, she took that pistol and blew a hole in her head. Dr. Faymore didn't miss a beat. There would always be someone to count the pills, even if it meant employing his common-law wife, a big-boned blonde who wheeled about town in a white Cadillac, or another pharmacist, who abused alcohol to the point of falling down drunk on the job.

Dr. Faymore's clinic supplied users as well as dealers. No sooner would people buy their drugs inside Faymore's clinic than many would resell them outside. During one two-and-a-half-month period, undercover narcotics officers made 77 illegal drug buys in the vicinity, resulting in 44 felony convictions. Still, Dr. Faymore remained in business. "Indict me or drop dead," he would tell prosecutors.

In person, Faymore was easy to like, self-deprecating, with more than a trace of black humor. As a doctor, he was a disaster. A decade earlier, he'd had to leave an Ohio hospital after colleagues stripped him of his surgical privileges. "His ability, his judgment and his dexterity did not improve," the hospital concluded. Once, Faymore even lost his medical license for illegal drug dispensing, only to regain it on a procedural error.

As long as he kept that medical license, his dreams remained alive. One wish was pure childhood fantasy: to build an immense castle for himself and his wife. Not just a big house, a castle. And sure enough, one day drug buyers who had gathered outside Faymore's clinic noticed a wall rising amid the distant trees. Foot by foot it grew, until it dwarfed all around it. So grand was its presence that it inspired rumors of equal proportion: bodies were buried out there, and the giant walls had secret compartments for jewels and cash. Faymore fed those rumors by paying construction workers with cash taken from paper bags. His money-handling practices carried over to his clinic, where police once found $100,000 in a paper bag stuffed under a table. The stories all added to the growing legend of Dr. Faymore, who one day would pass the hours in federal prison swapping stories with his cellmate, the Mafia don of Cleveland, James T. Licavoli.

But before society finally ridded itself of Faymore, he had one longing yet to be fulfilled: to find another hospital, one that would accept him. One that would give him respect. As long as he had that medical license, anything was possible. And then one day, just like his castle, his dream became reality. Faymore found a hospital that would not only let him admit patients but also give him back his surgeon's knife—and then some. To many in law enforcement, the doctor was an unconscionable drug pusher. To New London Hospital, he was something else. He was Dr. Leonard F. Faymore, chief of surgery.

About five miles down the road from Faymore's drug clinic, Dr. George Gotsis sat nervously in a Lorain County (Ohio) courtroom. Years earlier, Dr. Gotsis had taken a sacred oath of healing. Now, in the fall of 1975, he stood accused of conspiring to commit murder. According to prosecutors, Gotsis had offered a taxi driver $500 to kill his former boss, Dr. Denis Radefeld, chief of staff at Lorain Community Hospital. Gotsis did this, the government said, because he blamed Radefeld for Community Hospital's decision in 1973 to strip him of his surgical privileges.

The trial was just the latest setback in a medical career spinning out of control. Hospitals didn't expel physicians except for the worst of sins, and so it was with Dr. Gotsis, a blustery native of Greece. The hospital first became concerned after a random review of surgeries turned up irregularities in Gotsis's records. A more thorough investigation concluded that the doctor showed little respect for human life: he cut people open in "a great number" of unnecessary operations; he often diagnosed ailments incorrectly; he kept incomplete or inaccurate patient records; and he performed inadequate surgery.

One colleague, Dr. Ward V. Young, Jr., went so far as to say that Dr. Gotsis's careless medical care showed "contempt" for his patients. "It is inconceivable," said Dr. Young, "that he should be allowed to perform surgery." Others at Lorain Community said they had never seen a hospital investigative report so damning as the one on Gotsis.

Doctors who would later review Gotsis's record at another hospital concluded he was responsible for the abnormally high post-surgical infection rate of his patients. "The record as a whole," one doctor wrote, "shows a surgeon willing and anxious to operate at every opportunity with little or no regard for the medical necessity of the surgery, [or] possible complicating factors."

Even major corporations around Lorain County were angry at Gotsis for writing medical excuses for employees who didn't show up for work. The Lorain County Medical Society investigated one case where Gotsis signed a sick slip vouching that an absent Ford Motor Company employee had been hospitalized for a month as a result of assembly-line "neurosis." In reality, the employee had been serving a jail sentence for statutory rape. In February 1975, the medical society expelled Gotsis for unprofessional conduct, charging excessive fees, and falsifying medical-disability records.

To appreciate Gotsis fully, however, was to listen to him talk. Asked in 1980 why he had performed an elective sterilization procedure on a patient who had a staph infection plus vaginitis and cervicitis, took drugs, and had poor general hygiene, Gotsis replied, "Didn't have any choice, she would be pregnant next year. . . . The woman had five kids and drinks at the bars. . . . It was done like in Alabama. You sterilize the black girls, except this is elective. . . . It was something social, you elect to sterilize this person."

Horrible as Gotsis's conduct was, when he stood before a judge and jury on an attempted murder charge in 1975, he still retained his most prized possession: an Ohio medical license. This time, he would not lose his freedom, either. When a hung jury couldn't return a verdict on the attempted-murder charges, the government decided to drop its case. Gotsis was free to go.

It would take prosecutors another seven years to get their man. In February 1983, Gotsis was convicted of selling drug prescriptions to an undercover drug agent, a felony. Police, in calling him a major-league drug pusher, noted that Dr. Gotsis wrote between 10 and 25 percent of all drug prescriptions in Lorain County even though he was just one of 200 physicians practicing there. Upon sentencing, one cop said he expected to see a resulting drop in drug overdose deaths.

But in the years between his two trials, and before he went to prison on drug charges, Dr. George Gotsis still longed to resurrect his reputation by finding a hospital that would accept him on staff. The problem was that no hospital would take him. Except, that is, New London Hospital. And it not only took him, it would help make him chief of staff.

A strange place, this New London Hospital, with its Victorian turrets rising above a red-brick structure built almost 100 years earlier.

Originally a factory and later converted to an imposing personal residence, the structure looked less like a hospital than an ancient almshouse where, in the early years of this country, society hid its sick, poor, and insane. The almshouse wasn't so much a house of healing as a place to die. No one of status sought medical care in hospitals of that era, preferring treatment at home.

Although certainly no almshouse, New London did cast an eerie image for a hospital, particularly in the still of a rural Ohio night, with its cone-shaped towers silhouetted against a moonlit sky. And it was in darkness that many frightened patients first came to know New London Hospital, situated in the village of New London, population 2,400, about 60 miles southwest of Cleveland.

The willingness of New London to welcome medical rejects like Gotsis and Faymore—two future felons—added to the mystery of the hospital and its new management. If men like that were employed there, who else could be found wandering the hallways of New London? One doctor recruited by the hospital had been accused of overbilling Medicare in another state. He later left New London, only to be fired by a rural health clinic before ending up with a job in a state mental institution. "The minute [New London] found out that I was accused of overutilization, it's as if I had a signed contract in my hands," the doctor recalled with amazement. "Everybody has to have a flaw." The clear implication was that New London hired such people because they could be controlled.

Surely, that was an exaggeration. Or was it? New London Hospital in the late 1970s did seem to have characters too bizarre for anyone to believe.

- The administrator was a real-estate salesman with no formal training in hospital management. He was also a convicted felon and a motorcycle enthusiast who bragged about his White House and Pentagon contacts.
- The hospital psychologist, also a felon, arrived from Illinois after serving a jail sentence for defrauding that state's Medicaid program. He did counseling at Faymore's drug clinic.
- A surgeon who chaired the hospital's utilization review committee was banned from practicing medicine in Mississippi after failing a national licensing exam. Ohio allowed him to practice because of a reciprocity agreement with Texas, where the doctor held a valid license.
- The assistant administrator was a former Catholic priest who had

left the Church after marrying a divorced belly dancer named Saudi Arabia on a Mississippi riverboat. At one time, he headed the hospital's discharge-planning department, and he later did counseling at Faymore's drug clinic. In the early 1980s, he would be charged with selling cocaine but not convicted.

- One hospital doctor arrived after having been accused in another state of overtreating patients to make more money. Among the billings cited as unnecessary: 288 of 302 office visits, 597 of 609 injections, 285 of 298 laboratory procedures, and 276 of 296 physical-therapy sessions. And all those billings were for just one patient.

- The chairman of the board took his seat 10 days after his indictment for grand theft and having an unlawful interest in a government contract. Although eventually convicted of only a misdemeanor, he earlier was the subject of a *Cleveland Press* series revealing that he served as a top official in two charities that invested money in a jukebox and vending-machine concern, which, in turn, loaned money to Cleveland's top Mafiosi, including the legendary Angelo (Big Ange) Lonardo.

The background of hospital personnel on this quite remarkable roster was, of course, never even suspected by New London's patients. Most of them didn't come from the quiet villages along the nearby Vermilion River. They were not likely to be the local wheat farmers or merchants. They were, instead, visitors from afar, often shipped in after sunset by ambulances that traveled dozens—even hundreds—of miles before rolling onto one of the two country roads that bisect New London.

Patients came there because they often had no choice. They were old and poor, and they lived in nursing homes, some wretched, scattered across Ohio. In the early 1970s, an Ohioan, Mary A. Mendelson, wrote a scathing account of nursing home life, *Tender Loving Greed.* Her book was a call to arms for reformers, but while it won nationwide plaudits, many Ohio nursing homes remained a disgrace. Even doctors didn't like to visit them.

There was, however, one doctor who was willing, one who treated patients at nearly 30 nursing homes, in many of them as staff physician or medical director. That doctor was Leonard Faymore, and where others saw only despair, Faymore saw opportunity. There could be big money in getting these old people to a hospital where they could be tested and operated on. And Dr. Faymore knew just the place: New London Hospital.

Sadie Bronner, a 79-year-old widow, was one of Faymore's patients. She lived in a nursing home east of Akron in the northeast quadrant of the state. When it was decided that Mrs. Bronner needed surgery, an out-of-town ambulance company picked her up on the evening of June 18, 1978, but it didn't take her to any of the 15 area hospitals. Instead, it carted her through parts of four counties, apparently picking up a second patient in another city, Canton, before ending up at New London Hospital. The entire trip most likely took several hours.

And it was only the beginning. Over the next five weeks, this seriously ill woman would be packed into an ambulance six more times, bounced from county to county, before dying in a suburban Akron hospital at 6 P.M. on August 8. The Summit County Welfare Department lodged an angry protest—to no avail—with the Ohio State Health Department over Bronner's treatment. "Despite our efforts to maintain a cooperative relationship with [New London], there have been several incidents involving post-hospital needs that have had adverse effect upon patients," the department complained.

Bronner's case was particularly appalling. After operating on Mrs. Bronner's leg, New London returned her to the nursing home, whereupon it was found that gangrene had developed. So at 1:15 one morning, she was shipped all the way back to New London, where she underwent surgery again, this time to amputate her leg.

Three days later, New London told the welfare department that it was discharging Bronner to a general-care nursing home. County workers protested, saying she was too sick and needed more sophisticated medical care. But New London went ahead with its plan anyhow. The nursing home, quickly discovering that Bronner was too sick for its facility, transferred her to yet another nursing home. This home couldn't handle her, either, so she was sent to an Akron-area hospital that, ironically, had been bypassed for Bronner's initial visit to New London Hospital. There she died. "She was just a little old black woman who really didn't have anyone to care for her . . . and now she's dead," said Doris Combs, of the Summit County Welfare Department. New London blamed the welfare department for the foul-ups.

Had New London been a tertiary-care hospital, like Cleveland Clinic, Mrs. Bronner's nocturnal voyages might have made some sense. But it wasn't. New London didn't offer the latest innovative treatments. It didn't have the most sophisticated equipment. It wasn't affiliated with a medical school. New London was just a tiny rural hospital at 54 South Main Street that would have closed for good in 1974 had it not been bought by an out-of-town group headed by a felon from Cleveland and a former lawyer for Jimmy Hoffa, boss of the Teamsters Union.

Like many small rural hospitals, New London had once been run by a group of local doctors. But over the years, they died or left town, and by the early 1970s New London rarely had more than a handful of patients. In stepped the Clevelanders, who bought the hospital and then leased it to a nonprofit group they controlled.

The new proprietors had promised that New London would remain a community hospital, but area residents couldn't help noticing the unusual license plates that suddenly began to appear in town, plates that didn't begin with X, as was customary for the area. Under the new management, occupancy at the nonprofit hospital quickly doubled; hallways handled the patient overflow. The number of surgeries increased tenfold, and the sole operating room sometimes worked 12 hours a day, four days a week. "Surgeons change after three to four hours, [but] the nurses do not, and by midafternoon they are usually dead on their feet," the hospital confided to area health planners. Years later it was disclosed that patients frequently signed blank surgical-consent forms. Many failed to understand what they had signed. Nurse's aides also improperly assisted in surgery.

One doctor even charged that hospital staff meetings, required under the federal Medicare program, weren't held and that phony minutes were created as a cover. Perhaps nothing, however, symbolized New London's standard of patient care more than its use of cystoscopy. To check for urinary-tract problems, doctors insert a scope via a tube through the urethra and into the bladder. It is a common and relatively simple procedure. Yet when federal health officials reviewed New London Hospital, they reached a startling conclusion: "There were no cases reviewed in which this procedure was successful." No cases? If New London couldn't do one of those, what could it do?

It may not have mattered, because the government also found that many other procedures, tests, and admissions were apparently unnecessary. At one point, Medicare reviewers refused to reimburse the hospital for one-third of all claims submitted. In a confidential letter to the Ohio State Health Department, federal health officials wrote: "In almost all cases, the same laboratory tests and x-rays are ordered. . . . These studies and tests are performed in many cases on patients having no symptoms or complaints." Staff physicians, it was also found, sometimes owned companies that performed the diagnostic tests.

Government auditors singled out Faymore, who joined New London in 1974, for overtesting his patients. He and Gotsis, who arrived two years later, were responsible for admitting the great bulk of patients. Different in style and temperament, the two medical outcasts coexisted and little more: Faymore cool and calm, Gotsis emotional and quick to anger.

At one point, Gotsis became so disgusted with Faymore that he contacted a law enforcement official, accusing Faymore of surgical malpractice. "I'd be willing to testify in any kind of proceeding, anywhere, against Dr. Faymore," Gotsis said. In exchange, Gotsis wanted the agent to help him find a hospital in the Lorain area that would take him. Why couldn't he get hospital privileges on his own? the agent asked. "Due to personal and professional problems, I'm prohibited from practicing medicine in the area," Gotsis replied. In other words, only New London would take him. The deal never developed, and Gotsis never testified against Faymore.

The strange happenings inside New London Hospital were no secret to government authorities. Federal health officials certainly knew, but they weren't telling the public. The state of Ohio knew, but its regulators weren't saying anything, either. Many doctors around the state knew but, like the rest, kept silent. What they all knew was that New London Hospital was a dangerous place to be. And while they did nothing, patients kept coming.

In 1974, as New London Hospital's new managers were settling in, an old warhorse of Ohio politics, Republican James Rhodes, was gearing up for a return to glory. After serving as governor from 1963 to 1970, Rhodes was constitutionally barred from a third successive term, but three years later he was ready to retake his old job. He would not only win, he would go on to be reelected again in 1974, making him Ohio's governor for 16 years, longer than anyone else.

When it came to the practice of medicine in his state, Governor

Rhodes believed that doctors knew best and that medicine's problems weren't really the business of consumer groups or even government. As the state's chief executive for 16 years, Rhodes, a gruff and sometimes profane politician, had the time and power to make sure his philosophy prevailed in Ohio.

Take, for example, the Ohio Medical Board, a state agency with the legal responsibility to license and discipline Ohio's 27,000 doctors. Rhodes relished his role as an uncompromising advocate of law and order—he sent the national guard to Kent State University in 1970 to put down antiwar protests, which resulted in the killing of four students—but he held the medical profession to a different standard. Under Rhodes's appointees, it functioned as a private gentlemen's club, a place of dignified, quiet voices. Most appointees were in the image of Dr. Peter Lancione, a stern, gray-haired doctor who once said he thought the indefinite suspension of a doctor's license "seems to be an awfully harsh penalty for anything." Not surprisingly, then, after an Ohio doctor was caught dispensing nearly 4 million dosage units of addicting drugs in just three years, Lancione thought a three-month license suspension was more than enough.

Governor Rhodes amply demonstrated his contempt for consumer rights by filling the only consumer slot on the Ohio Medical Board with a crony of his, Walter Paulo. Then 77 years old, Paulo had once headed a company that bankrolled the production of "magic" milk, a product that purported to cure allergies, rheumatism, and asthma. The Ohio State Medical Association had no choice but to call these claims medical quackery, and the Ohio State Health Department once ordered Paulo to stop advertising it. Rhodes's other appointments weren't always much better. At one point, he tried to fill a position on the Ohio Medical Board with a podiatrist who had practiced in the state without a license, and who had signed his name in such a way as to suggest he was a doctor, which he wasn't. The legislature refused to confirm the nomination.

These, then, were medicine's traffic cops during New London's biggest years. Even when abuses were uncovered, very little was done about it. "It says something about the system," said an official of Lorain Community Hospital, "that after we found out all this about the guy [Gotsis]—and get him kicked out—that he gets turned loose on the rest of the world."

Over at the Ohio State Health Department, the Rhodes philosophy was very much in evidence as well. Under contract to the federal government, the health department was supposed to help ensure that federal dollars weren't going to substandard hospitals. How seriously did the department carry out this mission? "We don't like the word inspection," explained Sterling Gill, who in 1979 was chief of the department's Medicare certification division. "We consider ourselves surveyors and consultants." In this fertile soil, New London found its nourishment.

The health department did, in fact, receive much damaging information about New London, but somehow its "surveyors" never seemed to turn up enough to threaten its Medicare funding. It wasn't until the *Cleveland Press,* in 1979, published an exposé on the hospital that things began to change. Only then, under the glare of media attention, did the federal government decide to bypass Governor Rhodes's "surveyors" and send in its own investigators. They found the hospital seriously substandard and ultimately revoked its Medicare certification. Without federal reimbursements, business dwindled to nothing by 1980.

Later, as Faymore and Gotsis marched off to prison and their coworkers scattered across the country, it was hard for anyone who knew what had gone on at New London to believe ever again that medicine was properly regulated. For six years, society's castoffs had been herded into this hellhole, while informed government regulators and doctors' groups stood silently by. The cost in human life— and taxpayer dollars—was incalculable.

New London may just have been ahead of its time. In the years that followed, some hospitals would develop patient admission and dumping, like the case of Sadie Bronner, into a fine art. In the 1980s, more doctors than ever would discover the benefits of acquiring their own testing facilities and referring patients to them. Even attempting to overbill Medicare, as New London did, would become a widely practiced sport for many hospitals.

The medical community, embarrassed by what had happened at New London, found solace where it could. The hospital was an aberration, its spokesmen believed. They cited its lack of professional accreditation, which most hospitals in the country had. Nothing so bad, they suggested, could happen in an accredited hospital. They were wrong, of course, but that realization would have to wait.

The federal government made the best of it as well. Although it still had to rely on the Ohio State Health Department to oversee

Ohio hospitals, the government did have a backup system—something called the Professional Standard Review Organization (PSRO). But it was hardly an independent agency. In the spirit of political compromise, the government agreed to organized medicine's demands and let doctors review their own colleagues. Any problems, they would catch.

But like so many other regulatory illusions, this one never quite did what it was supposed to. In fact, had it not been so tragic, even the AMA might have seen the humor in its creation. Drs. Faymore and Gotsis, being members of the PSRO, were supposed to ferret out the same kind of abuses of which they were accused. "I know this sounds shady—sort of like letting the fox guard the henhouse," said the director for the regional PSRO. But as long as they held valid medical licenses, the director explained, there was nothing he could do. In later years, PSROs would be modified and given a new name, but ultimately, they would be no more successful.

Such was the state of hospital regulation in Ohio—and much of the nation—in the 1970s. In this environment, Dr. James C. Burt would later, under the protection of a large Dayton hospital, surgically redesign female genitalia, apparently with the conviction that whoever had created women did a lousy job. Dr. Burt also thought his rearranging of body parts would enhance a woman's sexual pleasure. In this environment, one of the worst serial killings in U.S. history would occur inside a Cincinnati hospital. And in this environment, it was no surprise that Ohio under Governor Rhodes became one of the first states to join Ronald Reagan's push in the 1980s to deregulate the health care industry by getting rid of health planning. Let the marketplace solve the problems of hospitals: this became the new rallying cry.

Meanwhile, in New London, as the 1980s took hold, the brick structure at 54 South Main Street stood nearly empty, waiting to be rescued. But after all the town folk had seen there, many weren't too happy to learn from the local papers that a nearby psychic from the "Temple in the Man" society had announced plans to reopen the hospital. One local woman even began a prayer vigil in hopes of blocking the new owners. In Ohio, and elsewhere, residents didn't have much else to protect them from inferior hospitals and the type of rogue physicians who had held sway in this tiny Ohio village.

13 | Midnight Fire

THE hour was late and the doctors desperate. They were members of the American College of Surgeons, distinguished and prosperous men meeting in 1919 at one of the world's grand hotels. Soon, however, they would act in a most unbecoming manner. The doctors had something to hide. And what better time to hide it than at midnight, when others were busy socializing or sleeping?

What led these men to a room deep inside New York's Waldorf-Astoria Hotel was a tale of noble intentions gone awry. It went back in part to one spring day in 1913 when Dr. Ernest A. Codman delivered a speech to some colleagues titled "The Product of a Hospital." He noted that industry measured results by the quality of its products. Yet hospitals, even the best of them, didn't bother to do the same for patient care. Many leading surgeons of the day wanted to change that. If agreement could be reached on what constitutes good hospital care, then all hospitals could be measured against that standard, the surgeons reasoned. Not only would this help hospitals improve themselves, but patients would have some way to assess which hospital was good and which wasn't.

The American College of Surgeons was founded, in part, to set such standards. The country badly needed such a program. In the early years of this century, many hospitals were little more than boardinghouses for the poor and sick, lacking in standardization, quality control, and the ability to translate scientific advances into healing. The College had high hopes of changing that. In April 1918, it began inspecting hospitals, with the expectation that at least 1,000 of them would pass muster in the program's first year.

The College's estimate fell shockingly short. On October 24, 1919, at that conference on hospital standardization at the Waldorf, it divulged its sorry tally: of 671 hospitals with 100 beds or more, only 89 had met the College's standards. Some of the nation's most distinguished hospitals had failed. Frightening as that was, the College still had an opportunity to turn bad into good. It could have warned potential patients which hospitals posed serious health risks. It could have, through public disclosure, further pressured those substandard hospitals to improve.

Instead, the College tossed its list of substandard hospitals into a hotel furnace. Better that than let the press get hold of it. The surgeons had let the genie out of its bottle, only to be frightened by its power. Now, on this day in 1919, they wanted it back in.

So ended medicine's first serious attempt to regulate hospitals. To be sure, self-regulation would improve steadily over the next 70 years, upgrading countless hospitals in the process. And by midcentury, inspections would become so detailed that a new group had to be formed to conduct them: the Joint Commission on Accreditation of Hospitals, an amalgam of medical groups that included the American Medical Association and the American Hospital Association.

Nevertheless, that furtive act of incineration at the Waldorf would for the next 70 years characterize the medical community's attitude toward the consuming public. Specifics about dangerously substandard hospitals remained a secret between the inspectors and the inspected, the privileged information of physicians and hospitals. State and federal health officials heartily endorsed this approach. Beginning with the passage of Medicare in 1965, government increasingly relied on the Joint Commission to identify substandard hospitals. Thousands eagerly sought Joint Commission accreditation because it kept most government inspectors from wandering their halls, made it easier to obtain financing for new construction, and provided other important perks. With government's blessing, accreditation became the industry's Good Housekeeping Seal of Approval.

Perhaps the Joint Commission's finest moment occurred in August 1987, when the *Journal of the American Medical Association,* a widely respected publication known universally as *JAMA,* printed a lengthy article extolling the successes of private self-regulation. "[T]he voluntary accreditation movement has been a consistent and persistent voice for quality in health care," the Joint Commission wrote. Hardly anyone disagreed. But then, few outsiders really knew what tales might lie inside the Joint Commission's secret files.

About a month after the glowing *JAMA* article, 68-year-old Nick Vigorito, semiretired and living at home, suffered a heart attack and was admitted to Parsons Hospital, a fully accredited facility in the heart of Flushing, Queens. After stabilizing Vigorito with drugs, Parsons moved him out of intensive care, allowing him to move about. A subsequent test signaled impending danger—including an irregular heartbeat—but according to doctors who later reviewed Vigorito's medical records, Parsons failed to react to that critical warning. Soon after, the hospital found him dead. The doctors called his hospital care grossly deficient. Mistakes, of course, happen in any institution or profession. But Parsons went way beyond that. Over the next six months, 72 other patients would die within its precincts. More than half were later judged to have received deficient medical care.

Meanwhile, 100 miles to the south in Philadelphia, the James C. Giuffre Medical Center was living through its own medical nightmare. Apart from a long history of using unlicensed and unqualified medical personnel, Giuffre had gotten so out of control that a doctor allegedly operated on a corpse, thinking it was alive. According to a board member of the hospital, the surgeon didn't realize the patient had died on the operating table, because he was tired and there was "a lot of blood."

Like Parsons, Giuffre was fully accredited. To patients, to government officials, to the medical establishment, that designation provided a comforting reassurance. But the Latinos who lived near the hospital weren't fooled. They had their own name for Giuffre. They called it *matadero*—Spanish for "slaughterhouse."

In the mid-1970s, Beth Birnbaum worked a block from Parsons in a nursing home that catered mostly to Jewish and Italian families of working-class backgrounds. Birnbaum, the daughter of a hospital official in another borough of New York, had the job of trying to mentally stimulate senile, or "confused," residents. Back then, this condition of the elderly was believed to be environmentally induced. If residents, for example, didn't know the time of day, it was only because they had no need to know it. As an antidote, Birnbaum talked frequently to her residents about the news of the day. She even tried to get them to publish an in-house newspaper.

Birnbaum's nursing home was bright and clean, each floor painted a different color. One obsessed employee went outside nearly every morning to make sure window shades were exactly even. The nursing home posed a stark contrast to Parsons down the block, which Birnbaum remembered as "small, cramped, hot, and dusty," without any air-conditioning.

Although Birnbaum's residents were relatively healthy, they did, from time to time, require some hospitalization. "When one of our residents was sent to Flushing Hospital, only five blocks away, we said goodbye," she remarked. "When one of our residents was sent to Parsons, we said goodbye and we meant it in a different way, because we knew that they would probably never return." Birnbaum was no doctor and she had no way of knowing exactly what went on inside Parsons. Still, there was something about the place that frightened her.

Birnbaum left the neighborhood in 1977, just as it was beginning to change. In the 1980s, wave after wave of Asian immigrants swept through, and the patients and the work force at Parsons reflected that change. Some families found comfort in the presence of hospital workers who spoke various Asian languages. Others, however, used the hospital as a human refuse heap. "Patients were dumped there . . . by families that didn't want any part of their mothers or fathers," said Ira Madin, a vice president at nearby Flushing Hospital.

The building, meanwhile, began to deteriorate. On July 9, 1987, visitors were shocked to find water "gushing out of the elevator" onto the first floor. Water also leaked from a ceiling over a nursing station. "Parsons was in complete disrepair," said Madin. Some rooms, he noted, had no call systems or patient monitoring equipment or private bathrooms.

Most hospitals, regardless of quality, generated a good measure of civic pride, and Parsons was no exception. When talk surfaced in the mid-1970s about closing the hospital, Birnbaum's nursing home circulated a petition to save it. "I was one of the few who refused to sign," she said, pointing out that other hospitals were nearby. Even now, years later, she wonders how many lives might have been saved had Parsons closed back then.

But it did not. And over the years, one of the most powerful groups in all of organized medicine helped to keep it open—the Joint Commission.

• • •

Philadelphia residents needn't have been patients at Giuffre Medical Center to know of its high-flying ways; they merely had to read the local gossip column. Entertainment and sports celebrities paraded in and out of Giuffre as if it were some trendy spa. They came because of one man: James C. Giuffre, after whom the hospital was renamed in 1978. Small in stature and with big glasses, Giuffre presided over this private, nonprofit, 228-bed hospital like the dictator of a banana republic. Once, when his personal car had a minor fender bender, he didn't want it fixed; he ordered hospital workers to get him an identical car by close of business that day.

Although harsh at times, Giuffre craved attention, whether working the cafeteria tables telling jokes, or collaring anyone from clerks to maintenance men to go watch him cut and stitch in the operating room. "Come on up," he would say.

If not master of the universe, Giuffre at least thought he was the center of it. Employees were encouraged to contribute through payroll deductions toward a $40,000 life-size statue of him. Upon its execution and delivery, the doctor placed his replica behind a roped retainer in the hospital lobby, complete with proper illumination. And as if that weren't enough, hospital officials were expected to pay tribute to Giuffre with Christmas gifts. "We had to stand around while he opened them. It could get very uncomfortable," said one of the gift-givers.

Giuffre's love of the spotlight attracted those who performed in it. Among the hospital's visitors and patients: Al Martino, Joey Bishop, Danny Thomas, Vic Damone, and Buddy Greco. Joe Frazier came to Giuffre to recover after fighting Muhammad Ali. John Travolta came to Giuffre for medical care while filming *Blow Out*. Most hospital artwork is calm and soothing, but Giuffre's cafeteria featured large posters of him posing with the likes of Frank Sinatra. His celebrity patients would beep him, and he would answer the phone. "The stars loved that," a friend said. And in return for always being around—Giuffre lived in private quarters inside the hospital—the doctor claimed the right to pass items about his famous friends to his favorite *Philadelphia Daily News* columnist, Larry Fields.

Some items were pretty wacky, such as the one in 1983 when Fields announced that Joe DiMaggio had come to Philadelphia to be inspected by a local proctologist.

The Yankee Clipper's end was in fine shape . . . so DiMaggio decided to visit his old pal, Dr. James C. Giuffre. Giuffre also insisted on checking out Joe's rear, confirming that it was in fine shape. All this poking, prodding and checking got DiMaggio hungry, so Doc Giuffre took him for lunch at Cou's Little Italy, where Joe ordered a hot sausage platter—until Giuffre slapped him on the hand, and said: "Eat that kind of stuff and you will have trouble with your backside."

Giuffre also kept the company of people who loathed the spotlight. One time he was awakened at 4 A.M. by a call from the Virgin Islands: an associate of Giuffre's Atlantic City pals had fallen from a balcony. Columnist Fields wrote what happened next:

Giuffre told the caller to bring his associate to Philadelphia as soon as possible. A private plane was chartered for $9,600 in St. Thomas to jet the ailing man to Our Town. Upon arrival, only a few hours later, the staff at Giuffre was ready for the emergency: two orthopedic specialists were there, as was a neurologist, a radiologist, a specialist in nuclear medicine, a neurosurgeon and two surgeons—Giuffre himself and his daughter.

The identity of this particular patient was never publicly revealed.

The best stories, however, were the ones the hospital didn't publicize, such as the party where Giuffre executives handed out envelopes of money to favored employees. The executives were later convicted of covering the payouts through phony expenditure claims. Then there were Giuffre's friends in the underworld, including two Mafia figures from New York who once attended a hospital Christmas party. Giuffre even acquired a few mob affectations of his own, insisting, for example, that his Lincoln Town Car be black— inside and out.

Giuffre employees were understandably queasy when one day a mysterious package arrived at the hospital. Inside was a goat, beheaded and gutted but still in possession of its hooves and fur. A hospital dietitian, not knowing why the package was sent, feared it was some underworld message and contacted a hospital supervisor. "I had no idea what it was, either, so we took it to the freezer," the supervisor recalled. The hospital later learned it was just a gift "from somebody."

Weird happenings were, in fact, rather common at Giuffre Medical Center. Consider the story of Heinz, a permanent resident of the hospital. Heinz was a dog. Ordinarily, hospital visitors don't hear barks echoing down the hallways. But Heinz belonged to Giuffre and, like his master, got first-class treatment. Hospital guards took him for walks. At dinnertime, when Doc Giuffre wasn't around, a guard sometimes had to load Heinz into the Lincoln Town Car, then drive him to South Philadelphia for his favorite sandwich. Once, after Giuffre took in a stray dog with an upset tummy, hospital dietitians were asked to cook the mutt a special meal of boiled meat and oatmeal. Hospital housekeepers cleaned up after the dog.

Giuffre liked to advertise his hospital as having a big heart. But not everyone would agree. *Philadelphia Daily News* reporter Robin Palley wrote an article about a man who went to Giuffre Medical Center complaining of a lump almost the size of a golf ball under his arm. In a sworn statement, the man said he was examined by a woman in a white coat, who concluded that the lump "was cellulite or fatty tissue deposit." Upon learning that the man had no medical insurance, the hospital told him to come back when he could pay for its removal. Many months later, the man made two unfortunate discoveries: the lump turned out to be Hodgkin's disease, and his examiner at Giuffre turned out not to be a doctor but, rather, a foreign medical graduate who had twice failed to qualify for a license in this country. The man later died.

For 17 years, Pennsylvania health officials knew that Giuffre repeatedly used underqualified or unlicensed medical personnel to treat patients—yet they allowed the hospital to remain open. The Joint Commission also found nothing to stop it from affording Giuffre Medical Center the full privileges of accreditation.

But if public and private regulators were content with their monitoring of the hospital, some Giuffre employees were not. On January 4, 1988, an anonymous letter was sent to the office of the president of Giuffre's board of directors. "As employees of Giuffre Medical Center we have had and tolerated enough," the letter began. It specifically demanded that two surgeons be suspended and that the suspension be announced publicly to the staff within one week. If not, the letter threatened to publicly release details about unnecessary surgery and other dangerous practices. It was signed "The Committee of 52," although the group most likely represented only a half dozen or so.

On January 13, 1988, the committee delivered on its promise. Now calling themselves The Committee of 55, the Giuffre employees sent

18 copies of a letter to the media and public officials. It read, in part: "Because most of our patients are poor, often near illiterate, and without families, they can be easily taken advantage of. They have had needless surgery, bad surgery, and concealed results. . . . There has been enormous waste of hospital resources and supplies." The letter also alleged a series of medical horror stories, complete with patient chart numbers.

The Committee of 55 took this desperate step because all the elaborate checks and balances designed to protect patients had failed. Where were those meddlesome government regulators, about whom medical groups complained so frequently? Where were the medical societies? Where were the peer review groups? Where was the hospital's board of directors? Didn't they know what was happening inside Giuffre? Because if they didn't, who did?

On June 6, 1986, Parsons Hospital opened its doors to inspectors from the Joint Commission. Hospitals usually regard such visits more as an irritation than as a menace. For one thing, the Joint Commission almost always told hospitals weeks in advance when it would arrive. Hospitals said they needed to know the date so their key managers could be present to answer questions. The greatest benefit, however, was that hospitals could use the time to fix up the place.

Insecure hospitals could even, for a fee, seek help from the Joint Commission on how to pass its inspection. This dual role of inspector and consultant invited abuse, critics said: hospitals might feel pressure, warranted or not, to hire the commission consultants as insurance against failing an inspection. The Joint Commission denied pressuring anyone.

When inspectors arrived on the doorstep of Parsons in June, the hospital supposedly was prepared for the visit. But if this was how Parsons looked on a good day, one could only imagine what went on when it wasn't expecting important visitors. The Joint Commission found the hospital dangerously substandard. It cited Parsons for inadequacies in nursing, surgery, infection control, dietetic services, emergency care, laboratory services, pharmaceutical services, radiology, rehabilitation, social work, and medical records. Inspectors specifically noted that blood was stored at improper temperatures, emergency drugs weren't available, outdated drugs weren't discarded, inappropriate people were administering drugs, and patients were victimized by bad nursing care.

Although Parsons was bad enough to flunk its inspection, the Joint Commission neither warned patients nor immediately revoked the hospital's accreditation. It chose a more leisurely approach, waiting nearly a full year before informing Parsons in writing that it had tentatively decided to revoke its accreditation. Even then, the accrediting body saw no need to rush. Month after month passed with still no action. Had its accreditation been pulled, government inspections would have resulted, which almost certainly would have forced the closing of the hospital. The Joint Commission, however, wouldn't even disclose publicly what it had found at Parsons.

Meanwhile, patients by the hundreds continued to stream into the hospital. About a year and a half after the Joint Commission found Parsons to be substandard, government inspectors—acting on a tip—visited the 100-bed hospital in Queens. They could hardly believe what they found: flies and roaches crawling in the food preparation area, soiled pans passed off as washed and sanitized, and dust so thick the inspectors could write their names on a table designated for sterilizing surgical equipment.

And that wasn't the worst. Drugs, including heart medicine, were prescribed but not given; treatment plans were poorly prepared and carried out late or not at all; patient exams were inadequate; no registered nurses were assigned to the intensive care unit or the emergency room; vital signs weren't checked; high-risk patients weren't given discharge plans; unqualified medical workers rendered medical care. A doctor evaluated a patient's complaint about his left leg by examining the right leg.

In the final analysis, government authorities faced the sobering conclusion that they had sanctioned the operation of a hospital where dozens of patients had died following substandard care. New York State could wait no longer. It ordered Parsons to close down in the name of public safety. At 8 A.M. on May 12, 1988, Parsons surrendered its operating license.

Even the Joint Commission, after two years of waiting, decided it had to act. At its fashionable headquarters inside Chicago's John Hancock Building—overlooking Michigan Avenue's Magic Mile, a neighborhood quite different from Flushing, Queens—the men and women of the Joint Commission made a decision that they did not regard lightly. Yes, they concluded, we must pull Parsons Hospital's accreditation.

They needn't have bothered, really. The hospital had already been closed for a week.

On May 12, 1988—the same day Parsons closed—Giuffre Medical Center was ordered by the Pennsylvania Health Department to stop admitting general acute-care patients. The order crowned the lengthy government investigation into allegations made by the anonymous Committee of 55.

Over the previous four months, many medical misadventures at Giuffre had been graphically chronicled in the press. According to the *Philadelphia Inquirer,* one 72-year-old woman whose bowel had burst through a surgical opening suffered the indignity of having her bowel hang outside her body for nearly three weeks before a plastic surgeon finally corrected the problem. Even veteran nurses were shocked, and tried to keep the exposed intestine clean and moist so it wouldn't die or become infected, the paper reported. One 50-year-old man accidentally had his spleen lacerated and his esophagus cut in two.

The 66 medical records reviewed by state investigators showed 56 postoperative complications, 29 unnecessary surgeries, and 12 patient deaths. Instead of first trying drug treatment on ulcer patients, doctors performed partial gastrectomies, in which sections of the stomach were surgically removed. "Patients were not given information about alternative treatments," the state said.

The state also found that in 13 of 35 selected cases, patients apparently had healthy organs removed, three of which were damaged during surgery. No one at the hospital bothered to review those cases. Finding 124 deficiencies at Giuffre, the state wrote: "There is no review of the acceptability of procedures undertaken. There is no review for justification of normal tissues removed. There is no review of procedures in which no tissue has been removed." Furthermore, the hospital allowed "an unauthorized, unqualified and uncredentialled" person to assist in surgery, the head of emergency services had no background in that area, physician assistants diagnosed and treated patients without physician supervision, and unexpected deaths weren't reported to the state medical examiner as required by law.

How might these deplorable deficiencies and abuses have been prevented? Three years before the Committee of 55 went public with its complaints, a Giuffre physician had written a letter to the Philadelphia County Medical Society alleging that the hospital was pushing unnecessary surgery. Whatever the society had done or not done, it wasn't enough. The society wouldn't comment. Pennsylvania health officials blamed their failure to protect patients on a prior administration, which they said had cut back the number of state hospital inspectors. Federal health officials, meanwhile, relied on the Joint Commission to correct the systemwide breakdown of quality assurance. The Joint Commission said its monitoring wasn't perfect.

One of Giuffre's longtime supervisors remembered the last days, when Dr. Giuffre's dream of a hospital with heart was crumbling around him. "Toward the end, he was getting very paranoid," the supervisor said. "He thought it was some major plot by his enemies." Then, one day, this wisp of a man, now in his 70s, walked into the same hospital cafeteria where he had so many times entertained people with jokes and stories. This time, something was clearly wrong. "He went in there and started rambling," said one hospital employee who witnessed the incident. The cafeteria fell silent. "Everyone knew he was incoherent." After 15 minutes, he turned and left. Even then, people were too stunned to speak.

Several months later, Giuffre left the hospital and his life-size statue forever, his reign of four decades over. Two years afterward, he died.

Giuffre Medical Center and Parsons Hospital were only two of many embarrassments for the Joint Commission. *The Wall Street Journal* reported that from January 1986 through June 1988, federal inspectors had found serious deficiencies in 156 accredited hospitals. And that represented only those discovered through spot checks and complaint investigations; a more comprehensive government survey almost certainly would have yielded a much higher figure.

The *Journal* found one accredited hospital where patients were moved into an operating room soiled by the fresh blood of previous patients; a bloody towel was used to wipe the operating table in between surgeries. In another, an inspector found that a neglected patient had developed an infestation of maggots in the mouth and nose. While the commission frequently claimed that it denied accreditation to 2 percent of hospitals it surveyed, the *Journal* reported that in 1986 and 1987 the figure was more like 0.3 percent.

Publicly, Joint Commission president Dennis S. O'Leary, M.D.— who came to the commission in 1986—dismissed the findings as inconsequential. "[N]either we nor you owe anyone an apology," O'Leary wrote in a Joint Commission memo. But privately, he apparently realized his group had to change to maintain its credibility. Since the *Journal* article, the commission has begun releasing the names of marginal hospitals, as well as those failing inspections. More accreditations are being revoked, although not nearly as many as some consumer groups would like. O'Leary is also working toward measuring not just how well a hospital meets standards but how patients actually fare during hospitalization. Many hospitals don't like these changes. One hospital executive told *Modern Healthcare* magazine, "I don't look forward to being beaten with a two-by-four that I helped buy."

Therein lies the problem: hospitals finance most of the Joint Commission's operation. Should the group get too tough, it could find its major political backers in the American Hospital Association and American Medical Association pulling their support. "It's a creature of the industry, so what's it going to do?" asked Art Levin of the Center for Medical Consumers. He thought it would be better to have no Joint Commission than an illusion of safety.

The federal government, meanwhile, flopped in its efforts to monitor surrogate inspectors. Until the late 1980s, the U.S. Health and Human Services Department's assurances that the Joint Commission was performing well were based on what it now admitted were inadequate samplings.

Given its failure with the Joint Commission, Health and Human Services could have, at the very least, aggressively used peer review organizations to weed out bad doctors inside hospitals. But it didn't. PROs review Medicare records for signs of poor care and waste. But until late 1989, the PRO in New York State had recommended sanctions for only a few physicians during its four-year contract with the federal government. Like the Joint Commission, the PRO had close AMA ties. The state medical society underwrote some of its start-up costs and appointed the PRO's policy-making board, according to *Newsday*. The PRO subsequently lost its contract, but PROs in other states generally weren't much better—and some were worse.

Contrast the New York PRO's timid regulatory effort with what researchers from Harvard Medical School found when they analyzed 1984 New York State hospital records: almost 7,000 patients died from negligent care. All told, nearly 4 percent of New York's hospital patients suffered some injury from their medical care, many resulting from drug complications and diagnostic mistakes. "[M]ost adverse events are preventable," the authors of the study wrote in *The New England Journal of Medicine.* Added Howard Hiatt, a professor of medicine at Harvard, "There's a big problem, and it isn't going to be dealt with with any simplistic approach."

When Dr. Giuffre departed the medical center that bore his name, he left a community of razor wire and rows of buildings either bricked up or burned out. Disease and early death were the realities of life in this North Philadelphia neighborhood. Giuffre Medical Center could easily have succumbed to the fear and scorn it had aroused among the local citizenry. But it didn't. And one reason was a man named William L. Vazquez.

The son of a barkeeper, Vazquez spent much of his later childhood in the South Bronx; the mean streets of North Philly were no mystery to him. When the Giuffre Medical Center faced legal, financial, and spiritual collapse, he turned his back on a secure future at a New Jersey hospital and gambled that he, with the right people, could save the hospital. "I couldn't believe that a community as needy as this would let it go," he said.

A public-relations firm probably would have recommended a quick name change, but Vazquez knew better; the scars of deception ran too deep. "We had to build credibility first," he said. Most important, Giuffre needed to reestablish the natural checks and balances that come with a strong governing board, administration, and physician staff. Under the old regime, all were rolled up into one.

Besides addressing the 100-plus deficiencies uncovered by state inspectors, Vazquez took down the glass restraining walls inside the hospital and put his security staff in blazers. He moved Giuffre's statue into a corner. Instead of visiting entertainers, Vazquez went to every community meeting he could find. Only then did he change the hospital's name to Girard Medical Center, after the thoroughfare that defines the neighborhood.

Girard may yet fail. Doctors don't want to come here. Patients have no more money than before. And Girard continues to lose money, although not nearly as much as in previous years. It is, however, building trust. Having William Vazquez at the helm may be enough to ensure quality patient care. But not every institution has a Vazquez or a committed board like Girard's. In those institutions, trust is no substitute for better laws more rigidly enforced, hospital investigators with no conflict of interest, and more public disclosure and accountability.

14 | Waiting

AT times, it seemed the moment would never arrive. Now, at 9:37 on the morning of March 23, 1988, Robert Johnson shifted his weight on a wooden bench inside a dark-paneled U.S. Senate hearing room. Johnson had waited seven years to tell his story to someone who mattered, and today he would get his chance.

Outside, Washington's cherry blossoms had just begun to celebrate the end of winter and the renewal of life. Johnson's mood, however, didn't fit his surroundings. Yesterday, he had visited the grave of his wife, Janice, and promised he would be going to Capitol Hill to tell her story.

It began one day in 1980 when Janice, the mother of two, discharged what looked to be a large blood clot. At the time, after missing several menstrual cycles, she thought she had been pregnant. Now, she fearfully hurried to a doctor. Robert was at his office when she called. "She was hysterical, crying and talking incoherently," he would say later. "I left the office for home immediately to console her, thinking that she had been told that she had miscarried. Although we had been married for over seven years, I had never seen her in that condition before."

Looking back, he could only wish it had been a miscarriage; instead, it was advanced cervical cancer. Her treatment began, and the next year became a blur of hope and disappointment. Three days after Christmas in 1980, Janice entered a Washington, D.C., hospital for the last time. By now, she had little appetite and complained often of stomach pains. There was more chemotherapy—

five uncomfortable days of it. And more narcotics to kill the pain. Her stomach swelled, and drug therapy caused mental confusion and hallucinations. She vomited frequently. As Janice's major organs began to shut down, her body bloated with water, and constipation became a problem. On her 51st day of hospitalization, she developed trouble breathing. Finally, just before dawn on the morning of February 20—one year to the day after her cancer was diagnosed—Janice Johnson's struggle ended.

Later that afternoon, doctors did an autopsy. In a final report, the physicians expressed concern about what they found: "This 35-year-old white female had yearly Pap smears which were negative for malignancy. This would appear to be quite unusual."

The doctors, of course, were right. Janice Johnson did not have to die.

Robert Johnson, now living in Florida, had returned to Washington to tell a Senate committee how erroneous Pap tests had killed his wife. Janice was no ignorant consumer. A former educator, she had worked as chief lobbyist for a large national medical association. "Janice knew all the cancer warning signs, and she methodically picked out every one of our physicians," Robert Johnson said. What made Janice's story particularly disturbing was that her Pap tests hadn't been analyzed by some commercial storefront lab, or even a doctor's office. Testing had been done by a hospital, a place where the sickest people depend on accurate lab work to ensure they will live to see the next day. Each year, hospitals run nearly 2 billion tests on patient fluids or tissue. "It is a place you would expect to be regulated, to have some standards," said Daniel Schultz, a Johnson family lawyer.

For years, Congress knew that shoddy medical testing was widespread. In 1979, one Senate committee had concluded that patients "cannot have confidence in clinical laboratory testing, despite its critical relationship to good health." Still, no real reform resulted. Robert Johnson wanted to change that. Now, another Senate panel had begun to reexamine labs, prompted by news accounts of profiteering and high error rates. Johnson made a strong witness: "If Janice's story can save but one life," he began, "then I can look my children in the eyes and tell them when they are old enough to understand that their mother did not die in vain. She, with the help of Congress, changed the laws to save thousands of lives."

Even under the best conditions, the job of analyzing Pap slides isn't easy. Using a microscope, an analyst must examine every single cell—sometimes hundreds—smeared onto a single slide. It is akin to looking at wall after wall of flowered wallpaper and having to inspect each flower for the slightest sign of irregularity. Under such conditions, the more slides an analyst reviews, the greater the likelihood that mental numbness will set in, allowing cancerous cells to slip through undetected.

For that reason, the field's leading professional group recommends restricting how many Pap slides any one analyst should read. A top limit of 80 to 100 patient slides a day is thought to be safe for someone working under perfect conditions. Unfortunately, Northern Virginia Doctors Hospital had processed Janice Johnson's Pap tests without following that guideline, and no outside agency intervened—not the hospital accrediting agency, not the state, not the federal government.

In the absence of any serious regulation, the hospital took a gamble: it built its Pap test program around a part-time, foreign medical graduate who had flunked her boards in clinical pathology. The hospital paid her little more than Burger King wages—$5.90 an hour—to search for cancer in her spare time. Although she held down another, full-time job, the analyst still found time to screen about twice the number of Pap slides that experts say can be accurately reviewed by a full-time worker. On any given morning, trays of Pap slides—sometimes 300 of them—were delivered for review. Speed was important "because we don't know what the next day [will bring]," the lab analyst said.

Under these conditions, it was not surprising that mistakes were made. A year apart, on two Pap tests in a row, this same overworked lab analyst failed to spot cellular abnormalities on Janice Johnson's slides. If Johnson's tests had been accurately read, she almost certainly would have lived. "The possibility of two blatantly clear positive Pap smears being missed—if any type of quality-control standards were being followed—is so remote it's mind-boggling," said the Johnsons' lawyer Schultz.

Those responsible for botching her tests hadn't even bothered to tell the Johnson family of their errors, Schultz charged. "The private physician, the gynecologists were informed; the laboratory knew." Worse yet, Schultz said, the hospital apparently made no effort to contact thousands of other women who had their Paps read there. "The laboratory technician may have been the bullet that killed Jan, but there were others who helped hold the gun," said Johnson. "Who was in charge of overseeing who?"

The problem of shoddy lab testing wasn't limited to this hospital, or to the Pap test. Other derelict hospitals practiced "kitchen cytology," where lab workers analyzed patient specimens at home, amid family distractions and nonexistent supervision. "That borders on fraud," one cancer specialist told *The Wall Street Journal*.

Regulation, meanwhile, was poor, even contradictory. A Minnesota hospital that couldn't accurately run kidney function tests was barred from testing interstate specimens but permitted to test in-state specimens. A Pennsylvania hospital was barred from performing a genetics test on New York patients but allowed to run them on Delaware patients. A Los Angeles hospital had a 55 percent accuracy rate on AIDS testing, yet state officials waited months before taking action against the lab.

Robert Johnson was particularly galled by the federal government's failure to impose work load limits on Pap test screeners and to require analysts to undergo proficiency exams. "How many more Janice Johnsons have been unnecessarily killed . . . due to either incompetence, fatigue, or lack of training?" he asked.

Some senators were clearly moved by the testimony of Johnson and others. "To the extent that Congress has contributed to this problem, we have to make some corrections," Senator William Cohen promised as he adjourned the hearings. Within months, Robert Johnson's dream of a tough federal law that would protect patients against shoddy medical testing became reality. Called the Clinical Laboratory Improvement Amendments of 1988, it passed with broad-based support in both parties. When Robert Johnson left Capitol Hill on that spring morning in 1988, he carried only hope. Now, the awesome legislative power of Congress was squarely behind him.

In the afterglow of victory, Johnson could hardly be faulted for failing to recognize that there were still powerful people who refused to accept his victory.

At 9 A.M., the gathering winter winds found no resistance on the flat, barren ground of Chicago's Pasteur Park. Years ago, this splotch of land held many trees, along with an old diner, a favorite among the medical workers who labored across the street in a giant complex of hospital buildings. Historical plaques further enriched this setting, established years ago as a green haven from the daily suffering that is part of every hospital. But eventually, the trees gave way to a helicopter landing pad, the plaques were stolen, and one Labor Day weekend the diner burned down. On this freezing December morning, the gateway to Pasteur Park was adorned with a solitary bottle of Richard's Wild Irish Rose, a high-alcohol slop marketed to the down-and-out wino crowd.

Like the park, the hospital across the street had not aged gracefully. Once, it had been one of the world's largest medical institutions. Now, a mixture of greenish mold and dirt nearly obscured the words "Cook County Hospital" carved in stone above the main doorway. Inside the foyer, a maintenance man swept away a carpet of cigarette butts, as three homeless people in various degrees of recline took shelter from the winter winds. In the main lobby, a small artificial Christmas tree stood near a glass bulletin board that held a framed certificate: "Joint Commission Accredited," it read.

On this day—a Friday in December 1989—hospital workers talked of Christmas and the weekend ahead. Over at the public-relations office, a call had just arrived from a Cook County commissioner: Three out-of-state politicians want to tour the hospital. . . . They will arrive at 10:30 A.M. . . . Answer their questions. . . . They want to know how you are coping. Because the county commission controlled this hospital's funding, the call signaled a red alert: key department heads were instructed to remain close to their stations. But when the visitors arrived two hours late, well into the lunch hour, anticipation had long since changed to annoyance.

The tour went ahead anyway, and the politicians enjoyed their walk back into history. There were old wood-backed wheelchairs, high institutional ceilings, and huge open wards that offered no individual bathrooms. Fans, both stand-up and ceiling models, were in abundance—a necessity, the guide explained, because the building had no air-conditioning. "During the summer we bring up ice water all the time, anything to make the patients as comfortable as possible," she explained.

The tour ended in the office of the hospital's medical director, Dr. Agnes Lattimer, who stated the obvious: the hospital building was too old and its treasury barren. Once, Cook County had hosted 4,000 patients; now, it rarely got 1,000. "Our hope is to build a new hospital," Dr. Lattimer said, her face brightening. Not a word was mentioned, however, about the unusual deaths that had occurred within the building—preventable deaths that had very nearly turned this warhorse of a hospital to glue.

By 2 P.M., the VIPs had departed through the emergency room door to a waiting car, and at least a few hospital workers began to relax, returning to thoughts of Christmas shopping and the weekend now just hours away.

Up on the seventh floor, amid cramped quarters, men and women in white lab coats darted from one refrigerator to another, as the last of Friday afternoon ticked away. They worked in a world of blood—frozen blood, liquid blood, blood platelets, blood plasma, red blood cells. A single unit of donated blood, researchers had discovered, could be broken down into its various components and used to treat multiple patients. Anemics might need only red blood cells, burn victims might need plasma, those with bleeding problems might need platelets. "We can keep the blood 42 days in the refrigerator," explained Augustine Mathews, the blood bank's technical director. "But if you freeze the red blood cells, you can keep it up to 10 years."

Because blood is always in short supply, it is big business. Several months earlier, the *Philadelphia Inquirer* reported the story of a blood bank in Appleton, Wisconsin, that had issued an emotional plea for blood, prompting the local citizenry to turn out in force. Donors, however, didn't know that the same blood bank was selling blood to another blood bank in Lexington, Kentucky, which then sold it to Fort Lauderdale, Florida, which turned around and sold it to hospitals in New York City. The brokered blood, after traveling 2,777 miles, was finally sold to New York hospital patients at $120 a pint.

Cook County's blood center wasn't a regular stop on the usual VIP tour—an odd decision, because the blood bank represented one of the most glorious moments in Cook County's history. A plaque on the laboratory wall told part of the story:

> Dr. Bernard Fantus, 1874–1940 . . . Through whose guidance and tireless efforts the first Blood Bank was originated and established at Cook County Hospital, March 15, 1937.

Dr. Fantus had helped make blood transfusions commonplace in America, saving countless lives in the process. Before blood banks, donors had to be called whenever a transfusion was needed. Samples from each donor had to be tested and sometimes retested. Often, patients died before the right blood type could be found. Dr. Fantus figured out a way to preserve blood in storage, as well as how and when to administer it. Cook County honored Dr. Fantus by naming its huge outpatient clinic after him.

It was no small irony, then, that this very blood bank—Cook County's pride and joy—triggered a state and federal investigation that nearly closed the hospital. And it all began when Atanasia Mendoza, a 62-year-old mother of six, checked into Cook County Hospital one April day in 1988 complaining of abdominal pains.

Blood-typing is a test so routine that most new patients barely give it any notice. And so it was with Mrs. Mendoza; soon after she was admitted April 22, a hospital worker drew a small blood sample to test for infectious diseases such as AIDS or hepatitis, and to determine blood type in case a transfusion became necessary.

The test is an essential precaution. Transfusing the wrong blood type could set off a potentially fatal chain reaction as antibodies attack and destroy the new red blood cells. Blood literally begins to clot in the bloodstream, while a continuing physiologic reaction damages the kidneys, leading to other organ failures. "If you don't give much of the incompatible blood, it will only give patients fevers or chills," said Dr. E. Shannon Cooper, who ran a hospital blood bank in New Orleans. "Whether you die depends on how much is transfused. It's a dose-related phenomenon."

Good hospitals employ elaborate safeguards to keep such mistakes from occurring—a necessity not only in blood banks but in all medical laboratories, because faulty tests can occur for so many reasons: a machine loses its calibration, testing chemicals lose potency or are used improperly, human specimens are inadvertently switched. Even if a test is performed properly, it may be misinterpreted. If quality controls fail, resulting in a transfusion of mismatched blood, there is yet another safeguard: monitoring a patient's temperature at regular intervals. A sudden rise will flag doctors to a possible transfusion reaction.

Mrs. Mendoza had every reason to believe she would be getting the best care available. Cook County was licensed by the state of Illinois, certified for Medicare by the federal government, accredited by the Joint Commission and also by the College of American Pathologists, the nation's preeminent laboratory peer review group. Soon after her arrival, Mrs. Mendoza underwent a noninvasive ultrasound test to rule out cancer. But when the test suggested the presence of pelvic masses, she was wheeled into surgery for confirmation that cancer was present.

The seventh-floor blood bank was ready when the call came: surgeons needed blood to transfuse into Mrs. Mendoza. Having already tested her blood type, the lab quickly selected some donor blood, putting it in a plastic canister for transport through a pneumatic tube. Exactly 26 seconds later, the blood arrived in the operating room on another floor. Surgeons went ahead and opened Mrs. Mendoza's body, but to their surprise, they found no cancer. They closed her and sent her to recovery.

Another surprise soon followed. Instead of getting better, Mrs. Mendoza mysteriously began to deteriorate. Worried that she might be bleeding internally, doctors returned her to surgery, where she was reopened. Again, they found nothing. Doctors were befuddled. What could be happening? The mystery remained unsolved until several weeks later, when doctors gave Mrs. Mendoza a second transfusion and medical tests showed that her first transfusion had involved mismatched blood. The damage, however, had already been done. Mrs. Mendoza died May 12.

Later that day, at 3:15 P.M., the hospital called the medical examiner with news of Mrs. Mendoza's demise. "Possible Hospital Misadventure," wrote the medical examiner, who would later call the death "a real freak occurrence." The hospital put on its best public face and told the media that its fail-safe system had somehow broken down. Not in years had there been such a peculiar happening, the medical examiner recalled.

That, at least, was what the public was told. Illinois health officials refused to release the findings of its inspection at Cook County. For many months, the federal government had nothing to say, either. Likewise for its surrogates, the Joint Commission and the College of American Pathologists. Meanwhile, as thousands of people continued to seek medical care at Cook County, state health officials knew—but didn't publicly disclose—that the hospital had failed to follow up properly on the transfusion death. Moreover, the entire place was unsanitary; authorities had found a dead animal and urine stench in one hospital passageway. But without fear of public disclosure or serious punishment, Cook County lacked the will to correct its problems quickly.

Nine months after Mrs. Mendoza got mismatched blood, this

"freak" mistake was repeated with the same outcome: death. The second victim, 46-year-old Dorothy Tharpe, died January 14, 1989, two days after she, too, got the wrong blood—the result of "three concurrent errors" in blood bank procedure, according to the Joint Commission. The hospital also failed to monitor the patient's temperature properly, which might have alerted doctors to a problem. Even the federal government, which had been relying on the Joint Commission to police the hospital, couldn't ignore this second laboratory death. In March 1989, its inspectors found that people at Cook County who "collect blood for transfusions are not trained or monitored, nor are they members of a permanent phlebotomy staff."

To prevent other deaths from mismatched blood, the hospital issued new guidelines designed to reduce the possibility that specimens would be inadvertently switched. Yet several weeks after these changes, nearly half of the blood requests were processed in violation of that policy. Far from being a "freak" occurrence, Cook County's blood handling made it a virtual certainty that someone would get mismatched blood.

"Housekeeping in the laboratory is poor," the Joint Commission reported. "Laboratory facilities are old, cramped and in poor repair . . . some techs are only minimally trained." Specimens were mishandled eight to ten times a month. "The potential for error remains high," the Joint Commission stated. Even the final safeguard—taking the temperature of patients soon after receiving blood—had been ignored in some cases. One patient showed an elevated temperature but continued to receive blood.

Sadly, the rest of the hospital wasn't in any better shape than the laboratory. Inspectors found poor infection control, medicine not being given as ordered, a medical staff whose credentials had not been checked, too few dietitians to ensure that patients got proper food, and a "desperate" shortage of nurses. Insects were so bad that food service workers had complained of bug bites for a full year. The cash-strapped hospital went so far as to reuse disposable, single-use breathing tubes for children.

The hospital's sorry condition shocked some doctors who had long regarded Cook County as an outstanding public hospital. "It consistently has some of the best mortality statistics of all the public hospitals," said Dr. Lynn J. Soffer of the Health Research Group, a patient advocacy organization. That was what made the findings at

Cook County so worrisome. If this hospital was one of the best, imagine the worst.

Only 15 miles or so to the north of Cook County Hospital is a two-story office building that houses one of the best-kept secrets in medicine: the College of American Pathologists. While the public is more familiar with other medical groups such as the American Medical Association, it is the College—better known as CAP—that is largely responsible for how medical labs are regulated in this country.

As the leading authority on laboratory testing, CAP helps shape state and national regulations governing the testing of everything from cholesterol to Pap smears to blood. Bankrolled by medical laboratories, CAP operates an elaborate program of proficiency testing for its members. It also inspects and accredits laboratories, hundreds of which are in hospitals.

Legislators love CAP because, like other such organizations, it provides the veneer of regulation at little or no government expense. CAP is the ultimate example of government buck-passing. First, Congress passes its regulatory responsibility for hospitals to the Joint Commission, a private group funded and run mostly by doctors and hospitals. Then, the Joint Commission passes much of its laboratory oversight to CAP, making the government twice removed from its responsibility to see that billions in tax dollars aren't being wasted on inaccurate medical testing.

CAP believes the public is well served by its efforts. "Clinical laboratories represent one of the most stringently regulated segments of the health care industry," a former CAP president told Congress. The families of Mrs. Mendoza and Mrs. Tharpe might disagree; Cook County Hospital's lab was CAP-accredited. CAP, however, refused to discuss how one of its labs got so bad. In fact, it won't publicly disclose its findings on any lab, for two basic reasons: CAP believes patients aren't smart enough to use the information properly, and labs might not voluntarily join CAP's peer-review program. Even so, many labs choose to ignore CAP, and thus are free of any outside monitoring.

Meanwhile, CAP's weak performance at Cook County had an eerie echo at another CAP-accredited lab, inside Charity Hospital in New Orleans. Around the time Cook County suffered its first fatal transfusion, Charity was suffering through its third such death in three years. Twelve times during one 21-month period, Charity had made blood-testing errors. Moreover, the hospital permitted unauthorized and unsupervised staffers to draw blood in violation of hospital policy, then failed to discipline those responsible. Charity, like Janice Johnson's hospital, also had too few people reading Pap smears. The result: a dangerous two-month backlog.

Poor lab work at Charity was no aberration. In November 1990, the Joint Commission reported that more than 1,000 of its accredited hospitals had achieved only partial or minimal compliance in their blood banks and laboratories, many of which were CAP-accredited. Yet *The Wall Street Journal* reported in 1987 that CAP had yanked its seal of approval from just one of 3,800 labs over the previous two years. The Joint Commission wasn't any tougher. According to the *Journal,* it couldn't cite a recent instance where a bad lab alone had cost a hospital its accreditation.

Poor lab work need not kill someone to be harmful. At Nassau County Medical Center, a CAP-accredited hospital on Long Island, New York, some 48 percent of doctors polled said lab response time there was "seldom adequate." On average, it took five hours to get results on routine lab work, compared with acceptable norms of one to three hours, according to *Newsday.* Even emergency lab requests took two hours on average, compared with acceptable norms of 15 to 40 minutes. "Ours is not a regulatory program," CAP says in its defense. Yet state and federal regulatory agencies continue to use CAP and the Joint Commission as its eyes and ears inside America's labs.

New York State is a major exception. "These programs are not regulatory, nor are they designed to be," complained Dr. Herbert Dickerman, New York's chief lab regulator. "The scheme lacks the crucial ingredient of public accountability—the assurance that laboratory services offered to the public are of the highest quality, and that those laboratories not complying with this standard will not be permitted to operate." Thus, New York conducts its own investigations and has uncovered everything from a hospital that released blood untested for AIDS, to another hospital that did TB testing in an old fish aquarium. Such shoddy lab work probably would have gone undetected and uncorrected in most states.

But even in New York, punishment isn't significantly harsh. In late 1988, the director of pathology at Franklin General Hospital on Long Island pleaded guilty to charges that he ran an unsupervised, unlicensed Pap smear lab. State investigators got onto Dr. Sidney Gellman's trail when a Nassau County woman sued her doctor for allegedly botching an abortion. The woman produced strong evidence to back her claim: she had twins. It later came out that Gellman had signed a lab report certifying that "products of conception" had been removed.

In the course of its investigation, the state accidentally discovered that for 15 years Gellman had run an uncertified Pap smear lab. The state charged Franklin Hospital with "aiding and abetting" Gellman and fined it $1,000. Gellman himself was fined $10,000. Half of each fine was suspended.

Franklin General didn't seem particularly upset with its errant pathologist. The hospital called the charges "technical violations" and permitted Dr. Gellman to continue working there.

Congress's passage of the Clinical Laboratory Improvement Amendments in 1988 was hailed as marking a new era in medicine. It didn't take long, however, for key segments of organized medicine to begin criticizing the new law. The Joint Commission, for instance, resented the implication that it hadn't done a good job policing labs. Its president, Dennis O'Leary, termed the new law an "unbelievable piece of legislation." He remarked, "This law is quite symptomatic of our chaotic environment—where people assume there is quality in the system and suddenly somebody finds a few horror stories—[and] Congress goes clear off the deep end. . . ."

As with any complex law, congressional passage is only the beginning. The law must be enforced, and the appropriate regulatory agency—in this case, the Health Care Financing Administration—still had to usher in specific rules to carry out the law's intent. The agency's knack for bungling important jobs, however, carried over into this assignment as well. Month after month passed with no new rules being issued. The first anniversary of the law's passage came and went. Still nothing. Although the 1988 law stipulated that key standards were to be implemented in January 1990, the government wasn't even close to meeting that deadline. When an angry Congress summoned HCFA to explain its tardiness, the agency claimed "difficulty in reaching a scientific consensus" on key regulatory points. Senator Barbara A. Mikulski of Maryland, who had helped lead the fight for lab reform, wasn't swayed. "Women are just as likely to die from misread Pap smears now as they were two years ago," she seethed.

Finally, in late May 1990, the agency published 63 pages of new rules. For the first time, Pap smear analysts—along with other key lab technicians—would be required to undergo proficiency testing. The American Medical Association responded predictably, saying the rules added unnecessary regulation that would drive up the cost of medical care.

Indeed, even supporters of the legislation thought some rules were poorly devised. Doctors and hospitals may have lost the legislative battle in Congress, but they saw HCFA as an easier target. Some 60,000 letters, most of them negative, flooded into the office of federal regulators, prompting them to say they would rework some of the rules. That, however, meant another delay. As 1991 got under way, federal health regulators still hadn't managed to carry out the will of Congress—not to mention the three-year-old dream of Robert Johnson.

He was still waiting. But one person who won't be around to witness the new law's impact is a 43-year-old man who checked in to a Minneapolis hospital for a heart transplant. This enormously costly procedure went well except for one problem: his transplanted heart mistakenly came from a donor with the wrong blood type. He died in October 1990 after his body rejected the organ.

15 | Dear Ann Landers:

ON Wednesday morning, April 26, 1989, millions of Americans awoke to find an unusual letter in their local newspaper. "I nearly killed someone last night," the letter began. The confession arrived courtesy of Ann Landers, the most widely syndicated columnist in America. The letter continued:

> I wasn't driving drunk. I am a tired, overworked nurse. The hospital where I work has a nurse shortage. Please, before you say, "So does every other hospital in the country," hear me out. We were told that because of the nurse shortage we had to work short-handed, even though we are terribly understaffed. Then a small hospital in this city closed its doors and many nurses became available. My hospital hired a few, then put on a hiring freeze. It cited budget problems. Now hear this! The hospital has just broken ground to build a multi-million-dollar parking garage that we could do without. Out of the clear blue sky, it formed a partnership with the library across the street to buy a building. The hospital has purchased several small hospitals and opened several health centers. I am not the only nurse around here who resents the way it spends money on things that do not enhance patient care.

The anonymous writer had reason to worry that her plea might go unheeded. By 1989, the nursing crisis had developed a bad case of overexposure. Although the shortage was very real, and ultimately tragic, some hospitals had begun to use it as a convenient excuse for the latest embarrassing foul-up—whether nursing-related or not.

Moreover, it played well from a public-relations standpoint because the crisis affected most hospitals, so it seemed devoid of bad guys. Now that women could find more professionally rewarding jobs in law, business, and medicine, who could blame them if they left nursing?

But in viewing the nursing shortage as some kind of natural disaster, some hospital managers avoided having to confront whether they were really doing all they could to solve the problem. Was that extra public-relations executive really necessary? Or the expanded advertising budget? Or the truckloads of financial inducements used to lure doctors? Couldn't that money have been used to lure more nurses or keep the ones they had? One Michigan State University scholar warned that too many hospital administrators had entered a sort of "moral twilight zone." Where blame cannot be precisely fixed, Associate Professor Leonard M. Fleck argued, "bad things happen to patients that can too easily be rationalized."

The distraught nurse in the Landers column, to be sure, was in no moral twilight zone. Right or wrong, she blamed her hospital bosses for pleading poverty to explain staff shortages while gorging on real-estate and construction deals. Her letter ended with this warning: "Maybe someone reading this will have a child in this hospital who will be given the wrong medication by a nurse who has worked too many hours and has too many patients. Just sign me—Tired and Discouraged."

The published letter bore no address. "We don't know where it came from," an aide to Ann Landers said several days later. "We destroy letters on the day they are printed, for the very reason that we want to protect people's confidentiality. Even if I wanted to, I couldn't tell you who wrote it."

Landers did proffer a bit of advice, however. She suggested that the nurse seek professional help, although not of the Freudian variety. "Go talk with the editor of the newspaper," she counseled. "When the common interest is not being served and lives are in danger because dollars are being put ahead of people, the public should be informed. A civic-minded newspaper will be keenly interested in your story, and I urge you to tell it."

Countless newspapers across the nation would, no doubt, publish such a story. More than ever, the troubled hospital industry needed the kind of outside scrutiny that the media provides. But as

Ann Landers would later discover, "civic-minded" can have more than one meaning.

Soon after the *Topeka Capital-Journal* newspaper thumped onto doorsteps across that city, people began to buzz about the Landers column. "Surveys have shown that Ann Landers is the best-read feature in the newspaper," said Peter W. Stauffer, executive editor of the newspaper, the only remaining daily in the Kansas state capital. That morning's column was particularly interesting, however, because the nurse's letter described events very similar to recent happenings in Topeka. She mentioned, for example, that a local hospital had just closed, freeing up a new pool of prospective nursing hires. That might be old Memorial Hospital, readers thought, the one down by the railroad tracks on the "wrong" side of town.

But what really caught the city's attention were the two sentences in the letter that mentioned the new parking garage and the partnership with the local library. To anyone who lived in Topeka, that description seemed uncomfortably specific. And right now, among the most uncomfortable Topekans were officials of Stormont-Vail Regional Medical Center.

Stormont-Vail, unlike Memorial, had prospered in the competitive 1980s, slicing its way through arcane government reimbursement formulas like a Super Bowl halfback through high school defenders. With nearly 400 beds, it had bulk and $34 million in surplus cash. Its corporate structure was a maze of joint ventures and profit-making units that sold everything from diet plans to rehabilitation services.

Stormont-Vail was a handsome success story in a city that tried but never managed to escape the look of a dreary farm town, forever in the shadow of nearby Kansas City, less than a two-hour drive away. Five decades earlier, Topekans had basked temporarily in the national spotlight as the home of presidential candidate Alf Landon. But the city also had the notoriety of a segregated school system that sparked the 1954 landmark case *Brown* v. *Board of Education*. But things were changing, and health services had become a thriving component of the new Topeka, led by the renowned Menninger Foundation. Stormont-Vail, no slouch itself, had in the previous year paid $38 million in wages, making it one of the city's largest nongovernment employers.

On this morning, however, Stormont-Vail officials had cause for alarm. It was the Ann Landers letter. The hospital was, as the letter stated, constructing a parking garage. Moreover, it had just struck an unlikely partnership with the local library to buy a medical building. Would readers make the connection? they wondered.

The answer came quickly. A friendly *Capital-Journal* reporter alerted the hospital's public-relations staff "that we would be getting news media inquiries." The hospital responded as though hordes of marauders were outside scaling the walls. By 8 A.M., Stormont-Vail had hastily assembled a SWAT team that included the chief executive officer; vice presidents of marketing and human resources, nursing administration, and community relations; and other top officials. Their job: assess possible damage and prepare a public-relations counterattack. The hospital would later say that over the next several days it spent 1,000 employee hours addressing the controversy.

Meanwhile, more than a mile away at the *Capital-Journal,* staffers were fielding calls from readers who "seemed to delight in putting two and two together and solving the puzzle," one editor observed. But the key question remained unanswered: was Stormont-Vail the hospital in the newspaper column? The mysterious nurse hadn't yet surfaced, and Stormont-Vail, ingeniously, did turn up evidence of a similar situation in a distant city.

The bad news came later that day in a phone call from a *Capital-Journal* editor to Howard Chase, Stormont-Vail chief executive officer. The syndicator for Ann Landers in Los Angeles, the editor confided, had confirmed that the nurse's letter was mailed from Topeka. Suddenly, Stormont-Vail wasn't the only local institution in the spotlight. Ann Landers had thrown down a public challenge in advising the nurse to seek out a "civic-minded newspaper." Would the *Capital-Journal* answer her call?

The paper would, indeed, but not in the way Landers might have imagined. In the following days and months, the issue would explode in a series of articles, columns, and letters to the editor. There was even an editorial cartoon showing a helicopter whirring above an agitated citizenry, as one resident cried, "Run for your lives! It's Ann Landers."

The hubbub must have taken many Topekans by surprise. They, weren't accustomed to the kind of hospital politics and controversy more common in cities like New York. What little they did know about Stormont-Vail was mostly what the hospital wanted them to know. Key discussions about money and hospital care were placed out of bounds for most Topekans, even though they could claim something many other cities could not: Topekans owned Stormont-Vail. It was their hospital. They had helped build and pay for it.

Ann Landers and her anonymous correspondent had managed to bring to public attention an issue that many hospital administrators preferred to keep safely locked in their bottom drawers. That issue, in a word, was accountability.

Stormont-Vail dates back to a two-story frame building more than 100 years ago, at a time when some Kansas farmers still lived in sod houses and Topeka had a population of just 15,000. Surgeons back then often did their cutting early in the morning to avoid the afternoon heat, while a designated swatter killed flies that buzzed in through open windows. Although newspapers in 1927 called Christ's Hospital "the best and most up-to-date hospital in this part of the country," the Great Depression bled it dry, eventually forcing its merger in the late 1940s with another hospital, thus becoming Stormont-Vail.

It was an exciting time for the hospital industry—soldiers returning home from war, the beginning of the Baby Boom, and the suburbanization of America. Hospitals quickly discovered, however, that they couldn't handle the new demands being placed upon them, so Congress in 1946 passed what became known as the Hill-Burton program, originally authorizing $75 million a year for hospital construction.

Stormont-Vail wanted badly to expand, but "there was some reluctance to use those funds because of fear of government involvement in hospital operations," recalled Balfour S. Jeffrey, a longtime hospital director. Stormont-Vail went ahead anyhow, helping itself in 1949 to $1.2 million in federal financing. Its virginity now a thing of the past, the hospital even asked the city of Topeka for matching funds. But before the city could float a bond issue for the hospital, it had to own the facility. So Topekans bought Stormont-Vail for the price of a bond issue, then leased back the facility, including land and equipment, to hospital officials—at $1 a year.

It wasn't the last time Stormont-Vail would seek taxpayer help for building projects. Nor would it be the end of other forms of government support. Stormont-Vail, for instance, was nonprofit and paid no property or income taxes, although several profit-making subsidiaries did pay taxes. Federal funds also accounted for the single largest chunk of hospital revenues, in the form of Medicare and Medicaid payments.

But for a hospital so quick to romance the public for assistance, it could turn surly when that public wanted to know what it got in return. Its managers, at times, ran the place as if they were building the stealth bomber. Board meetings were strictly off-limits. So were minutes of those meetings.

"We are a private company," explained John Glassman, a hospital vice president and fundraiser. A lean, towering man, Glassman was not atypical of the new hospital executive: his background wasn't in health care. The hiring of nonmedical people, in and of itself, wasn't bad, though it did have its pitfalls. Some disturbing insights into such practices figured in Pulitzer Prize–winner Paul Starr's account of how one hospital hired an executive from the maker of Clorox bleach, who viewed the doctors in her hospital as salesmen marketing a line of diagnoses to the public. The salary of that executive could have been used to hire several nurses, Starr noted.

Glassman wasn't so crassly commercial; his experience was in politics. But he embraced the idea that if hospitals were to survive, they must be run like most "private" corporations; that is, privately. "I know there's a lot of pressure to open these things up, but I think you run into all kinds of management problems [if you do]," he said. Lawsuits and personnel, for example, need to be discussed privately. Although public agencies get around that problem by restricting such matters to private executive sessions while keeping the rest of the meeting open, Glassman said, "Our board would not agree to that."

Even asking for names of hospital board members made one feel like an unwelcome visitor who has just soiled the living room carpet. "Well, we just don't give out [the names of] our board of directors to anyone," said Mistee Leighty, a hospital spokeswoman. The hospital later relented; but forgotten, whenever convenient, was the simple fact that Stormont-Vail, as a nonprofit institution, was supposed to operate in the public interest.

How long public institutions remained unaccountable to the public depended largely on how eager news organizations were to scale barriers set up to keep them away. By most accounts, barrier-climbing wasn't a popular pastime at the local daily in Topeka. "It wasn't that it was just a small-town newspaper," said Mary Beth Markley, who worked at the *Capital-Journal* in the 1970s and later joined *The Wall Street Journal.* "It was that it had no toughness. It was feature-oriented."

The *Capital-Journal* did at one time have a national reputation for photography. (When President Gerald Ford occupied the White House, his daughter Susan served a photo internship at the paper.) But its reporting had been largely lethargic. The *Capital-Journal* certainly had capable journalists. Institutionally, however, it lacked the one ingredient that makes bread rise in the news business: curiosity.

The *Capital-Journal* had many reasons to be curious about Stormont-Vail. Not only was the hospital city-owned, but its board of directors made decisions that deeply affected Topekans, in terms of both cost and quality. By 1989, health care consumed nearly 12 percent of the average worker's compensation—a 500 percent increase in just two decades, according to one estimate. Phone company workers got so mad in August of that year that they walked off their jobs in many parts of the country—not over wages but over a company plan to cut costly health coverage.

Aggressive coverage of the hospital industry was particularly important in the 1980s because of "unprecedented innovation and experimentation," said Jeff Goldsmith, a widely respected health care analyst. Unfortunately, Goldsmith argued, the media did a less than stellar job, depriving the industry of a chance to learn from its failures. "An aggressive, investigative press could have saved the health care industry a lot of money, headaches, and poor acquisitions," he said.

While some big-city dailies did aggressively probe hospitals, often the best reporting on health care in the early 1980s came from small business publications—the first to recognize hospitals as major businesses rather than as friendly neighborhood charities. Although nearly two-thirds of the nation's hospitals were nonprofit, only a handful of newspapers covered nonprofit groups as a regular beat. Moreover, editors tended to assign hospital coverage to reporters interested in science or technology. Thus, the paper got insightful stories when hospitals pioneered the use of a new drug or medical procedure, but it failed to realize the stranglehold that rising medical prices had on the economy, and why those costs were so high.

Linda Quick, a southern Florida health planner, complained that civic pride still got in the way of good reporting. She angrily recalled an editorial some years back by a southern Florida newspaper that helped galvanize support to block the closing of a small, poorly run, unneeded hospital. "They said we must save the 300 jobs," Quick said. "Those 300 jobs weren't worth the price society had to pay."

Had the *Capital-Journal* carried a reputation for muckraking, that nurse might have skipped writing Ann Landers and gone straight to local reporters. That she didn't "exemplifies good judgment," said Gloria O'Dell, managing editor of the weekly *Topeka Metro News*. Why? "Look at the paper's coverage of the hospital," O'Dell suggested. "Judge for yourself."

The *Capital-Journal*'s coverage did, in fact, illustrate Jeff Goldsmith's view of the press in the 1980s. The newspaper first wrote about the Ann Landers letter on Thursday, April 27, the day after the letter appeared, which basically told readers that a statement from Stormont-Vail would be forthcoming. The next day, however, brought a journalism professor's worst nightmare: a 21-paragraph story that uncritically reprinted word for word the hospital's press release, minus two short, inconsequential sentences. The story even retained the hospital's emphasis of certain words. Not surprisingly, the hospital had nothing but kind words to say about itself.

The article didn't include a single interview with anyone. No nurse, no hospital worker, no community leaders, no health care experts. Just the hospital press release. So much for balanced reporting. That wasn't all. The next day, Saturday, the *Capital-Journal* ran a 22-paragraph story under the headline STORMONT PRESIDENT TO GIVE LANDERS ADVICE ABOUT LETTER. Again, the paper quoted just one source: Howard Chase, the hospital's president and CEO.

Topeka's newshounds, if not curious, were at least polite. In an internal log kept by Stormont-Vail on the controversy, the hospital PR staff crowed: "News media expressed appreciation at [the] openness of [Stormont-Vail] and Mr. Chase's accessibility." The hospital later refused without explanation to release to the public copies of hospital inspection reports prepared by outside agencies. So much for openness.

When it was the *Capital-Journal*'s turn to speak in its own voice, executive editor Peter Stauffer wrote a Sunday column summing up his reporting philosophy: "As editor, I am eager to hear from the author of the letter. I'm certainly interested in our hospitals. But that nurse will have to have some evidence to support her charges. So far, nobody has shown up and I doubt that anyone will." The invitation had been issued, but the paper didn't exactly leave the porch light on.

Weeks later, the newspaper published a series examining Stormont-Vail, but readers needn't have bothered to read beyond the main headlines: HOSPITAL-LIBRARY PACT USEFUL, FRIENDLY . . . STORMONT MAJOR HEALTH PROVIDER . . . FINANCE A KEY TO HEALTH CARE . . . STORMONT-VAIL DIVERSIFIES IN EVOLVING HEALTH INDUSTRY.

Again, the series included no substantive quotes from competitors of Stormont-Vail or outside health care experts, nor any attempt to assess the impact of Stormont-Vail's spending practices on declining health care standards and rising health care costs. Hospital spokeswoman Mistee Leighty found the series very pleasing. "It puts [us] in a very positive light," she noted.

Also left unsaid in all this coverage was one fact readers might have wanted to know: the same family that owned and operated the *Capital-Journal* played a major role in building and running Stormont-Vail. Not only was the Stauffer family a major donor—the hospital library carried the Stauffer name—but in 1985 the newspaper's editor and publisher, John Stauffer, had served as the hospital's chairman of the board. At the time of the Ann Landers column, Stauffer was president of Stauffer Communications, the newspaper's parent company, and a regular hospital board member. His nephew Peter was the paper's executive editor.

John Stauffer wasn't the only news executive to be seduced by a hospital that painted itself with civic virtue. But no matter how well intentioned these news executives may have been, the question remained: what happens when the interests of their readers and the interests of their hospital collide? One publisher solved this dilemma, the *American Medical News* reported, by passing confidential quality-of-care problems to his reporters, much to the consternation of the hospital. But the hospital also found that it gained a public-relations advantage by telling the public how it was solving the problems—most of which centered on a very high cesarean rate.

John Stauffer said that he never confused the two corporate hats he wore. Still, readers will never know how his paper's coverage might have differed without the Stauffer family's close ties to the hospital. Might the paper have fought to attend closed board meetings? Might it have probed the hospital's management more deeply? There were, for sure, a number of interesting topics to explore, such as:

- Why the hospital's fundraising foundation had performed so poorly. Instead of raising money, it lost $241,000 in one two-year period. In fiscal 1987, for example, the foundation raised only $124,122, while spending $127,836 in salaries and $69,275 in professional fundraising fees.
- Why the hospital, a nonprofit entity, paid its CEO more than many other comparable hospitals, about $210,000 in 1988. His two assistants together earned another $250,000. In contrast, the head of the New York City Health and Hospitals Corporation—which runs about a dozen hospitals—earned just $129,000 in 1988.
- How competition between Stormont-Vail and its chief competitor, St. Francis Hospital, had affected the cost and quality of care. Both did open-heart surgery, for example, even though they were within blocks of each other and were, according to some national standards, underused.

Peter Stauffer of the *Capital-Journal* said he really hadn't thought much about whether his paper should be allowed into hospital board meetings. He also said there wasn't much he could do about his family's hospital ties. "What am I going to do, ask that they give back our donation?" he remarked.

As for the Ann Landers column that had started everything, Stormont-Vail denied that it could have hired more nurses and that it provided poor care. Not that the hospital had all the people it wanted. About a month after the Landers letter appeared, the in-house hospital newsletter listed nearly two dozen nursing positions that needed filling.

What support Ann Landers may have lacked at the *Capital-Journal* was more than offset, however, by mail she received. About a month and a half later, she published an entire column of letters from nurses around the nation. Among their comments: "Our hospitals care more about the landscaping than patients" . . . "The hospital I work for recently spent $300,000 to decorate the lobby, but the nurses are keeling over from exhaustion" . . . "We are so short of nurses . . . They fired guards here to save money and the vandalism went wild. Meanwhile, they put in a new computer system and commissioned an artist to paint murals."

This time, Landers skipped her advice about seeking out the local press. Had she known, however, about the exploits of a feisty man named Clarence Pennington, she might have reaffirmed her faith in the Fourth Estate.

• • •

Reporters at the *Review Times,* a daily paper in Fostoria, Ohio, had just enjoyed a good laugh. It was the summer of 1987, and they were amused by what a woman said she had seen over at a large steel storage tank on the edge of town. "It was right over there," Clarence Pennington said one afternoon two years later, in between sips of hot soup at the local country club. "You can see it through the trees." He gestured at a distant white tank filled with soybean oil. "It wasn't white then, it was unpainted, and beginning to rust. So this woman drives by and spots what she thinks was an image of Jesus and a child's head. My reporters thought it was funny. I said write the story."

Pennington, in his 60s and with a soft round face, had the look of a man who knew how to enjoy himself. As publisher of the *Review Times,* circulation 7,500, he realized that what passes for news in rural Ohio might fall short somewhere else. He never expected that the Associated Press would put this local story on its wire. It did, and soon calls began coming in from as far away as France. "*Time* magazine did a story, Dan Rather and CBS sent a crew here. We had cars stretching bumper to bumper for a mile and a half, waiting to get a look." Pennington chuckled. "We even had artists coming in to paint the image."

Excitement like this rarely came to Fostoria, an old railroad and factory town seemingly misplaced amid the flat agricultural fields of northwest Ohio, where in the fall, open trailer trucks scatter sugar beets along the road as they rumble by town. Clarence Pennington, although he wasn't a Fostoria native, grew up in working-class towns like it along the hilly banks of the Ohio River. And while he appreciated the occasional humor of small-town life, he had another, more serious side that revealed itself when he handed out copies of the Constitution and "The First Amendment Handbook" to those who visited his modest office at the top of a dim stairway, just around the corner from Bill's Men's and Boys' Wear and a half-dozen or so empty storefronts. A former railroad brakeman and World War II seaman, Pennington wasn't ashamed to admit that he harbors a low threshold of indignation.

It was this side of Pennington that brought him face-to-face with another kind of news story—one involving Fostoria City Hospital. And like the rusting tank, it began small and ended up a national story, ultimately ensnaring the Ohio Supreme Court and the Ohio legislature while pitting major newspapers against the political muscle of the Ohio Hospital Association. Before it was over, it would cost Pennington's *Review Times* countless subscribers, advertising, and many tens of thousands of dollars in legal fees. Or, as he put it, "about 40 percent of my bottom line." But it was a battle worth fighting. "If a publisher isn't going to accept this kind of First Amendment dispute as part of doing business," he said, "then we might as well be running a pickle factory."

Technically, the battle was over Pennington's insistence that his reporters be allowed to attend Fostoria City's board meetings and to examine nonpatient records. But it was more than that. "The larger issue here is the attitude of health care professionals all over the United States," Pennington said. "They want the public to believe that medical procedures are too complex for health care recipients to understand; they say trust us. I say bullshit."

More than just a newspaperman, Pennington was also a business manager, and in that role, too, the hospital industry angered him: each year, he had to pay more and more for employee health coverage. "We aren't going to control medical expenses until the people who pay the bills have more than enough information about what they are paying for."

Pennington found out how difficult it was to do just that in early 1986, when he squared off against the management of Fostoria City. It was the quintessential community hospital—70 beds, located in a residential neighborhood with neatly cut lawns bordering its property. While big-city hospitals were fighting to keep out murderers and crack-heads, Fostoria City Hospital had lesser concerns. ALL VISITORS: SHIRTS & SHOES REQUIRED, a sign advised.

Although much smaller than Stormont-Vail, Fostoria's operating structure was similar in that it was city-owned but leased at little or no cost to a nonprofit group. It also shared Stormont-Vail's penchant for secrecy. That practice may have played well in Topeka, but it didn't in Fostoria. Each time the hospital's governing board met, Pennington sent a reporter. Each time, that reporter would be ordered to leave. And each time, Pennington would mention this affront in his newspaper. Pennington once gathered some of the city's corporate leaders, including the mayor and the hospital's chief of staff, then marched into the board meeting. All were asked to leave. The trustees even threatened to call the police to eject the hospital's chief of staff.

No matter what the hospital's reputation, such conduct by a public institution was out of order, Pennington believed. Even worse, Fostoria City had a blemished record for quality. In the early 1980s, the hospital suffered the ignominy of losing its professional accreditation due to poor care—a rare event, indeed. Moreover, one of the people running the hospital when those deficiencies occurred had left, only to return as chairman of the hospital's governing board.

Frustrated, Pennington filed suit in September 1986, hoping the courts would force the hospital to open up. The legal battle wouldn't end for more than two years. "In Fostoria, the hospital is the biggest institution in town," said David Marburger, a media lawyer with Baker & Hostetler, a big Cleveland firm that Pennington hired to wage his legal fight. "It wasn't just this hospital vigorously fighting accountability, it was the Ohio Hospital Association."

Although nearly 30 years younger than Pennington, Marburger matched up well with his client; he was a bulldog advocate who worked up a genuine dislike for those who trampled on the First Amendment. Once, when a reporter client was about to enter a room for a legal deposition in an unrelated matter, Marburger passed along his final instructions: "Now, this lawyer is going to introduce himself and probably say some pleasantry," he advised. "Don't even acknowledge him."

"You mean don't say anything?" the reporter asked.

"Don't even say hello," he replied.

Marburger had passion, all right, but he also knew the law, having won several successful battles to make Ohio hospitals more accountable. In the legal fight against Fostoria City Hospital, however, Pennington and Marburger initially met only with failure. First, a state appeals court declined to take action, saying the newspaper had to go through lengthy trial court proceedings, which could have taken months, even years. The next step was the Ohio Supreme Court, but it upheld the lower court decision by a four-to-three decision.

Undaunted, and with the editorial backing of the state's large daily newspapers, Pennington led a personal crusade in the Ohio legislature, successfully getting lawmakers in October 1987 to strengthen the state open-records law. Armed with tougher legal language, he went back to the Ohio Supreme Court, where one year later he finally won his victory.

At a subsequent ceremony in Boston, Massachusetts, Pennington and his tiny paper received the prestigious First Amendment Award from the Associated Press Managing Editors group, beating out papers 50 times the size of his.

The war, however, was costly for both sides. Wayne Moore, Fostoria City's administrator, looked back sadly at the battle that had been waged around him. "It's cost this hospital tens of thousands of dollars in legal-defense money that should have been spent on health care for those who need it," he complained. Although the old board is gone, along with its policy of secrecy, the new board must contend with a hospital that now loses money, in part because of the bad publicity Pennington's fight stirred up.

So far, Pennington hasn't found any major scandals or medical misadventures inside the hospital, but that doesn't mean the battle wasn't worth fighting. The public is better informed now, and that alone acts as a safeguard against the hospital losing its way sometime in the future. "I am willing to stand on what I did," Pennington said. "Maybe you are going to hurt that small hospital, but what about the rest of society?"

Pennington and Marburger both knew perhaps better than others how high the stakes can be when hospitals lack proper oversight. When Marburger wasn't battling Fostoria Hospital, he was successfully waging another legal fight that forced a Cincinnati hospital to open itself to public inspection.

This wasn't just any hospital—it was Drake Memorial Hospital, scene of one of the worst serial killings in U.S. history. Month after month in the 1980s, a nurse's aide murdered one patient after another. Dozens of these murders might never have been discovered if not for the Cincinnati media. Later, when the media wanted to examine how those deaths had gone undetected for so long, the hospital tried to keep them out, saying such outside investigation would be harmful. "Well, deaths are going to harm their competitive standing," Marburger said sarcastically.

It is no surprise that public accountability has failed to become a hot-button issue inside America's hospitals. Because neither the government nor the medical community demands it, hospitals can all too easily block legitimate inquiries from the press, and from patients as well. But in allowing such an important institution—one that holds the power of life and death—to operate in a climate of secrecy and impunity, society steers a perilous course that exposes patients to needless risks, not the least of which are hospital psychopaths.

16 | Lessons from the Grave

POLICE sergeant Robert Edgar didn't remember much about the day except that it was sunny and pleasant. He and several other men were standing next to a freshly dug hole, a small village church on one side, the rolling hills of Maryland horse country on the other. In a moment, they would haul to the surface a coffin that held the body of Martha Moore. Although this 44-year-old woman had apparently died of a heart attack, the men witnessing her exhumation in a Prince George's County graveyard now believed she might have been murdered.

Edgar felt vaguely uneasy. Relatively new to homicide investigation, he had been put in charge of what would become a tangled, complex case. He would ultimately become angered enough by the politics involved to quit homicide and join another police division. But that wasn't what was on Edgar's mind that day as he stood under a peaceful autumn sky in this tiny cemetery. "It's kind of strange," he would say later, "pulling someone you know from the grave."

Edgar wasn't the only cop who had known Martha Moore, a friendly, outgoing employee of Prince George's General Hospital. The nature of police work meant that anyone not chained to a desk in headquarters eventually ended up at the hospital. Maybe there was a stabbing victim to interview or a drug dealer cut down by gunfire. "Every policeman knew who Moore was, because she worked in the admitting part of the hospital," Edgar observed.

If not for a coincidence of timing, Edgar wouldn't even have been in Maryland. A solidly built, six-foot-one-inch, 35-year-old ex-Marine, he was poised to follow the dream of many young men who grew up in Queens: to become a New York City police-man. But the city's financial crisis of the 1970s had forced him to look elsewhere. After working awhile with the Baltimore police force, he joined the Prince George's County Police Department.

Even veteran detectives would have been baffled by this case. The alleged crime hadn't occurred in a back alleyway, tenement house, or drug den—turf that homicide investigators knew well—but rather in a maze of sophisticated gadgetry and alien terminology. Police now had reason to believe that Martha Moore had been murdered in Prince George's Hospital, not while working as a hospital staffer but while lying in an intensive care unit as a patient.

Edgar had no murder weapon to work from, no motive, and no witnesses. Also, his investigators were bucking a health care system that wasn't keen on either self-scrutiny or confronting a bureaucratic logjam that led one investigator to seek assistance from the highest levels of the Reagan administration. Those who worked the case, which dragged on for years, would always remember certain moments. For Edgar, one was Martha Moore's exhumation. For the assistant prosecutor, Jay Creech, it was the "violent smell" that exploded from Moore's coffin when they broke its air seal. For others, it was the sheer magnitude of the case, because Moore wasn't the only alleged victim. Somehow, investigators believed, a serial killer had been attacking and sometimes killing patients at Prince George's Hospital for more than a year without detection.

If that was true, then this case would raise disturbing questions that went far beyond a simple homicide investigation. Why, for instance, did the hospital take so long to uncover and report these alleged attacks? And what did that say about the ability of the hospital's internal-review committees to investigate any suspicious death, whether by murder or by medical mistake? One federal health investigator said that what had happened inside Prince George's should serve as a warning to hospitals everywhere—yet that warning, he suspected, was being largely ignored. As Martha Moore's remains were loaded for transport to the morgue, Edgar could only hope that they would yield that one bell-ringing clue which had thus far managed to elude him.

By the time Moore's grave was opened, Edgar had devoted 19 months of his life to the case. It all began early on the evening of March 18, 1985, when several representatives of Prince George's

Hospital arrived at the headquarters of the Prince George's County Police Department. For more than a week, members of the hospital staff had been quietly conducting a detailed review of medical charts to learn why an epidemic of cardiac arrests had been plaguing the intensive care unit. Now, they had come to the police because their findings pointed toward the possibility of foul play. The ramifications of such acts—if true—were so great that the hospital delivered its findings in person to the chief of police and deputy chief, among others.

The report didn't come as a total surprise. The day before, police had received an anonymous call alleging suspicious deaths inside the hospital. Buttressed by the hospital report, police officials were convinced they had to act now, and to run the investigation they turned to Robert Edgar. His orders: get down to the hospital, find out what he could, and report back to the chief with preliminary findings the next day.

At 8:30 P.M., Edgar arrived at Prince George's Hospital. He would not return home for days. Feeling slightly overwhelmed by what he had heard, Edgar patiently began reviewing the medical-chart audit that had prompted the hospital to contact the police. After midnight, he interviewed three employees of the intensive care unit where the deaths had occurred. They expressed suspicion about one particular nurse who was on duty at the time of many of the deaths. It was this nurse whom the hospital had recently placed on administrative leave pending completion of the chart audit. After a long night of interviews, Edgar drove to the police station, where at 9:30 A.M. he interviewed Dr. Joseph Colella, the director of the intensive care unit.

The evidence thus far suggested that on the evening shift, 3:30 P.M. to midnight, someone in the ICU had been giving patients unauthorized doses of potassium chloride, an electrolyte that can, in high doses, disrupt the heartbeat—but also, unfortunately, a substance that doesn't show up in an autopsy. By now, Edgar and his squad of detectives understood that the ICU was divided into two eight-bed units and staffed by a total of 10 or so nurses. Each nurse, upon reporting to work, selected a patient to care for. Because ICU patients were gravely ill, no nurse took more than two patients at a time.

Edgar's probe faced several major obstacles. Potassium chloride, the suspected murder "weapon," was a stock item in the ICU; sick patients who lose too much potassium must have it replenished or face the risk of an irregular heartbeat. Not only was the potassium chloride stored in an unlocked medication cabinet accessible to anyone in the vicinity, but vials of the chemical were sometimes kept at a patient's bedside when frequent doses were required. Moreover, as many as 18 to 20 people a shift typically passed through the ICU, from physicians to housekeepers to clergy. Any one of them, conceivably, could have administered the potassium chloride. Even the hospital pharmacy did its part to muddy the waters: for a time, it foolishly supplied the ICU with potassium chloride and saline in vials of the same color, increasing the possibility that a nurse might mistakenly grab the wrong fluid.

Hospital employees first began in the fall of 1984 to suspect something bad was happening in the ICU. Two nurses approached ICU management with their concerns that Jane Bolding, a nurse in her late 20s, had taken too much responsibility in the unit. One went so far as to note the frequency of cardiac arrests on Bolding's shift. Later, other hospital employees began to notice the high number of ICU heart attacks.

Edgar, after interviewing Dr. Colella, decided it was time to interview Jane Bolding. Shortly after noon, Prince George's detectives arrived at Bolding's home in nearby Washington, D.C. They waited as she made several phone calls and walked her dogs in a park across the street. Then, just before 1 P.M., she climbed into the backseat of a charcoal-gray Plymouth police cruiser for a ride to the police station.

About 23 hours later, without benefit of sleep, and after lengthy questioning without her lawyer present, Bolding signed a statement admitting to criminal behavior in the ICU. A judge later ruled that police had violated Bolding's constitutional safeguards in obtaining that statement, and threw it out. But even before the judge made his ruling, prosecutors knew the "confession" was shaky at best. Without it, investigators would have to pursue the case armed with little more than their suspicions.

Lacking a solid confession, Edgar realized he would have to prove this case the hard way. His first job was to find experts to help him interpret the medical records. Since autopsies on suspected victims, such as Martha Moore, would lead nowhere, the medical charts constituted the only hard evidence he had. Edgar tried calling several hospitals that had once investigated suspected murders, but they "didn't want to get involved," he recalled.

One logical resource was the federal Centers for Disease Control in Atlanta, but it also declined to help. Edgar speculated that the CDC, having recently assisted a Canadian hospital in investigating patient murders, had decided that to do it again would be just too costly and time-consuming.

Even Prince George's Hospital, which had brought its suspicions to police, turned mysteriously uncooperative. "A lot of reputations were at stake," Edgar said, noting the hospital's close ties to the local political establishment. The hospital forced police to subpoena key records. Hospital lawyers also sat in on police interviews with nurses, Edgar said, instructing them not to answer such innocuous questions as what constituted a low or high potassium level and what they would do if they found one. "What I learned is that they don't really give a shit," Edgar seethed. "Here they are, health care practitioners, and they won't even answer questions they knew we needed." Hospital officials declined to be interviewed about the case.

David Hatfield, a now-retired detective who worked with Edgar, said that when medical experts were finally located, his superiors didn't want to pay to fly them in. "They said, 'Try to find somebody locally.' " But local medical schools, including one with connections to Prince George's Hospital, declined to help as well. Although it was a local murder case, Hatfield even turned in desperation to the Armed Forces Institute of Pathology at Walter Reed Army Medical Center in Washington. But after looking through the records, the best the hospital could offer was that "we should have someone look further," as one investigator said.

Angrier than ever, Hatfield decided he had to do something dramatic. Because he had close friends in the Republican party he was able to arrange a meeting with what he called "very high officials" in the U.S. Department of Justice. "I knew we were doomed within our own little infrastructure," he said. Hatfield declined to say whom he contacted, but one police source said it was the attorney general himself, Edwin Meese. Later, as the investigation progressed, one of Meese's top aides called in for updates.

Finally, Edgar and fellow detectives got some good news: the Centers for Disease Control had, under pressure, changed its mind. Hatfield's end run had gotten his team on the scoreboard at last.

It was November 1985 when Dr. Jeffrey J. Sacks of the CDC was approached by his boss and asked if he wanted to investigate some suspicious deaths at a Maryland hospital. In addition to looking the part of a scientific sleuth with his full beard and glasses, Dr. Sacks was ideally suited for the assignment. Earlier, he had probed suspicious heart attacks in a Georgia hospital's ICU, as well as an unusual cluster of deaths at a nursing home in the St. Petersburg, Florida, area.

Although licensed to practice medicine, Sacks derived more pleasure from his other work as a medical epidemiologist. "The epidemiologist does not believe that disease strikes at random," he said. He pointed with pride to the father of modern epidemiology, John Snow, a 19th-century English physician. When cholera swept through London in the mid-1800s, Snow refused to accept the common belief that the disease was passed through miasmas, or bad vapors. According to Dr. Sacks, London was then served by two waterworks on the Thames: one obtained its water upstream, and the other did so downstream after sewage had been discharged into the water. By observing who succumbed to cholera, Snow traced the disease to a public well, known as the Broad Street Pump, in Golden Square, which was fed by the downstream waterworks.

An epidemiologist, however, always had to be wary of false association. For example, Snow's findings seemed inconsistent with the fact that workers in a particular brewery served by the diseased water supply hadn't developed a high incidence of cholera. But, according to Dr. Sacks, it was ultimately discovered that "the workers there did not drink water at all on the job but were given free beer."

Dr. Sacks accepted the Maryland assignment, and on December 2, 1985, he arrived in Prince George's County to conduct a quick initial assessment. "We don't want to commit a lot of time and resources to what may be a nonproblem," he explained. Sacks interviewed hospital employees. He read the morgue book to get a feel for the pattern of deaths occurring in the hospital. He also studied the operator logbook, which recorded every Code Blue, the hospital's method of signaling a cardiac arrest.

The logbook in particular disclosed a frightening pattern. From January 1984 to March 1985, the operator had paged twice as many cardiac arrests as in the period after that, from March through December. Moreover, Sacks noticed that Code Blues were skewed toward the evening shift, particularly in the last few hours before midnight. He later learned that many of these episodes of cardiac arrest had occurred after the lights had been turned off.

After a week in Prince George's County, Dr. Sacks gathered up his files and returned to the CDC in Atlanta. Upon further analysis by CDC staff, it was decided that Prince George's Hospital did indeed have a serious potential problem, and that Sacks had better return quickly to conduct a full-scale investigation. Soon after the new year, Dr. Sacks, accompanied by another CDC physician and two Ph.D.-level analysts, arrived in Maryland for what would be a long and exhausting probe into the unknown.

Dr. Sacks first had to find a place to set up shop. Most of all, he needed a lot of room. Police investigators wanted to rent an office but said they couldn't get government authorization to pay for it. The only alternative was Prince George's Hospital, which had an empty patient care floor. The idea of running a sensitive investigation within earshot of a possible murderer didn't appeal to investigators Edgar and Hatfield. Not only might their conversations be overheard, but their records, analysis, and reports might too easily fall into the hands of people who might not want to see the hospital or themselves embarrassed. With no other option, however, they tried to make the floor as secure as possible. Hatfield obtained specially designed secure locks, and Edgar did his best to monitor who went in and out.

Dr. Sacks began with two basic questions: was there, in fact, an epidemic of cardiac arrests any time between 1983 and 1985; and if so, was there an association between these episodes and any one nurse? To help out in the investigation, Sacks persuaded the Maryland Department of Health to loan him two physicians and two nurses. Together, they developed a method of abstracting key information from patient medical charts.

First, the team went through the ICU logbook and identified 2,219 admissions to the hospital from 1983 to 1985. These patient names were placed in a computer and alphabetized, as a prelude to obtaining their full medical records. Even with the state's help, however, Sacks's team was too small to properly analyze so many records. As a solution to that problem, Sacks hired and trained 32 nurses from the D.C. area, carefully excluding anyone currently working at Prince George's Hospital. Most weren't told the exact nature of the project.

With so many people involved, Sacks worried that some nurses might deviate from their instructions. Consequently, he designed an intricate system to catch any errors, willful or not, that could undermine his probe. Nurses in one room abstracted medical records on pink sheets of paper, which they placed in sealed envelopes. The same records were then passed to nurses in another room, who abstracted them again on green sheets. A supervisor then opened the envelopes containing the pink sheets and compared them against the green sheets. Dr. Sacks followed that up by personally comparing many of the forms himself.

"Even then," Sacks later explained, "we were still concerned that the quality of our data might not be high enough." For that reason, he randomly pulled 290 charts so they could be analyzed a third and fourth time. Finally, the colored sheets were delivered to a computer room, where Sacks had four keypunchers waiting. Two punched in the green sheets, and the other two did the pink. The computer checked to make sure both sets matched.

The police watched Sacks with amazement. "I'm not sure you could have picked anyone better than Jeff Sacks," said David Hatfield. Robert Edgar thought he was the hardest-working man he had ever met. One weekend, Edgar ordered Sacks out of the building. "I said Go to your brother's or something." (Sacks's brother lived in the neighboring county.)

From this original screening, which took several months, 302 records were isolated because they involved a death or cardiac arrest. These were then subjected to an intense study focusing on what medicines, procedures, and intravenous lines the patients got, how sick they were, and who cared for them. Finally, from all this meticulous work, there emerged a distinct picture. "We found that there had been an epidemic of cardiac arrests and that there appeared to be an association with one nurse," Sacks said.

Sacks's work was far from over, however. "We wanted to see if this was a false association." For example, if someone suggested a connection between the number of telephone poles in a country and the incidence of heart disease, "that would be what we call false association," Sacks said. As protection against that, he set out with an even more elaborate scheme to test hypotheses that might explain why one nurse had been associated with more heart attacks than others:

• Did the nurse panic and call a code when it wasn't necessary?
• Did the nurse get patients who were undergoing an unusual procedure or getting unusual medication?

- Did the nurse handle more patients than other nurses?
- Did the nurse record information better than other nurses?
- Did the nurse care for sicker patients?

To answer those questions, Sacks picked the best nurse abstractors and released the rest. This time, he needed to abstract more detailed medical information from the hospital charts. Again, each chart was reviewed independently by two different people in two different rooms at two different times.

Sacks took these abstractions back to the CDC in Atlanta, where he assigned codes for particular words. "There's more opportunity for error if you use words," he explained. "If somebody spells 'penicillin' with one *l* and somebody [else] spells it with two, the computer won't recognize it as the same thing." Once the CDC staff keypunched the data, Sacks arranged to have an independent contractor do the same so the two sets of results could be compared. This second phase of analysis, Sacks said, found nothing to shake his original conclusions.

As a next step, Sacks brought in a consultant doctor from another part of the country to study the records of 103 cardiac-arrest patients and make clinical judgments about their care. More analysis followed. Finally, on October 8, 1986, about 10 months after that winter day when he had first shown up in Prince George's County, Dr. Sacks issued his report.

One specific nurse, he found, had cared for 65 percent of the cardiac-arrest patients on the evening shift during the epidemic period, and her patients were atypical of those one might expect to have a cardiac arrest. "[On] the evening shift we would have expected 31 arrests. Eighty-eight were observed. The probability that this was due to chance was . . . one in one hundred trillion. It's roughly the equivalent of randomly choosing one second from all the time that life has been on earth."

Throughout the study, the nurse in question was identified only as Nurse 14. But investigators knew her, and knew her well. She was Jane Bolding.

Although Bolding had once confessed, under duress, to criminal behavior in the ICU, she now denied that she had ever tried to harm anyone. Even with Dr. Sacks's study, prosecutors lacked direct evidence that she had either committed crimes or had the motive to do so. Nonetheless, she was charged with three counts of first-degree murder and seven counts of assault with attempt to murder, allegedly by injecting five patients (some of them more than once) with unauthorized doses of potassium chloride.

At Bolding's 1988 bench trial, the prosecution produced doctors who testified about the unexpected nature of certain cardiac arrests in the ICU, some of which were apparently linked to potassium chloride. Still, the government's case mostly revolved around Dr. Sacks.

After the prosecution rested, Judge Joseph S. Casula dismissed all charges against Bolding for lack of evidence. "Sacks' testimony," Casula said, "did not and could not demonstrate that the defendant caused the cardiac arrests in the ICU during the epidemic period nor could he rule out the possibility that someone else may have been responsible for the cardiac arrests."

Dr. Sacks, of course, had never claimed otherwise.

While epidemiologic studies have their limits in a courtroom, they can identify suspicious death patterns and save lives. For years, scientists have asked hospitals to do more than just investigate each suspicious death, as they are supposed to do in regular mortality and morbidity conferences. "Such conferences look at trees—I suggest you look at forests," said Dr. Sacks.

On July 25, 1985, two articles in *The New England Journal of Medicine* implored hospitals to be more vigilant in spotting serial killers who might be stalking their patients. One study focused on a pediatric intensive care unit in San Antonio where 42 children died between April 1981 and June 1982. Investigators there found "a significant association between the presence of Nurse 32 and death and cardiopulmonary resuscitation." That nurse, Genene Jones, is now in prison for the assault and murder of patients. "[S]urveillance of deaths and cardiopulmonary resuscitation may allow early recognition of similar problems in other hospitals," the authors of the study concluded. A companion piece analyzed the association between one nurse and infant deaths inside a Toronto hospital. It, too, recommended that hospitals "implement a system for monitoring the occurrence of deaths by time and place within the hospital."

Dr. Sacks followed those articles with his own plea for new safeguards. In February 1988, he coauthored an article in the *Journal of the American Medical Association* that called the cardiac arrests at

Prince George's Hospital "an example of how an epidemic can continue undetected for 15 months in the absence of epidemiologic surveillance that looks at patterns as opposed to clinical reviews of individual patients." After noting that five published studies of unexplained deaths or cardiac arrests had found a clustering in the night hours, Sacks concluded, "We believe that the time has come for hospitals and other health care facilities to implement epidemiologic surveillance systems. . . ."

To be sure, America's hospitals face far greater problems than those posed by serial killers. Even so, hospitals do provide an ideal setting for someone bent on causing serious harm. One of the most prolific serial killers of the century was nurse's aide Donald Harvey, who confessed to killing dozens of patients in Kentucky and Ohio hospitals in the 1970s and 1980s. Harvey is serving a life sentence for his crimes.

More recently, nurse Richard Angelo was sent to prison after a jury in December 1989 found him guilty of killing four patients and assaulting a fifth in Good Samaritan Hospital on Long Island. Earlier that year, at Lenox Hill Hospital in Manhattan, police reported that someone had injected a potentially lethal muscle relaxant into the intravenous bags of two surgery patients. That case remains open.

The nursing shortage hasn't helped matters. Hospitals desperate for help are less vigilant than they should be in screening out bad nurses. The same is true for many temporary-staffing agencies that supply big-city hospitals with nurses and nurse's aides. Even more disturbing, Dr. Sacks suspects that hospitals have largely ignored suggestions in scientific journals to develop methods for spotting clusters of unusual deaths. "My impression is that things haven't changed very much," he said in early 1990.

Hospitals are failing in other patient safeguards as well. At decade's end, the Joint Commission on Accreditation of Healthcare Organizations said its inspectors had found roughly 2,200 hospitals that fell short in monitoring what happened to patients in special intensive care and coronary care units. In the aftermath of Richard Angelo's arrest, the New York State Health Department fined Good Samaritan Hospital for the poor recordkeeping that had made it nearly impossible to determine Angelo's role in other deaths. The state also criticized the hospital for failing to review deaths in a timely fashion. The hospital has since agreed to conduct more extensive background checks on its employees.

Even when hospitals suspect foul play, they may try to ignore it. The Texas hospital that employed baby-killer Genene Jones suspected that it might have harbored a criminal, but it didn't convey its concerns to police. In Columbus, Ohio, the local prosecuting attorney's office blasted Ohio State University Hospitals for failing to investigate promptly and aggressively seven suspicious incidents involving patients. Five suspicious deaths weren't even discussed in mortality and morbidity conferences, the prosecutor charged in 1986. "The unusually long delay between incidents and investigation . . . adversely affected any hope to uncover admissible evidence," the report stated. Although police had a suspect, Dr. Michael J. Swango, he was never charged with any hospital crime. Dr. Swango later went to work as a paramedic in Illinois, where he was convicted of poisoning his fellow paramedics. But that didn't stop him, either. After his indictment for that crime, he managed to get a job as an emergency room physician in Norwalk, Ohio.

And how did Ohio State University Hospitals feel about its handling of Swango? When the Cleveland *Plain Dealer* broke stories of Swango's ties to the hospital, management decided this time it would act swiftly and decisively. A top hospital official, according to the *Plain Dealer,* spent $78 buying up copies of the newspaper around the hospital so patients wouldn't see the stories and become upset. "They thought there would be a general panic," a hospital source told the paper.

The newspaper also reported that when the Ohio State Medical Board came to the hospital to investigate the Swango matter, it was ordered to leave the building. No charges were ever filed against the hospital.

Epilogue | Showdown

ON September 1, 1990, the nation's medical community began carrying out a program so obviously sensible that it was almost unfathomable why it hadn't been instituted decades earlier. At Congress's insistence, hospitals, health maintenance organizations, and state licensing bodies were now reporting to a national data bank the names of doctors disciplined for major incompetence or misconduct.

From the standpoint of patient safety, the data bank appeared to have no downside. For years, patients and hospitals alike had been victimized by doctors who were drug-impaired, dishonest, or well-meaning but incompetent. A doctor who got in trouble in one state could simply move to another. Usually, however, it never came to that; a troublemaker just switched hospitals, sometimes in the same city. So long as errant doctors left quietly, neither hospitals nor medical societies did much to stop them.

With the data bank, hospitals could still give staff privileges to risky doctors, but at least they would be doing it with their eyes open. For such a noble concept, however, the program angered many patient advocates. And for good reason. The data bank had one major flaw: access. Hospitals could tap into it to protect themselves from potential financial liabilities. So could medical societies and group medical practices. Excluded from this process, however, were patients themselves—the very people the data bank was supposed to protect, the people whose lives were on the line. Once again, doctors backed by government had decreed that patients and their families weren't smart or responsible enough to use the information wisely.

Which doctors are good and which aren't has long been one of the most closely guarded secrets in all of medicine. Even before the data bank, good hospitals knew who had better surgical successes and who was more inclined to operate unnecessarily. They just didn't share it with John or Jane Doe, the patient, who lacked the clout to make them. The medical community, however, overplayed its hand. Had it provided good services at reasonable cost, had it not been so wasteful, its secrecy might have gone unchallenged. Instead, medical costs doubled in the 1970s, then doubled again in the 1980s. John and Jane Doe, who had comprehensive medical coverage, were largely immune from these developments. But their employers, who had to cover the rising premiums, weren't.

For years, companies failed to fully realize the leverage they had over hospitals. Health benefits managers rarely got the ear of busy CEOs, who often sat on the boards of hospitals and shared in the civic pride these institutions engendered. But as more corporate profits disappeared into the sinkhole of medical costs, CEOs could no longer ignore the huge cost disparities among hospitals. They began demanding that hospitals justify their costs. "Buy cheap!" became the new corporate rallying cry—a defensible policy so long as everyone accepted the notion that all hospitals provided care of equal quality, or that quality couldn't be measured, or that hospitals wouldn't cut quality to win cheap contracts.

But knowledgeable people inside medicine and out knew the fallacy of those notions. They also realized that, sooner or later, corporate America would discover the secret that high-quality care need not be more expensive; in fact, it was often cheaper. And when it did, medicine would face its biggest challenge ever. By the 1980s, ugly confrontations had already begun to surface. Chrysler Corporation had the means and stature to accuse certain doctors at hospitals in the Kenosha, Wisconsin area of lousy care. An angry Wisconsin State Medical Society met with Chrysler to demand an explanation but left unsatisfied. "They stonewalled us," complained the medical society's Jim Paxton. The society, which as a matter of policy refused to disclose the disciplinary records of its members, now found the tables turned—and didn't like it.

It was a minor skirmish, however, compared to what was happening in Cleveland, Ohio. The corporate community there wasn't after a few bad doctors. It had a plan that, if successful, might shut down entire hospitals and cripple the lucrative surgical practices of many Cleveland doctors. Just as important, hundreds of thousands of

Clevelanders would for the first time learn which hospitals were more likely to cure them and which were more likely to kill them. This was no skirmish. It was a revolution waged over the very essence of how medicine is practiced in this country.

At 5:30 P.M., the bar section of Pat Joyce's Tavern was filling quickly. Located near Cleveland's federal building and police station, the bar had long been a favorite watering hole for federal agents, cops, and midlevel bureaucrats. That winter evening early in 1983, Thomas Quinn, a rumpled, chain-smoking reporter for the *Plain Dealer,* the city's big daily, was lucky enough to grab a small table. In a few moments, he would meet a source who had promised to guide him toward a startling story.

Quinn's source didn't like to be seen with him in public, but the crush of humanity near the bar would provide adequate cover. Quinn had first been introduced to this middle-aged man by another reporter months earlier. The source had approached the *Plain Dealer* to ask that it investigate local hospitals and doctors. He said he worked for a company that had access to medical records, and what he saw inside Cleveland's hospitals—huge disparities in cost, utilization, and mortality—both angered and frightened him. Fearing that the medical community had the political muscle to kill any private effort to expose its misdeeds, the source chose to go public through the *Plain Dealer.*

Cleveland hospitals had over the years become quite smug, even pompous. While the city struggled to overcome fiscal mismanagement, a Rust Belt economy, and bad jokes, Cleveland hospitals knew mostly success stories. Much of that traced to famed Cleveland Clinic, where foreign heads of state often came for medical care. The clinic also made house calls; when Iraq's Saddam Hussein needed a medical specialist (several years before the Persian Gulf war), the clinic sent him one. The clinic's prestige rubbed off on other hospitals in the city, which began to see themselves as part of an emerging medical mecca, a potent economic force that could propel the city's economic recovery.

That many employers saw them as just the opposite—a yoke of ever-increasing costs—didn't slow the hospitals' public-relations machines. When an outside consulting firm found overuse of hospital services, the Greater Cleveland Hospital Association, unaccustomed to bad press, tried to suppress it. The association took more radical action when one of its own committees recommended the elimination of hundreds of unneeded hospital beds. As soon as the explosive report hit the desks of member hospitals, an urgent call went out from association headquarters: destroy all copies of the report immediately; the public must not learn its contents.

Quinn's source, besides leaking to the paper the first of these suppressed studies, was providing a road map to show the *Plain Dealer* how it could document the hospital association's best-kept secrets. All the while, the source feared that the medical community might learn of his role and get him fired—possibly even threaten him physically. "These are powerful people," he would say in his more worried moments. Although perhaps overblown, the source's concern led Quinn to playfully assign him a code name—Sore Throat—which he used in all his notes.

Tonight, inside Pat Joyce's bar, Sore Throat was his usual nervous self. "The hospital association is trying to track down who leaked its report," he said. As he drained his cocktail, worry quickly evolved into anger. "There's a new federal program beginning later this year called DRGs. They say it's going to rein in Medicare costs, but the smart administrators will know how to beat it." He asked Quinn to remember the phrase "DRG creep," used to describe how hospitals might manipulate Medicare codes to get more money.

Quinn, however, wasn't particularly interested in vague predictions; he wanted hard data. Sore Throat had several times mentioned that he had a source with access to death rates inside Cleveland hospitals. "When can we get it?" Quinn asked. Sore Throat said to be patient. "Let's see how you handle what I've already given you." The conversation ended like so many others with Sore Throat—a few more tantalizing crumbs but no main course. Quinn would have to wait for that.

It would be nearly six months before Quinn and another reporter wrote their first stories in 1983. But once they started, they didn't quit for six months. The stories chronicled a panoply of hospital problems, including corruption, conflicts of interest, and raw mortality data suggesting that patients were five times more likely to die at certain heart surgery units than at others. The paper also reported that Greater Cleveland hospitals kept patients in their beds 26 percent longer than the national urban average, subjected them to 21 percent more surgeries, and had 20 percent more beds.

The articles did not go unnoticed in Cleveland's corporate suites.

Committees were formed and strategies formulated. Still, hospitals weren't about to make any major concessions. When one major corporation naively approached a hospital to discuss rising medical costs, it was rebuffed with a condescending, two-hour lecture that ended with this message: we don't need you.

Then, one day, Cleveland business discovered an intense, wiry Minnesotan who preached an end to subservience. Stop looking to others for help, he told corporate America. You alone have the power to reform the nation's hospitals. His name was Walter McClure.

Like other Americans in 1957, Walter McClure was deeply moved and worried by the Soviet launching of Sputnik. Hoping to serve his country, he decided to become a physicist. "By the time I emerged 10 years later," he observed, "two things had happened: the country had too many physicists, and I discovered I was unhappy."

After working several years in a government lab, McClure wanted out, but nobody, he said, wanted "a used physicist." Conjecturing that human behavior might be, for him, a more satisfying field than nuclear physics, McClure in 1969 joined the Minneapolis think tank Interstudy, which was seeking to reform medicine through a new concept called health maintenance organizations.

McClure knew nothing about the subject, but as a theoretician, he was attracted to the unknown. With Interstudy's help, HMOs were quickly becoming the darling of medical reformers, an alternative to the costly fee-for-service concept, the foundation of Blue Cross and Blue Shield coverage plans. Fee-for-service rewarded volume; the more services or procedures you sell, the more money you make. HMOs, on the other hand, believed that doctors in a group practice could be controlled and induced to provide only necessary services. In theory, the more efficient an HMO, the lower its costs and the more clients or contracts it could secure. Even the federal government encouraged tens of thousands of elderly Americans to join Medicare HMOs. Some states set up welfare HMOs for poor people.

McClure, however, became increasingly worried by what he saw. "HMOs were beginning to act like Blue Cross in drag," he said. "Instead of competing on quality and efficiency, they were competing by adding benefits. You find out what your competitor is doing, price just a little lower, and add benefits so people will shift. If there were any savings, they weren't passing them along; they were using it to buy the HMO in the next town. They weren't acting like we thought." Only years later did the public learn that some HMOs had endangered lives by reducing quality in search of profits.

McClure knew that when it came to health care, "buying cheap" wasn't good enough. One must also, as he put it, "buy right"—in other words, reward efficiency and quality. By quality, he meant sick patients getting better; by efficiency, quality care for less money, not less quality for less money. "When you ask quality providers to earn less on each patient, there is only one way to reward them—send them more patients," McClure concluded.

The quickest way to do that, he reasoned, was to persuade the purchasers of group medical care—employers, unions, and government programs—to develop a system to identify the high-quality, efficient hospitals and send them patients. An individual patient, McClure argued, didn't have the resources or clout to get that information. But a unified corporate community did. Once they got that data, they could direct their employees to the most efficient, high-quality hospitals. And employees wouldn't lose their freedom of choice, either. They could still go to an overpriced hospital—or even a substandard one—but they would have to pay more money to do so.

By the time McClure's Buy Right strategy crystallized, he had already left Interstudy to form his own think tank, the Center for Policy Studies. He had his theory. Now he had to spread the word. In coming years, he would make hundreds of speeches in cities across America. His message didn't always take hold. "It's easy to invent the Pill," he acknowledged. "The difficult part is to convince the Pope."

A defining moment in Powell Woods's professional life occurred when he opened a piece of mail containing two cassette tapes sent to him by a colleague. The tapes bore the words of a man who claimed to have found the solution to the nation's health care crisis. Woods had been around long enough to regard such statements with great skepticism. As vice president of human resources at Nestlé Enterprises, Woods knew how inflexible and resistant to change the medical community could be. He also had spent years listening to people spout theories on how to tame the health care monster. All these theories had one thing in common: none worked.

Yes, Woods thought, he would listen to the tape anyhow. As a leader of the local health care reform movement, it was the least he could do. The movement couldn't have found a better leader. For openers, Woods had worked in a Cleveland hospital for a year; he didn't particularly like it, but he did get to know how hospital types thought. Apart from his easy smile and nonthreatening manner, Woods was also a master communicator. A former linguistics professor, he had learned early on, for example, that when confronting doctors the worst faux pas was to be too deferential. In the wild, that was tantamount to a wounded animal letting a predator spot it. Any headway then was virtually impossible.

Woods took the cassettes to his car that evening. On his way home, he popped them into his tape player and listened. And listened. Four times he listened, and each time, he was swept away by the simplicity of its message. The speaker was Walter McClure, explaining his Buy Right strategy to a group of Canadian doctors.

This, Woods concluded, was one man he must meet. Quickly, he arranged a meeting with McClure where other health reformers in Cleveland could talk to him as well. When McClure arrived, he began with an announcement: "I am going to keep talking until someone interrupts me. Don't expect me to stop, because I am not that way." An hour and a half later, he stopped. Woods was stunned. "I don't use the word 'genius' lightly, but he is one," Woods would say later. "I can be a pretty good evangelist if you give me a good idea. I decided right then that I was going to do whatever I could to get [McClure's] idea going in Cleveland."

McClure had the message and strategy; Woods had the political skills to carry it out. It was time to get to work. If all went well, Cleveland's hospitals would never be the same.

Cleveland City Hall sits at the top of a hill overlooking Lake Erie. Over the years, it has hosted many a celebrated ruckus, a reflection of Cleveland's surly political scene. Its public politics have been chronicled in great detail in the media. Almost nothing, however, has been written about the private political decisions made in the secrecy of a building several blocks from City Hall. The squat structure, which for years flaunted a filthy marble facade, carries no sign indicating what goes on inside.

Known simply as the Union Club, the building is the exclusive preserve of Cleveland's gentry and corporate elite. More than 100 years old, the club reeks of status, from its grand marble staircase to its vigilant attendants, mostly men of color. Hanging from the walls are solemn portraits of corporate leaders, lighted just enough to set them off against the deep-maroon carpets and dark-paneled walls. Not until the 1980s did the club admit its first woman. In the late 1970s, Mayor Dennis Kucinich so disliked the Union Club, which he suspected of sabotaging his administration, that he mockingly held his own "Union Club" meetings in a greasy-spoon diner on Cleveland's working-class West Side.

While the real Union Club serves dinner and drinks, most business is completed over breakfast. "It's said that by the time people get to work at 9:30 A.M., all the important decisions in town have already been made," said Brent Larkin, editorial-page editor of the *Plain Dealer*. Thus it was that at 7:30 on the morning of March 14, 1989, about 35 of the city's top 50 CEOs, who formed a leadership group called Cleveland Tomorrow, were seated around a horseshoe table at the Union Club. They had gathered to hear Powell Woods tell them why they should endorse a high-stakes gamble to pressure Cleveland-area hospitals into making radical reforms. Woods was nervous. Two of the city's top 50 CEOs were from Cleveland Clinic and University Hospitals; if either showed up and caused trouble, he might lose his health care battle before the first shot was fired.

A lot of preparation had gone into just getting this far. One didn't simply call up 35 tycoons and ask them over for a Danish and coffee. Woods first needed someone to sponsor his presentation. He found that person in John Morley, president and CEO of Reliance Electric Company. Earlier, spotting Morley at a party, Woods had handed him the McClure cassettes. Morley, too, had been mesmerized. Even though he sat on the board of a major Cleveland hospital, he was to take the lead among local CEOs in trying to reform the medical community.

Woods knew that at the Union Club meeting he had to be at his evangelistic best. With so many people and ideas competing for the attention of CEOs, he had to shake them, and shake them hard. He also knew that executives were fearful of backing any idea that might make them vulnerable to attacks in the press by the medical community. As one executive explained, "In any battle against hospitals in this country, the CEOs lost every time; the hospitals and doctors portray themselves as Mother Teresa, and corporations come off as trying to extract an extra buck out of human suffering."

Woods's plan was to turn that perception upside down. McClure's Buy Right strategy gave corporations the high ground of quality. Either the hospitals joined them, or they would have to defend bad care. As McClure often preached, "Quality needs to be the first word out of every employer's mouth."

Finally, Woods's turn came to speak. "We have—in our community and in our nation—a very serious problem," he began. Imagine, he said, if a law were passed that forced everyone to buy a Chrysler and that someone else would pay 80 percent of the price. "With virtually unlimited demand and no competition, prices would rise steeply and quality would be an unknown, since there would be no motivation for its measurement and no meaningful comparisons would be available. We might have good quality, we might not; the point is we would not know. Both of these things are exactly what has happened to medical care. . . . We must stop overpracticing medicine, and we must begin measuring clinical outcomes."

Until now, Woods explained, the only reason companies could give employees for selecting one provider over another was to increase corporate profits by decreasing medical costs. In most minds, less expensive care was not top-quality care. And that had limited persuasive value, especially when applied to oneself or one's family. But, Woods added, if companies could provide a kind of *Consumer Reports* on local hospitals indicating which of them provided quality care, then employees might listen.

Woods's 20-minute talk didn't specifically discuss tactics. But he did mention that a corporate war chest of $150,000 had been raised for an explosive project already under way that would boost the Buy Right campaign. Later, as word of this project leaked to hospital administrators, tension between business and doctors would escalate to new levels.

But for now, Woods left the Union Club with hope; his message had clearly gotten through. Still, the CEOs of Cleveland Clinic and University Hospitals hadn't attended the breakfast. Were they just busy, or plotting some counterattack? Woods wondered. No matter; he would find out soon enough. The time had come to knock on the doors of a few hospital administrators.

Powell Woods didn't relish the prospect of a bloody showdown with local hospitals. As he made the rounds explaining Buy Right, he hoped to enlist their help in squeezing out the wasteful, low-quality providers. But that appeared unlikely. "Hospitals are truly populated by fine, caring people," he once said to a group of fellow businessmen. "But no hospital will ever self-destruct even if that's the best thing it can do for the community."

A central tenet of Buy Right was that institutions behaved as they were rewarded to behave. The current system, for example, rewarded hospitals that spent lavishly on high-tech equipment, heart surgery units, and fancy doctors' offices. Without these "prestige" items, hospitals couldn't attract the top doctors who brought in revenue-producing patients. Hospitals that economized by sharing equipment were penalized. Buy Right would make hospitals stop competing to lure high-admitting doctors and begin competing to offer the highest-quality care at the lowest prices.

As encouragement for hospitals to change their ways, business collectively had to steer employees to "approved" hospitals by making them pay more for going elsewhere. The idea of being subjected to some sort of quality-care test was unpleasant to hospital administrations, but many questioned whether business could unite long enough to pull it off. Even so, Cleveland hospitals were clearly worried by reports that corporations were already involved in some powerful, unpublicized project that might embarrass them. "They knew something was going on, and they didn't like it," said one health reformer. One hospital executive asked Woods bluntly, "Are you really doing this?"

Woods confirmed it, but when possible he avoided discussing what he and his associates called "the hidden hammer." As one corporate boss had told him, "The best use of the hammer is not to use the hammer." Just knowing it was there would suffice.

The idea for this sensitive project went back to early 1988, when Dale Shaller, an analyst in Walter McClure's think tank, took a call from Don Flagg, Woods's predecessor at Nestlé. In the early days of rebellion against soaring medical costs, no one had pushed harder for reform than Flagg. He had also had the good sense to recognize that while Cleveland's CEOs disliked rising medical costs, they weren't focused enough for a showdown confrontation. After preaching conciliation, and getting snoozed out of auditoriums, Flagg turned provocateur. One year, he delivered 45 speeches, most of them aimed at shocking Cleveland's CEOs into action.

On this day, Flagg was angry and frustrated. "Nothing is happening here," he complained to Shaller. "We've got to do something."

Flagg had in mind a bold and risky plan that might persuade Cleveland's business community to begin its assault on the medical community. But if it backfired, relations between business and hospitals might be so damaged that any lasting reform would be impossible.

Flagg had called to enlist Shaller's help. His reasoning was this: What if there existed a medical center so well known for its excellence that no one could ever impugn the quality of its care? And what if that medical center also had a reputation for efficiency and low costs? Wouldn't it make sense, Flagg said, to compare Cleveland hospitals, with their hyperinflated medical-care costs, against that center of excellence? Cleveland's costs would then look obscene, and Cleveland doctors couldn't invoke quality as a justification. Even before he called, Flagg knew, of course, that such a center existed: the Mayo Clinic in Rochester, Minnesota.

Shaller liked the idea. If corporations could be found to fund the study, Shaller would help direct it. Soon, money began pouring in. By then, some 13.6 percent of corporate payroll costs were going to health care. Moreover, corporate insurance premiums were rising between 20 and 30 percent a year.

With money in hand, researchers in the fall of 1988 began analyzing corporate claims and federal mortality data on 33 Cleveland hospitals. Besides accuracy, secrecy was of the utmost concern. Corporate leaders had nightmares of waking up one morning to find leaks from their study on the front page of the *Plain Dealer.* Another political problem involved the Mayo Clinic, whose cooperation was required. Mayo didn't want to brag or embarrass other hospitals, particularly Cleveland Clinic, its powerful but friendly rival to the southeast. But by the time Mayo fully realized the study's implications, it was too late to withdraw. Cleveland's medical community could only wait and hope for the best.

The hammer came down with full force on the morning of January 4, 1990. Shaller had flown to Cleveland to deliver the study's results at a breakfast meeting at the Union Club, regarded by both sides as neutral territory. Thirteen people attended, including the president of the Cleveland Academy of Medicine and leaders of the Greater Cleveland Hospital Association.

Shaller could hardly have envisioned himself in such a setting. Not that long ago, he and his wife had been living among peasant farmers in the highlands of Guatemala. Backed by a scholarship, Shaller was studying the practicality of peasants using sand and clay stoves to cook their food. Today, he stood among Cleveland's ruling elite in their private club, about to deliver a high-voltage shock to the local medical community.

Corporate leaders opened the tense meeting with some reassuring words. "We have been making a concerted effort to limit the visibility and general knowledge of this study," one executive said. He underscored their success at keeping the study's contents out of the media.

As Shaller awaited his turn to speak, he knew full well why such preliminaries were necessary. The findings were powerful. Earlier, when he had presented them to a select group of CEOs, "jaws dropped," as one business leader said, as they learned that they could fly their employees to the Mayo Clinic for treatment and still pay millions less than if they sent them to local hospitals. The study's bottom line: the average per-capita hospitalization charges were 50 percent higher in Cleveland. Moreover, the study cited data suggesting large differences in quality. One Cleveland hospital had 23 percent fewer deaths than expected for its type of patients, while another had 21 percent more deaths than expected.

Shaller, who had given this presentation before, confidently began laying out the grim figures. At one point, while he was using slides to illustrate cost differences, Dr. Ronald Price, who was then president of the Cleveland Academy of Medicine, spoke up firmly: "Let's see that medical back slide again."

Was this the beginning of a counterattack? the business coalition wondered. Shaller complied. The slide showed that hospitalization for a back problem in Olmsted County, Minnesota, cost on average $3,844, compared to $6,845 in Cleveland. "Now," said Dr. Price, pointing at the slide, "we don't know, do we, if that patient in Olmsted County had to go back three or four more times for treatment?"

A business coalition member rose to the challenge: "And neither do we know, do we, if the Cleveland patient came back for more treatment?" And isn't that, he asked, why Cleveland's medical community needs to develop a way to measure treatment success? The assembled group nodded.

The meeting was a watershed. During the last two years, Cleveland's business community had organized the purchasing power of 350,000 employees, which it promised to direct to the highest-quality low-cost hospitals. Either the medical community could help business pick those hospitals, or business would do it on its own. Buy Right proponents further stipulated that they didn't want endless discussions on how to define quality. Earlier, the Greater Cleveland Hospital Association had proposed its own plan to measure quality, but business regarded it as a ruse to delay action—a charge denied by hospitals.

Nevertheless, as 1990 began, a scenario few would have predicted began to unfold in Cleveland: two bitter adversaries, business and the medical community, working hand in hand toward a common goal. In particular, it took courage and wisdom for the hospital association, individual administrators, and doctors to set aside their short-term self-interest for the greater good.

"When we decided to do this project, a lot of my colleagues thought I was out of my mind," said C. Wayne Rice, president of the Greater Cleveland Hospital Association. "They said, 'You will lose your job over this. There are going to be losers.' " Even so, Rice said, the association independently concluded that something had to be done. As one hospital administrator confided, "This project is doing more to upgrade the quality in my institution than anything I have seen in 30 years." Not only did doctors and hospitals agree on a method of measuring patient outcomes, they were also allowing an independent firm to gauge patient satisfaction. Corporations, for their part, promised to help find a way to channel some of the savings from Buy Right into coverage for the uninsured or underinsured.

By mid-1992, program organizers will find out just how well their strategy has worked. Then, they plan to begin distributing quality and cost findings to corporations and their employees. In deference to the medical community, businesses don't plan any formal release of data to the media. But that's a moot point. "I don't think 350,000 employees can keep a secret, and we will be sharing it with them," Woods said.

If all goes well, Buy Right proponents envision similar programs taking hold in as many as 200 cities over the next five years.

Buy Right is but one vision of the future, a reform strategy that relies not on federal intervention but on the marketplace. It isn't flawless. Not every community has Cleveland's committed corporate and hospital leadership. And even if corporations realize huge savings by eliminating waste, there's no guarantee they will fulfill their promise to share savings with the un- or underinsured. Also, what happens to patients not covered by corporate policies who end up in a low-quality hospital? Although these flawed institutions will likely be forced to close eventually, who in the meantime will protect unsuspecting patients?

A humane society recognizes that government, too, has a role to play in driving the dishonest, incompetent, or wasteful medical provider from business. Patients need the protection of better laws, better regulation and enforcement, truly independent investigators, and public disclosure of more than just the most flagrant abuses. Patients, taxpayers, and hospitals need the protection of an insurance system that doesn't leave 30 million–plus Americans without the ability to pay for their medical care. The federal Medicare program—the single largest buyer of hospital care—could reform hospitals virtually overnight if it followed Cleveland's lead and reimbursed only hospitals that could prove their high quality and efficiency. Unfortunately, Medicare continues to channel money into wasteful, poor-quality hospitals.

Meanwhile, the prospects for broad reform aren't good. *The Washington Post* reported that health care lobbyists made up the fastest-growing lobbying group in early 1991. Although they represent a discordant chorus of conflicting interests, they help to perpetuate the nation's patchwork health care system. The American Hospital Association, for example, plans to spend $1 million—part of it going to a public-relations firm run by Carter White House spokesman Jody Powell—just to learn how to lobby better and look better in public. As one congressional aide told the *Post,* "The lunches lobbyists are offering and the money they are spreading around is incredible. In six years up here, I've never seen anything like it."

Compounding the problem is weak leadership in the Department of Health and Human Services. "For the last decade, health policy has been run largely out of the OMB [Office of Management and Budget]," said Dale Shaller, now an independent consultant. It is, in other words, budget-driven, not policy-driven. The last two secretaries of HHS have been avuncular physicians who lacked the will and vision to stand up to White House politics. Neither man seemed to recognize that the lax regulation of hospitals, purportedly designed to save taxpayer dollars, has, in fact, cost billions in soaring medical expenses.

Nevertheless, McClure and others like him have hastened the day when hospitals will be held publicly accountable for their performance, when life-and-death medical decisions can be made by patients on the basis of hard data, not blind trust. With mainstream medical groups at least discussing quality measures, it's hard to imagine a return to the days when hospital inspectors burned the names of substandard hospitals so the press wouldn't learn their identities.

No one has fought longer and harder for openness in the medical profession than Dr. Sidney Wolfe, who along with Ralph Nader founded Public Citizen Health Research Group in Washington, D.C. "In the near future, doctors and hospitals no longer will be able to hide the details of who . . . is not doing a good job behind a shield of anonymity," said Dr. Wolfe, a native Clevelander.

Much has changed since the summer of 1973, when Wolfe sought to publish an innocuous consumers' directory listing doctors, their training, and their payment practices. Back then, the Maryland State Medical Society implicitly threatened doctors with loss of their medical licenses if they cooperated. Providing information "that would point out differences" among doctors was illegal, the medical society concluded. Two years later, Wolfe tried to compare infection control policies among D.C.-area hospitals, but the local hospital association urged its members not to cooperate. In 1976, Wolfe's group began demanding the release of hospital mortality data on Medicare patients. Nearly a decade of resistance later, Medicare finally agreed.

Time and time again, hospital administrators and doctors have argued that releasing quality data would "mislead" consumers. Dr. Wolfe called that patronizing, and false on its face. "It is only without the facts that consumers can be misled," he said. Since Public Citizen began publishing rates for cesarean section, the number of those often unneeded and potentially dangerous surgeries has finally begun to drop.

Still, there remains much that patients don't know. State medical boards don't routinely publish the names of disciplined doctors. Hospital inspection reports aren't always made public. Moreover, several years after the Joint Commission on Accreditation of Healthcare Organizations announced that it would develop quality measures, it still hasn't fully implemented them, nor has it decided whether to release them publicly when it does. Even so, one Joint Commission board member was forced to admit in 1989, "Disclosure is here. The cat's out of the bag. Now it's just a matter of degree."

In the meantime, consumers should realize that while it may be easy and reassuring to believe that most hospitals and doctors are equally good, it is also foolish and dangerous. The mystique of infallibility from which doctors and hospitals benefit so greatly has survived too long, at the expense of patient care. Consumers should not be afraid to pointedly probe the backgrounds of their physicians and hospitals, including their financial relationships. They should make use of what little information they have, such as which local hospitals fare well and which fare poorly in federal Medicare mortality studies. They should avoid underused open-heart units, where surgeons don't get the practice they need to achieve superior results. Corporations, on the other hand, should realize that it is morally indefensible to steer their employees to medical providers that compete only on the basis of cost without regard for quality.

Dr. Floyd Loop, one of the nation's preeminent heart surgeons, once said that surgical outcomes should be disclosed openly, just as "a restaurant posts its menu outside its door." In his view, surgeons and hospitals aren't all that different from toasters. Some work well, some not so well; some, it should be added, are even downright dangerous. Prudent shoppers should know the difference.

It may be somewhat discomforting to think of doctors and hospitals along the same lines as household appliances. And trivializing, besides, when one considers how much is at stake for medical consumers. Yet that, of course, is exactly the best argument for holding health care to the highest standards of quality and efficiency, and for insisting on public disclosure of all data needed to make informed choices. Only then will trust be justified and patients and their families finally cease to be victims of medicine's great white lie.

Notes

PROLOGUE: A FINAL RESTING PLACE

Details of Hinnant's murder come from Steven Smith's murder trial, from interviews with his prosecutor, James Kindler, and from articles about the murder published in *The New York Times, Newsday,* the New York *Daily News,* and the *New York Post. The State,* a Columbia, South Carolina, newspaper, reported many details of Hinnant's personal life, particularly an article by Claudia Smith Brinson, "Murder Victim and Suspect: Different Paths Lead to Tragedy" (January 15, 1989), p. 1-A.

Historical notes on Bellevue were provided by Lorinda Klein, Bellevue's special-projects coordinator, and various Bellevue brochures. Descriptions of sections inside Bellevue are based on author's observations.

13 *One of the . . . and prisoners:* Klein interview.
14 *It is here . . . corridors:* For a good description of Bellevue's emergency room, see Edward Ziegler, *Emergency Doctor* (New York: Ballantine Books, 1987).
14 *Over the next . . . psychiatric care:* Interview with Joint Commission on Accreditation of Healthcare Organizations.
14 *accused of . . . syringes:* Harrison J. Goldin, New York City Comptroller, "Audit Report on the Operation, Practices and Procedures for the Purchase of Disposable Products. July 1, 1985–June 30, 1989" (March 20, 1989), pp. iii–iv. Also, Goldin press release, March 30, 1989. The audit report notes that some of the discrepancies might only be the result of missing records.
14 *and ordered . . . registrations:* Bellevue blamed the state for bureaucratic delays in issuing registration renewals. Bellevue said the problem was partly resolved so that ultimately only 10 nurses were affected.

14 *In 1988 . . . City hospitals:* David E. Pitt, "Hospital Police: No Guns, No Respect, Lots of Trouble," *New York Times* (March 27, 1989), p. B1.

14 *The new year . . . bedside drawer:* Frank Bruni, "Patient Chases Bedside Bandit Down Hospital Hall," *New York Post* (January 4, 1989), p. 4.

15 *In the 1870s . . . of graft:* Klein interview.

15 *New York City's . . . in 1985:* Interview with Fred Winters, New York City's Health and Hospitals Corporation.

15 *During that time . . . he said later:* Interview with Durbin, and a Bellevue official who declined to be named.

15 *The self-assured . . . soup van:* Brinson, "Murder Victim and Suspect."

16 *In a letter . . . creatures:* Ibid.

16 *The main elevators . . . hallway:* Author's observations.

17 *Nearly a . . . psychiatric ward:* Klein interview.

17 *Bellevue officials . . . century-old legacy:* Ibid.

18 *Three months earlier . . . hospitals:* Pearson mailed the letter in response to an article, written by the author, that had appeared in *The Wall Street Journal.*

19 *Tonight, a . . .* Things Past: Interview with an employee of the Penine Hart Gallery.

20–21 *If only . . . murder:* Winters said that in 1989, the year of Hinnant's murder, Bellevue had 71 security guards, down from 91 in 1988.

21 *So Bellevue . . . came:* Klein interview.

21 *When you mix in . . . licensure:* "Media Tip Sheet," American Medical Association (March 8, 1991).

22 *a decade . . . more:* Interview with the investigator, Richard Kusserow, inspector general of the U.S. Department of Health and Human Services.

22 *In a report, the group described . . . "grim":* United Hospital Fund, "The State of New York City's Municipal Hospital System" (fiscal year 1989), p. 1 of introduction.

22 *"They are . . . Hospitals:* Michael Specter and Howard Kurtz, "Overlapping Epidemics Plague New York City Hospitals," *Washington Post* (February 11, 1990), p. A1. Andrulis was also quoted as saying, "New York is clearly the most dramatic example of this social disaster. But the poverty, the lack of basic health care and the financial neglect that have caused this crisis can be found in any city in the nation."

22 *numb to . . . overtime:* David Zinman, "The Diagnosis for NCMC," *Newsday* (May 29, 1989), p. 7. Overtime hours were for 1988.

22 *"Everybody . . . what you do":* Ruth Landa, "In B'klyn, Another Hospital Is Sickly," New York *Daily News* (October 28, 1988), p. 4. An attempt was made by telephone to verify the quotes with Blutstein, but she declined to comment.

23 *In 1988 . . . older:* Report by the Island Peer Review Organization, Focused Quality Review of Parsons Hospital. This group studied the

deaths at the request of the New York State Health Department. The contents of this report were first reported by the author in "Prized by Hospitals, Accreditation Hides Perils Patients Face," *Wall Street Journal* (October 12, 1988), p. 1.

23 *Yet there . . . city:* Interviews with New York State health officials.

23 *But the . . . 13:* Lucette Lagnado, "They Didn't Have to Die," *New York Post* (January 6, 1989), p. 1.

23 *The chief . . . woman:* The hospital said prosecutors found that no crime had occurred.

23 *One month . . . somebody!":* Lyle Harris and Joel Siegel, "Hosp Guard Attacker Shot," *New York Daily News* (February 5, 1989), p. 7.

24 *Metropolitan . . . beds:* Howard W. French, "Crack Filling New York Hospitals with Frustration, Fear and Crime," *New York Times* (May 10, 1989), p. A1.

25 *Since the . . . far-reaching:* This percentage provided by the American Hospital Association.

25 *More than . . . assignments:* American Hospital Association. Overall, about 40% of the nation's hospitals use temporary nursing services; *AHA News* (August 13, 1990), p. 4.

25 *Some exhausted . . . shifts:* See Chapter 9.

25 *Even so . . . shortages:* The Secretary's Commission on Nursing, Department of Health and Human Services, reported in December 1988 that "in every region of the country, between 10 and 32 percent of hospitals have had to limit elective admissions temporarily" due to the nursing shortage.

25 *In New York . . . researchers:* Troyen A. Brennan, Lucian L. Leape, Nan M. Laird, Liesi Hebert, A. Russell Localio, Ann G. Lawthers, Joseph P. Newhouse, Paul C. Weiler, and Howard H. Hiatt, "Incidence of Adverse Events and Negligence in Hospitalized Patients," *New England Journal of Medicine* (February 7, 1991), p. 370.

25 *Fifty-one percent . . . units:* These statistics were first reported by Michael L. Millenson of the *Chicago Tribune.*

25 *Forty percent . . . costs:* Editorial, "Educate Healthcare Buyers on Relationship of Quality to Cost," *Modern Healthcare* (December 22, 1989), p. 22.

25 *Eighty-nine . . . overhaul:* Associated Press citing survey commissioned by *Health Management Quarterly* (February 14, 1989).

25 *Nearly one . . . concerns: Los Angeles Times* poll.

25–26 *About one . . . compromised:* Health Care Investment Analysts, Inc., Baltimore, Maryland.

26 *Nor can . . . Luke's:* Press release, New York Health Department, "Hospital Enforcement Actions" (July 24, 1989). St. Luke's declined to comment.

27 *Some patients . . . tubes:* Laurie Goodstein, "Hospital's Deadly Problem," *Newsday* (May 1, 1989), p. 4.

27 *Chicago's Cook . . . tubes:* See Chapter 14.

27 *Detroit Receiving . . . died:* Patricia Anstett of the *Detroit Free Press* reported that no autopsies were done on the 22 patients who died.

27 *Elderly patients . . . increases: Journal of the American Medical Association* (October 17, 1990), p. 1981.

27 *Most patients . . . Chicago:* 1987 data; Center for Medical Consumers, New York, New York.

27–28 *But in . . . year:* The 7,000 figure is for 1984.

28 *"You will never . . . regulators:* Associated Press (January 26, 1986).

28 *After one . . . snapped:* Ibid.

28 *"What sense . . . president:* "Providers Link Health with Human Services," *Hospitals* (January 5, 1990), p. 34.

28 See Chapters 5 and 6 for a full discussion of hospital payments to doctors.

29 *By 1990 . . . unsuccessful":* "The Complexities and Perplexities of Cost Containment," *American Journal of Public Health* (November 1989), p. 1477.

29 *In* The New *. . . environment":* David Kinzer, "The Decline and Fall of Deregulation," *New England Journal of Medicine* (January 14, 1988), p. 112.

PART ONE: CUTTING CORNERS, PLUGGING HOLES

Chapter 1: Footprints in the Sand

33 *At midmorning . . . room:* Background on Mathew is from "Findings of Fact, Conclusions of Law and Order," Maryland Board of Nursing, RO88056 (December 19, 1989).

34 *Yolanda Holland . . . checks:* Background on Holland is from "Findings of Fact, Conclusions of Law and Order," Maryland Board of Nursing, LP22617 (February 1, 1990).

34 *Barbara Dugger's . . . unit:* Background on Dugger is from "Order for Emergency Suspension of Nursing License," Maryland Board of Nursing, LP20632 (September 15, 1989).

34 *With one . . . crack:* The nationwide vacancy rate is for 1989, the most recent year available. There is some evidence that the vacancy rate may have declined in late 1990 and 1991 due, in part, to the economic recession.

35 *One midsized . . . annually: All Care Nursing Service Inc. et al.,* v. *Bethesda Memorial Hospital Inc.,* Case No. CV 88-8568, U.S. District Court, Southern District of Florida, West Palm Beach Division; deposition of Sue Bradford, director of nursing for Delray Community Hospital. Unless otherwise noted, all depositions and affidavits cited in this chapter and the following two chapters are from this case.

35 *nearly 125,000 . . . 1988:* Secretary's Commission on Nursing (December 1988), p. 4.

35 *By the late . . . aides:* American Hospital Association.

35 *In Cleveland . . . weeks:* Doug Lefton, "Prescription for Worry, Nursing Shortage Affects Health Care for the Elderly," Cleveland *Plain Dealer* (June 25, 1989), p. A1.

35 *Florida's Palm . . . counting:* Affidavit of John Pisarkiewicz, Jr.

35 *They didn't know . . . care:* Depositions, affidavits.

35 *If they . . . painter:* The *Boston Business Journal* reported a raid by the Immigration and Naturalization Service on one temporary agency that had between 30 and 35 illegal aliens. The housepainter reference is from *All Care* v. *Bethesda.*

36 *"You need . . . a nurse":* Faron deposition. All of Faron's comments are from his deposition.

36 *One night . . . verdict: Northern Trust Co.* v. *County of Cook,* Case No. 84-2234, 481 N.E. 2d 957 (Illinois Appellate, First District, 1985). Also, interview with attorney who represented the family.

36 *In 1989 . . . nurses:* Health Care Financing Administration, inspection report (survey date: March 31, 1987).

37 *And there it . . . Beginning":* Aussler, in her deposition, indicates that this was the ad. The telephone number was All Care's.

38 *"There's a . . . hour":* Aussler's recollection of conversation.

38 Many conversations involving All Care workers are reconstructions based on depositions. The wording is sometimes modified to reflect how those conversations probably occurred.

38–39 *One area . . . Medex:* Deposition of Sue Bradford, nursing director at Delray Community Hospital. All Bradford quotes are from her deposition.

39 *"Every three . . . services":* Bailey deposition.

39 *"Our Xmas . . . 1990":* STAT Nursing Services.

39 *John Roylance . . . played:* All quotes from Roylance and details on his activities are from his deposition.

40 *Palm Beach . . . schoolteacher:* Details on Nedermier's murder are from interview with Palm Beach police, interview with Lemont's prosecutor, articles published in the *Palm Beach Post,* and Clifford L. Linedecker and William A. Burt, *Nurses Who Kill* (New York: Windsor Publishing Corp., Pinnacle Books, 1990).

41 *Soon, her . . . office:* From Aussler's statements and author's observations, this route appears to be the most logical.

41 *Aussler said . . . Monahan:* Monahan said she didn't reimburse people for travel expenses until they had worked for six weeks.

CHAPTER 2: IMPOSTORS

42 *Julie Monahan's . . . income:* The $6-million figure is from Monahan's affidavit.

42 *Monahan said she . . . muumuu:* Monahan interview. At first, Monahan declined to be interviewed. She later answered some questions, but her lawyer, Helen McAfee, terminated the interview. In some instances, McAfee answered questions for her.

42 *With only so . . . Carolina: All Care* v. *Bethesda,* deposition of Sheila Ripley Brubaker. Also, Monahan said she targeted economically depressed areas.

43 *All Care . . . lodging:* Monahan said she charged her workers $40 a week for lodging.

43 *An overnight . . . exams:* Monahan couldn't be reached for a response to this allegation.

44 *Even so . . . phones:* Monahan said only one person worked the 4 P.M.–to–1 A.M. shift.

44 *"You had . . . anymore":* Seibert deposition.

44 *Monahan subsequently . . . place:* Monahan said that Aussler, soon after arriving in Florida, befriended a taxi driver who often drove her around.

44 *On another . . . later:* Aussler deposition.

45 *Becky Seibert . . . toilet:* Seibert's recollection of the conversation.

46 *With hospitals . . . share:* The JFK figure is from an affidavit given by Julie Crick, director of nursing at JFK.

46 *"Where's that . . . here":* Aussler's recollection.

47 *"I got . . . done":* Monahan said she was shocked to hear Aussler say she was too tired to give medicine to patients. "I wasn't her shadow," Monahan said. "Did All Care send her out when she was too tired to do her job? I have no idea. I just can't believe she would do that."

47 *Hospital officials . . . it:* Bradford deposition.

48 *Then, ignoring . . . Worth:* Monahan's lawyer declined to comment on that allegation.

48 *"Can you . . . premises":* Seibert's recollection of the conversation.

49 *Eventually, Seibert . . . facilities:* Seibert deposition.

50 *Brubaker would . . . daughter:* Department of Professional Regulation, investigative report.

51 *No reputable agency . . . employees:* Brubaker deposition. Also depositions of other workers, and interviews with lawyers representing the South Florida Hospital Association. Another law firm, representing two Palm Beach County hospitals, made similar allegations in one of their related court filings.

51 *But John . . . LPN:* Roylance deposition.

51 *That called for . . . uncovered:* Details on Bethesda's discovery were provided by lawyers representing the South Florida Hospital Association and in depositions from former All Care workers.

52 *At least . . . exams:* Roylance deposition.

CHAPTER 3: THE PERFECT FILE

53 *"The perfect file . . . created":* All Brubaker quotes are from her deposition. Monahan told an investigator for the Department of Regulation that she fired Brubaker on June 16, 1988, because she refused to acknowledge her personal problems. According to the investigative report, Brubaker "was evicted from the home she shared with Monahan's daughter."

54 *Brubaker said . . . schools:* Tracey Marino also said in her deposition that she had created false documents. "I changed dates on health certificates," Marino said. "And they changed names on licenses, nursing licenses . . . Something happened and Julie was afraid that she was going to get in trouble . . . and we went through the files and . . . I whited out dates and typed in new dates or wrote in new dates and put false signatures on there."

55 *In the ultimate . . . folders:* Brubaker said it was her understanding that three folders were selected. Monahan, in an affidavit, said government regulators had found problems with two All Care workers. She said, "[I]n January of 1988, when HRS met with All Care Nursing Service, it was discovered that Becky Black's [Seibert] endorsement number had expired. In this regard, [Monahan] immediately informed Becky Black that she needed to proceed to Jacksonville to obtain licensure." Monahan also said that HRS had told her that "Georgia Jesse's endorsement number had expired. Immediately [Monahan] informed Georgia Jesse of this and indicated to her that she would not be permitted to fill any further shifts until her license was renewed and completely intact."

57 *After a few . . . place:* The exchanges that follow involved more than one questioner.

58 *According to William . . . records:* Dunaj interview.

59 *Some feared . . . hiding:* Whiteman affidavit.

59 *The state . . . aides:* John Marino, a spray-painter, said in a deposition that he posed as a nurse's aide. His wife, Tracey, named others who were sent out on jobs for which they weren't qualified.

60 *As for Sharon . . . profession:* Monahan, in an interview, suggested that the author contact two of Aussler's former employers, Prestige Nursing Service and Palms of Lakewood. A Prestige spokesman said he wasn't "completely happy" with Aussler's work. A spokesman for Palms of Lakewood, a residence for senior citizens, said Aussler only worked for

him a short time but was a "fine" nurse. "She did confide in me . . . that she said she was in fear of reprisals" for her role in trying to expose some scandal, the spokesman added.

60 *As the year . . . charges:* Interview with Lisa Bassett.

60 *Four of . . . risk:* "Patients Are in Danger," *RN* (October 1988), p. 32.

61 *"The so-called . . . medications":* Priscilla Scherer, "When Every Day Is Saturday: The Shortage," *American Journal of Nursing* (October 1987), p. 1284.

61 *"The powerlessness . . . drowning":* Karen Emra, "Does the Nursing Shortage Change the Rules," *RN* (October 1988), p. 32.

62 *"The result . . . called":* "Maryland RNs Push for Bill to Bar Unsafe Assignments," *American Journal of Nursing* (August 1986), p. 962.

62 *Atlanta's Physicians . . . attended:* Health Care Financing Administration, "Statement of Deficiencies and Plan of Correction" (survey date: January 31, 1989, and February 1, 1989).

62 *When Crawford . . . leaving":* HHS Inspector General, "Hospital Best Practices in Nurse Recruitment and Retention" (November 1988), p. 10.

62 *More than . . . nurses: Modern Healthcare* (September 1, 1989), p. 16.

62 *About one . . . foreign-trained:* Howard W. French, "Dire Need for Nurses Is Perplexing to Hospitals," *New York Times* (May 22, 1989), p. B1.

62 *"Filipino nurses . . . complain":* *RN* (September 1988), p. 61.

62 *"They're . . . exploited":* Stephanie Saul, "Two Probes Focus on Recruiting of Foreign Nurses," *Newsday* (August 25, 1985). p. 20.

63 *The future . . . education:* "States Lack Resources to Train New Nurses," *AHA News* (June 25, 1990), p. 4.

63 *Detroit Receiving . . . temps:* "Statement of Deficiencies and Plan of Correction" (survey date: February 5–7, 1990).

63 *Twenty-two . . . deaths:* Michigan Department of Public Health press release (February 9, 1990).

64 *"People of . . . Avenue":* Heidi Evans, "Quick Rx for Lincoln," New York *Daily News* (October 28, 1988), p. 5.

CHAPTER 4: "THE COMPELLING URGENCY TO EASE HUMAN SUFFERING"

65 Most details of Murphy's surgery are from proceedings before the North Carolina Pharmacy Board, interviews with board investigators, articles published in the *Charlotte Observer,* and news releases from Charlotte Memorial Hospital.

66 *Already the . . . needed:* Advertising budget is from *Charlotte Observer* (April 16, 1989), p. 1A.

66 *He was . . . odd:* For an excellent profile of Dr. Robicsek, see Kathleen

Coleman, "Robicsek Lives with Lots of Heart," *Business Journal* (February 1, 1988), p. 8.

67 *Between the months . . . men):* Details on the infection are from: Hoffman, Fraser, Robicsek, O'Bar, and Mauney, *Journal of Infectious Diseases* (April 1981), p. 533; *Ledbetter* v. *The Sanger Clinic,* Case No. 78 CVS 4670, Superior Court, County of Mecklenburg, State of North Carolina.

67 *"I'm delighted . . . disappointments":* Coleman, "Robicsek Lives with Lots of Heart."

69 *Days later . . . me":* Karen Garloch, "Surgeon Robicsek: 'I Feel Fate Set Us Up,' " *Charlotte Observer* (February 7, 1988), p. 12.

69 *Immediately . . . nation:* Explanation of how UNOS operates provided by K. Straw, UNOS spokeswoman.

69 *Besides damaging . . . fluids:* For a good description of open-heart surgery, see Jonathan L. Halperin, M.D., and Richard Levine, *ByPass* (New York: Times Books, 1985).

70 *"I have . . . that":* Interview with work.

71 *"We don't . . . flood":* Interview with Phillips, deputy director of the Division of Facility Services, Department of Human Resources.

72 *"We started . . . notch":* Interview with Cosgrove.

73 *A vigilant . . . 1989:* Health Care Financing Administration "Statement of Deficiencies and Plan of Correction" (survey date: February 23, 1989).

73 *In 1989 . . . responsibility:* "JCAHO Accreditation: Top Trouble Spots for Hospitals," *Hospitals* (August 5, 1989), p. 34.

73–74 *In early 1989 . . . areas:* HCFA "Statement of Deficiencies" (survey date: January 31, 1989).

74 *The shortage . . . recruit:* "Coming Up Short: Hospitals Seek Workers," *Medicine & Health* (June 12, 1989), pp. 1–4

77 *In March . . . procedure:* Associated Press (March 22, 1985).

81 *HHS said . . . investigation:* Letter to author from Clarence J. Boone, Health Care Financing Administration (July 19, 1989). It said in part, "Our records do not contain a survey of Charlotte Memorial Hospital."

81–82 *When* The Wall *. . . anecdotes":* David Burda, "JCAHO Dismisses Article," *Modern Healthcare* (October 21, 1988), p. 9.

82 *When families . . . "offensive":* Joe Calderone, "Doctors' Union Blasts Hospitals," *Newsday,* July 24, 1986, p. 17.

82 *Many hospitals . . . violations:* Author interviews.

82 *"That . . . volumes":* Interview.

83 *"There was . . . pharmacy":* *The Charlotte Mecklenburg Hospital Authority* v. *North Carolina Board of Pharmacy,* Case No. 89 CV 00731, Superior Court, Wake County.

84 *In 1990 . . . standards:* The deaths occurred at Bryan Memorial Hospital in Lincoln. For more information about the incident, see "FDA:

Warning Flags Should Have Alerted Bryan to Solution," *Evening Journal* (October 5, 1990), p. A1.

84 *One study . . . warned:* Lesar, et al., "Medication Prescribing Errors in a Teaching Hospital," *JAMA* (May 2, 1990), p. 2329.

84 *"Our vision . . . suffering":* Charlotte-Mecklenburg Hospital Authority, 1988 Annual Report.

84 *The American . . . worse:* AHA news release (December 19, 1990).

CHAPTER 5: THE PEOPLE-PUSHERS

85 *Weekend nights . . . Stadium:* Interview with Howard University Hospital spokesman.

85 *The twin dormer . . . County:* Author's observation.

85 *Mrs. Dempsey had . . . changes:* Unless otherwise noted, Mrs. Dempsey provided all details about herself and her sister in an interview.

86 *More than . . . forgotten:* Rayford W. Logan, *Howard University: The First Hundred Years* (New York: New York University Press, 1969).

87 *On one . . . Jaguar:* Author's visit, January 17, 1991.

87 *Two years . . . cash:* Interview with Kevin E. Lofton, executive director of Howard University Hospital.

87 *Its inner-city . . . billed:* Ibid.

87 *When the . . . clinic:* "Pay Freeze Rejected by Nurses; Howard U. Workers Fear More Dismissals," *Washington Post* (June 7, 1990), p. D1.

88 *"It's very . . . understand":* Interview with Norman Brooks.

89 *"We are . . . own":* Interview with Jacqueline Tillman.

90 *"The pace . . . be":* Interview with Sandra Butcher.

90 *"It's not . . . longer":* Interview with Lynn Lewis.

91 *"Honestly . . . you":* Lewis's story is supported by another social worker who attended the meeting.

91 *"I tried . . . Psalm":* "Poor, Elderly Patients with No Place to Go Burden City Hospitals" (November 23, 1990), p. A1.

92 *"Patients . . . patient?":* Interview with Kathy C. Forrest.

93 *Friday admissions . . . weekend:* Walt Bogdanich, Thomas J. Quinn, "Too-Long Hospital Stays Cost Millions," Cleveland *Plain Dealer* (August 14, 1983), p. A1. Hospital administrators blamed doctors for these admitting practices.

93–94 *Moreover, despite . . . care:* "The Increased Needs of Patients in Nursing Homes and Patients Receiving Home Health Care," *New England Journal of Medicine* (January 4, 1990), p. 21.

94 *Among many . . . worsening: Hospitals* (February 5, 1990), p. 14.

94 *These patients . . . hospitals:* "Medicare Curbs Aren't Harmful, Researchers Say," *Wall Street Journal* (October 17, 1990), p. B1.

94 *One day . . . care:* Transcript of the meeting, held May 1, 1987; provided by New York Statewide Senior Action Council Inc.

95 *"Very often . . . compliance":* Interview with Bonnie Ray.

95 *Almost two years . . . years:* Interview with John Cremo of Senior Action Council.

95–96 *"Some hospitals . . . caseloads":* Interview with Susan Haikalas.

96 *But since public . . . safe:* "Limited State Efforts to Assure Quality of Care Outside Hospitals," GAO (January 1990).

96 *"Time and time . . . hospital":* Interview with Sandra Butcher.

97 *"We aren't talking . . . bleeding":* "Despite Federal Law, Hospitals Still Reject Sick Who Can't Pay" (November 29, 1988), p. A1.

97 *One congressional . . . hospitals:* Health letter, Public Citizen Health Research Group (May 1991), p. 1.

97 *Even when . . . die there: American Medical News* (January 28, 1991), p. 2.

97 "We are talking . . . bad": Interview with Gerard Anderson.

PART II: THE NEW ETHICS

CHAPTER 6: ON THE THRESHOLD

101 Much of Inspector General Kusserow's background is from a lengthy interview with him and from material provided by his office.

101 *"Richard . . . Schweiker":* This is Kusserow's recollection of his conversation with Newhall.

103 *"We tried . . . Office:* For a superb analysis of the harm that came from the overzealous cutting of management and oversight budgets in government, see Jeff Gerth, "Regulators Say 80's Budget Cuts May Cost U.S. Billions in 1990's," *New York Times* (December 19, 1989), p. A1.

103 *"I make . . . barked:* Kusserow speech (New Orleans, May 1988).

103–4 *When doctors . . . bipeds":* Interview, *Internist* (January 1987), p. 26.

104 *"If I'm . . . me":* Interview, *Medical World News* (April 27, 1987), p. 53.

104 *"I'm no . . . you":* Kusserow speech, published in *Caring* (June 1985).

104 *Kusserow . . . motivation":* "Report on the Inspector General of the United States Department of Health and Human Services" (November 1990), p. 3.

104–5 *In June . . .* Medicine: Donald W. Simborg, M.D., "DRG Creep, A New Hospital-Acquired Disease" (June 25, 1981), p. 1602.

105–7 All quotes from Simborg, except those from *The New England Journal of Medicine,* are from an interview with him. The interview also provided details on his professional life.

106 *But with . . . inspired:* "Comments on a Health Care Financing Admin-

istration Regional Office Report on New Jersey's Diagnostic Related Group Prospective Reimbursement Experiment," letter from U.S. General Accounting Office to Sen. John Heinz (June 15, 1983).

108 The Richmond Heights Hospital story was first reported in Walt Bogdanich and Thomas J. Quinn, "Trustee Deals Cost Hospital," Cleveland *Plain Dealer* (December 18, 1983), p. 1.

109 *One Las Vegas . . . itself:* "Hospital Links with Related Firms Can Conceal Unreasonable Costs and Increase Administrative Burden, Thus Inflating Health Program Expenditures," GAO (January 19, 1983), p. ii.

CHAPTER 7: BURIED SECRETS

111 The story of this GAO investigation is based largely on what are called GAO workpapers. These documents are particularly enlightening because they were prepared by GAO employees as a contemporaneous record of their inquiry. To augment the documents, the author also interviewed the chief GAO investigators, Daniel R. Garcia and Ken Brake, along with their supervisor, Thomas G. Dowdal. In some instances, brief conversations are reconstructed from notes taken by GAO investigators.

112 *As he . . . history:* Garcia said it was one of the biggest GAO "findings" in its history.

112 *Fortunately for . . . examinations:* Garcia interview.

113 *To gauge the . . . regions:* "Need to Eliminate Payments for Unnecessary Hospital Ancillary Services," GAO (September 30, 1983).

113 *Dowdal later . . . rates:* "Excessive Respiratory Therapy Cost and Utilization Data Used in Setting Medicare's Prospective Payment Rates," GAO (September 28, 1984); "Medicare's Policies and Prospective Payment Rates for Cardiac Pacemaker Surgeries Need Review and Revision," GAO (February 26, 1985); "Past Overuse of Intensive Care Services Inflates Hospital Payments," GAO (March 7, 1986).

113 *In 1980 . . . cost reports:* "Evaluation of the Health Care Financing Administration's Proposed Home Health Care Reimbursement Limits," GAO letter to Rep. Sam Gibbons (May 8, 1980).

115 *"You'll never . . . mistake":* Brake's recollection of the conversation.

116 *"[Auditors] go back . . . investigators:* Laura Miller, "Overcharges to Medicare Found in Texas," *Dallas Morning News* (June 2, 1985), p. 1A.

119 *If accountants "had . . . angrily:* Tuma would later say in an interview that his comments were either taken out of context or inaccurate. He said Blue Cross hadn't used subcontractors since 1973. His statements are directly contradicted by GAO workpapers. Workpaper page numbers BA-11 through BA-19 are a record of an interview that three GAO staffers had with Tuma on January 15, 1985. In those papers, Tuma is recorded as explaining how he went about hiring subcontractors to

help his staff perform the audits. Page BA-13, for example, states, "California Blue Cross used a total of 6 subcontractors to assist with the base year audits. Mr. Tuma explained that he selected national, regional, and local firms in order to avoid accusations of favortism [sic]." Each page of the summary is signed by the GAO staffer who prepared it, and initialed by Garcia, indicating that he had reviewed its contents for accuracy.

119 *"I'm sure . . . suppose":* Miller, "Overcharges to Medicare found in Texas."

120 *One reason . . . investigators:* Olenick said through a spokesman that it is difficult to confirm or deny quotes from conversations that took place so long ago. Olenick also told the GAO that capital costs were included partly because HCFA had little time to implement DRGs.

121 *The AMA's . . . hospitals:* Details about the Paracelsus investigation are from "Fact Sheet on the Paracelsus Investigation," Office of the Inspector General, Department of Health and Human Services (n.d.).

122 *By decade's end . . . 1980s:* Inspector General's Office.

123 *"Dan, I've . . . said:* Garcia's recollection of his conversation with Dowdal.

125 *At 10:05 . . . announced:* Stark hearing transcripts.

126 *By 1984 . . . vote: Politics in America* 100th Cong. (Washington, D.C.: CQ Press, 1987), pp. 117–118.

127 *A freeze would . . . industry":* Miller, "Overcharges to Medicare."

128 *A clearly . . . bedpan":* Spencer Rich, "Medicare Is Said to Be Saving on Bookkeeping, Losing in Overpayments," *Washington Post* (June 15, 1990), p. A23.

CHAPTER 8: KEYS TO THE KINGDOM

129 *"Congress has . . . said:* This is Brooks's recollection of her conversation with Nicholson. Both were interviewed.

130 *Upon a patient's . . . payment:* Health Data Institute, "National DRG Validation Study" (September 1987), p. 7.

131 *It wasn't . . . either:* Brooks interview.

131 *Not surprisingly . . . bungling:* Interviews with six present and former employees of the Office of the Inspector General of HHS.

131 *Strokes surfaced . . . abuse:* Brooks interview and HHS Inspector General, "Semiannual Report to the Congress, October 1, 1987– March 31, 1988," p. 40.

132 *The final . . . problem:* Brooks interview.

132 *"Suddenly those . . . staff":* Interview, *Journal of AMRA* (March 1986), p. 25.

133–34 *"We've got . . . on this":* Brooks's recollection of the conversation.

134 *When Kusserow and . . . oh my"*: Ibid.

135 *"[But] there . . . mission"*: Kusserow speech (New Orleans, May 1988).

135 *Kusserow's concern . . . abusers:* "Comments on a Health Care Financing Administration Regional Office Report on New Jersey's Diagnostic Related Group Prospective Reimbursement Experiment," GAO letter to Sen. Heinz (June 15, 1983).

136 *"I was told . . . point"*: Kusserow interview.

136 *"Some doctors . . . said: Journal of AMRA,* p. 25.

136 *One of . . . Carson's:* Simmons's recollection of the restaurant discussion.

137 *So began his . . . 1980s:* HHS Office of the Inspector General.

137 *They eventually . . . room:* Interview with IG investigators.

139 *"I am surprised . . . percent"*: Robert Pear, "Twenty Percent of Claims for Medicare Termed Faulty," *New York Times* (February 11, 1988), p. A1.

139 *"[T]he spanking . . . coding"*: Editorial, *Modern Healthcare* (February 26, 1988), p. 22.

139 *At no time . . . creep:* No one interviewed in the Inspector General's Office could recall an instance.

139 *Whether he . . . 1988:* HHS Office of the Inspector General.

139 *Apart from . . . organizations:* Ibid.

CHAPTER 9: SACRED HEART

140 *At 7:45 A.M. . . . California:* Interview with Covington.

140–41 *Midway between . . . named):* Author's observations, and Eugene L. Menefee and Fred A. Dodge, *History of Tulare and Kings Counties* (Los Angeles: Historic Record Company, 1913).

141 *"Sister Angela . . . surgery"*: Committee minutes, Department Directors' Meeting (August 18, 1987).

141 *"The organizational . . . unknown"*: Facility Assessment Survey (May 27, 1987), pp. 1–2.

142 *Not only . . . industry:* Connie Siffring, assistant administrator, Fresno Community Hospital, reference letter, December 30, 1986.

142 *"She is . . . trendsetter"*: Ibid.

142 *Covington's limited . . . past:* Covington interview.

142–43 *On these nights . . . courage:* Interview with Covington's husband, Stanley Sidicane.

143–44 *Although sharing . . . hospitals:* American Hospital Association, *AHA Guide,* 1987 edition, p. B13

144 *"What are . . . office"*: Covington's recollection of the conversation.

144 *"He only had . . . over":* Interview with Mona Andres.

145 *"I don't . . . anymore":* Ibid.

145 *Later, in 1982 . . . found: Ramona Andres* v. *Sacred Heart Hospital and Wallace Flemming,* Case No. 32490, Superior Court of California, County of Kings, Second Amended Complaint, filed September 20, 1982.

145 *In January . . . question":* Catholic Health Corporation, "Facility Assessment Survey," reviewer Jane E. Poe (May 27, 1987).

146 *Instead of . . . patient: United States of America, ex rel. Janet M. Covington and Stanley H. Sidicane,* v. *Sisters of the Third Order, et al.,* Civil Action No. 87-632 EDP, United States District Court, Eastern District of California. Also, depositions from coders and others affiliated with Sacred Heart Hospital that were taken in connection with *Janet Covington Sidicane et al.,* v. *Sisters of the Third Order et al.,* Case No. 374447-1, Superior Court, State of California, County of Fresno. Sharon K. Flores, a coder, said multiple attestations, usually two, were prepared only a small percentage of the time (Flores deposition). Jody Willhite, also a coder, said it happened 5 percent of the time (Willhite deposition). Mary Quilty, who sometimes worked with the coders, estimated that multiple attestations were prepared in up to 10 percent of the cases (Quilty deposition). All three denied that Sacred Heart at any time tried to defraud the Medicare program.

147 *"I would take . . . trash":* Quilty deposition.

147 *"There was . . . department":* Margaret Meyer deposition.

147 *In May . . . diagnoses:* Deposition of Kaye Mickelson, senior vice president, western region, Catholic Health Corporation.

147 *Moreover . . . Covington:* Covington's allegation is backed by Mario Rocha, Sacred Heart's director of finance, who said he was told of the overpayments early in 1984 (Rocha deposition).

148 *Blue Cross . . . the problem:* Interview with Michael Chee, spokesman, Blue Cross of California, Woodland Hills, California.

148 *"I need . . . stuff":* Covington's recollection of conversation.

149 *And once . . . room: Sidicane* v. *Sisters,* amended complaint, p. 17, Case No. 374447-1.

150 *"My daughter . . . out' ":* Quilty deposition.

150–55 Wybaillie provided details about his background.

151 *"They are . . . itself":* Covington's recollection of conversation.

152 *The IG's top . . . began:* Interviews with four IG employees.

153 *Sacred Heart . . . mistakes:* Interviews with two lawyers representing Sacred Heart.

153–54 *In truth . . . hospitals:* Interviews with IG officials.

154 *With Wybaillie . . . witnesses:* Covington said IG investigators told her this. Her account is supported by a government investigator who requested anonymity.

154 *Then . . . reimbursements:* Chee interview. The IG had earlier criticized an insurance company serving as a Medicare administrator (known formally as fiscal intermediary) for failing to collect interest on other Medicare overpayments. IG, "Semiannual Report to the Congress, April 1, 1987–September 30, 1987, p. 36.

154 *Moreover, Medicare's . . . either:* July 6, 1988, letter from Joseph Tuma, Director of Provider Audit for Blue Cross of California, to HHS.

155 *"The hospital . . . manipulation":* "Special Report," *Medicine & Health* (August 28, 1984).

156 *When Blue Cross . . . overcharges:* "Health Beat," Blue Cross and Blue Shield Association (February 1991).

156 *Many hospitals . . . Orlando:* "Hearing on Health Care Fraud and Revenue Recovery Firms," Permanent Subcommittee on Investigations (June 20, 1990).

CHAPTER 10: CANDY FROM STRANGERS

160 *By 1987 . . . world:* Rochelle Jones, *The Supermeds: How the Big Business of Medicine Is Endangering Our Health Care* (New York: Charles Scribner's Sons, 1988), p. 42.

160 *"We peaked . . . something":* Gandy deposition, *Monroe* v. *HCA.* All Gandy quotes are from this deposition.

161 *"Pat . . . St. Francis":* Gandy deposition.

161 Joyner quotes are from two sources: an interview and his deposition taken in *Monroe Medical Clinic, Inc.* v. *Hospital Corporation of America, et al.,* Case No. 87-851, Fourth Judicial District Court, Parish of Ouachita, State of Louisiana. HCA has declined to be interviewed about matters raised in this pending lawsuit, which is scheduled for trial in August 1991.

162–63 *"Boy, this . . . bury them":* Joyner's recollection of conversation.

163 *"Admit patients . . . me":* Gandy admits sending the note.

164 *"This is . . . people":* Interview.

164 *"Pat Gandy . . . wives":* All Keller quotes are from an interview.

165 *Reynolds told . . . seemed":* Joyner deposition. Reynolds declined to be interviewed.

165 *"I need . . . word":* Keller's recollection of conversation.

166 *Reynolds later . . . hospital:* Reynolds deposition, *Monroe* v. *HCA.* Reynolds also said that he never approached doctors to relocate their practices; they always approached him, either directly or indirectly, he said.

166 *Reynolds . . . anyone:* Reynolds deposition.

166 *Undaunted . . . clinic:* Reynolds, in his deposition, acknowledges

making the offer. "I'm sure I probably said at that point whatever type of construction arrangements for a new building had been made for North Louisiana Clinic, HCA would probably have an interest in doing that for you also."

166 *"We'll take care . . . back":* All of Wolff's statements are from his deposition, *Monroe* v. *HCA.* Reynolds also said in his deposition that he had persuaded a pediatrician to relocate her practice next to North Monroe by paying her mortgage on her old building, a deal similar to the one given to North Louisiana Clinic.

167 *David Glover . . . years:* Glover deposition, *Monroe* v. *HCA.*

167 *Reynolds said . . . $190,000:* Armstrong, in an interview, said he believes that HCA gave him a $60,000 lump sum payment to help defray the cost of his move. He said HCA also paid him a $5,000 monthly subsidy on a commercial building he owned. Even before the payments, Armstrong said, he had become "disenchanted" with St. Francis. He pointed out that St. Francis had denied his request to allow fathers into the c-section birthing room. "A nurse told me that my leaving got more done at St. Francis than had ever been done."

167 *"We want . . . for this":* This quote and others involving the *CHEST* controversy are based on Joyner's recollection of his conversation with Reynolds. Reynolds declined to be interviewed, and his deposition did not address Joyner's accusations.

168 *Although not . . . payments:* Reynolds deposition. In that deposition, he was asked, "Why did you decide to pay them the money? Just to keep them happy?" Reynolds answered, "Basically."

169 *And what were . . . needed?:* One study found that doctors working for a health clinic chain ordered far more lab tests when they got paid bonuses to increase their clinics' revenues. Ron Winslow, "Physicians Offered Incentives at Clinics Prescribed Far More Lab Tests, X-Rays," *Wall Street Journal* (April 12, 1990), p. B4. For other studies and background on this topic, see Michael Waldholz and Walt Bogdanich, "Doctor-Owned Labs Earn Lavish Profits in a Captive Market," *Wall Street Journal* (March 1, 1989), p.A1.

169 *"How should . . . interests?":* Jones's recollection of a conversation with his father. Jones's comments are from his depositions and interviews.

170 *Then I . . . administrator":* Reynolds said Jones never complained to him about the hospital making payments to doctors.

173 *Apart from some . . . decisions:* Many details about Gary Jones are from an interview and his deposition, taken in *Monroe Medical Clinic* v. *Kerry L. Anders and Patrick Gary Jones,* Case No. 86-3410, Fourth Judicial District Court, Parish of Ouachita, State of Louisiana. Anders declined to be interviewed.

173 *According to Henry's . . . patient list:* Grubbs deposition, *Monroe Medical Center* v. *Anders.*

174 *North Monroe also . . . brother:* "Physician Income Guaranty Agreement" between North Monroe Community Hospital and Patrick Gary Jones, M.D. Also, "Contract for Construction and Sale of Medical Office Building," HCA Realty Inc. and Jones and Anders.

175 *The Ouachita (Parish) . . . committee:* Letter from Priscilla Perry, M.D., president, Ouachita Medical Society, to Dr. Jones (April 27, 1989).

175–76 *Even Henry's . . . so on:* Details of payments are from Glover deposition, *Monroe v. HCA.*

176 *As the list . . . against:* Ronstrum's comments are from an interview.

CHAPTER 11: CAVEAT EMPTOR

177 *The tiny, Swiss . . . sneaky:* Interview with Nagra salesmen.

177 *In his eight . . . Nagra:* Unless otherwise noted, the descriptions of Kane's activities are from a transcript of his testimony in *United States of America* v. *Russell Furth,* Case No. CR H-85-271, United States District Court for the Southern District of Texas, Houston Division.

177 *This posed . . . correctly:* Interview with Linda Lattimore, former assistant U.S. attorney, Houston, Texas.

177 *McShane wasn't . . . either:* Details of McShane's involvement in the investigation are mostly from his testimony, along with that of Dr. Michael Spinks and Russell Furth, *U.S.* v. *Furth.*

178 *Until now . . . criminality:* Interviews with employees of the HHS Inspector General's Office.

180 *One nonprofit . . . hospital:* KHOU-TV News, Houston (November 4–November 7, 1985).

180 *"I grabbed . . . it":* Walt Bogdanich and Michael Waldholz, "Hospitals That Need Patients Pay Bounties for Doctors' Referrals," *Wall Street Journal* (February 27, 1989), p. 1A. Bogdanich conducted the interview.

180 *The freewheeling . . . costly:* KHOU-TV reported that a study by 50 Houston corporations had found that local hospital patients pay 20 percent more than the national average (November 4, 1985).

181 *"I can admit . . . there":* Spinks testimony, *U.S.* v. *Furth.*

184 *In this atmosphere . . . contract:* Bogdanich and Waldholz, "Hospitals That Need Patients."

185 *Although 36 . . . violators:* HHS Inspector General, "Financial Arrangements Between Physicians and Health Care Businesses: State Laws and Regulations" (April 1989).

185 *Hospital officials . . . Doctors":* ABA Forum on Health Law, San Francisco, California (May 4–5, 1989).

185–86 *"CEOs are . . . record":* Hospitals (March 20, 1990), p. 77.

186 *Minneapolis lawyer . . . patients:* Fruth, in an interview, provided details of the bondholders' meeting.

186 *Lewisburg Community . . . staff: Alfredson* v. *Lewisburg,* Case No. 88-311-II, Court of Appeals of Tennessee, Nashville, Amicus Curiae Brief, American College of Radiology, on behalf of appellant, David Alfredson, M.D.

187 *In 1988 . . . there:* "Physician Partners Speed Cure of Ailing Hospital," *Hospitals* (November 5, 1989), p. 56. Dr. Dumenigo told *Hospitals* that he informs his patients of his investment. "I tell them, 'I have invested a little bit at Victoria. I am therefore in a position to solve whatever problems you bring to me about the care you receive there.' "

187 *By the late 1980s . . . payrolls:* Bogdanich and Waldholz, "Hospitals That Need Patients."

187 *"If you have . . . hospital":* Ibid.

187 *For example . . . physicians: United States of America* v. *Kensington Hospital et al.,* Case No. CV-90-5430, United States District Court for the Eastern District of Pennsylvania.

187 *"Physicians are . . . hospitals":* "Confessions of a Worried Doctor," *Yankee* (February 1986), p. 84.

187 *Unless . . . sold":* Waldholz and Bogdanich, "Doctor-Owned Labs Earn Lavish Profits in a Captive Market," *Wall Street Journal* (March 1, 1989), p. A1.

187–88 *In this legal . . . Michigan: Health First Inc. and BCN* v. *Bronson Methodist Hospital,* Case No. CV 89 1191, U.S. District Court, Western District of Michigan, Southern Division. James Falahee, Jr., general counsel for Bronson Healthcare Group, declined to comment on the lawsuit. For an excellent look at payments by HMOs to doctors, see Mark Lagerkvist, "The Dark Side of HMO Plans," *Asbury Park Press* (February 24, 1991), p. A1.

188 *Is it any . . . state?:* Ron Winslow, "Rival Operations Competitive Anomaly: Consumers Pay More in 2-Hospital Towns," *Wall Street Journal* (June 6, 1990), p. A1.

188–89 *The Reagan . . . Office:* Jeff Gerth, "Regulators say 80's Budget Cuts May Cost U.S. Billions in 1990's," *New York Times* (December 19, 1989), p. A1.

189 *Those placed . . . last:* "Special Consumer Survey Report" (February 1990).

PART III: ABSENT WATCHDOGS

CHAPTER 12: A GATHERING OF FELONS

193 *Yet this . . . veins:* State of Ohio ex rel. *White* v. *Leonard Faymore, et al.,* Case No. 87292-81, Court of Common Pleas, Lorain County, State of Ohio, Decision and Opinion of the Court, Judge Joseph F. Diver.

193 *An area . . . Ohio":* White v. *Faymore,* Written Closing Arguments, Gregory A. White, Prosecuting Attorney, Lorain County.

194 *Not only . . . job:* Interviews with Ohio Pharmacy Board investigators and various government investigative reports.

194 *During one . . . convictions:* White v. *Faymore.*

194 *"His ability . . . improve":* Walt Bogdanich, Walter Johns, Jr., "Investors Take Over Hospital; Doctors, Methods Under Fire," *Cleveland Press* (April 6, 1979), p. A1.

194 *Faymore . . . bags:* White interview

195 *Doctors who . . . patients:* Ohio State Medical Board, "Report and Recommendation in the Matter of George P. Gotsis, M.D." (1983).

196 *"Didn't have . . . person":* Ibid.

196 *Police, in . . . there:* The Journal (February 15, 1983), p. 1.

197 *"The minute . . . flaw":* Interview by author.

198 *Although eventually . . . murderer:* Bogdanich, Johns, "Investors Take Over Hospital."

201 *"I'd be willing . . . Faymore":* Conversation based on a government investigative report.

202 *Take, for example . . . doctors:* Details on the Ohio Medical Board are from a series of articles: Bogdanich, "The Weak Pulse of Medicine's Enforcer," Cleveland *Plain Dealer* (February 10–16, 1980), p. A1.

203 *It wasn't . . . change:* Bogdanich, Johns, "Investors Take Over Hospital."

204 *In this environment . . . job:* Letter to the Ohio Medical Board from Public Citizen (June 14, 1988).

204 *And in . . . planning:* Alma Kaufman, "Committee Tries to Set Up Group to Replace MHPC," Cleveland *Plain Dealer* (February 10, 1982), p. B1. Kaufman wrote, "Gov. James A. Rhodes was the first in the nation to accept federal permission to remove regional planning groups . . ."

CHAPTER 13: MIDNIGHT FIRE

205 *The hour was . . . manner:* The details of what occurred at this meeting are from American College of Surgeons, "The College's Role in Hospital Standardization," February 1981 bulletin.

206 *To be sure . . . Association:* For a detailed look at how the Joint Commission operates, see Bogdanich, "Prized by Hospitals, Accreditation Hides Perils Patients Face," *Wall Street Journal* (October 12, 1988), p. A1.

206 *Perhaps the . . . self-regulation:* James Roberts, Jack Coale, Robert Redman, "A History of the Joint Commission on Accreditation of Hospitals," *JAMA* (August 21, 1987), p. 936.

207 *About a . . . Queens:* Island Peer Review Organization Inc., "Focused Quality Review" (1988).

207 *Over the next . . . care:* Ibid.

207 *Apart from . . . alive:* Giuffre's longtime use of unlicensed and unqualified personnel was reported in a superb story by Robin Palley, "Giuffre: A 17-Year Epidemic of Violations," *Philadelphia Daily News* (March 24, 1988), p. 13.

207 *They called . . . "slaughterhouse":* Interview with William L. Vazquez, CEO, North Philadelphia Health System.

207 *In the mid-1970s . . . backgrounds:* Beth Birnbaum provided details about her background in an interview and in correspondence.

208 *"Patients were . . . fathers":* Interview with Ira Madin.

208 *On July 9 . . . station:* New York State Health Department, "Statement of Deficiencies" (survey date: July 9, 1987).

209 *Once, when his personal . . . day:* Unless otherwise noted, details about Dr. Giuffre are from interviews with officials who worked with him.

209 *John Travolta . . .* Blow Out: Interview with Anthony Stinson, who supervised the hospital's nonmedical functions.

209 *"The stars . . . that":* "James C. Giuffre Dies at 78," *Philadelphia Daily News* (April 27, 1990), p. 4.

210 *Then there . . . party:* Interview with hospital official who attended the party.

210 *"I had no . . . somebody":* Interview with the supervisor.

211 *At dinnertime . . . sandwich:* Stinson interview.

211 *For 17 . . . open:* Palley, "Giuffre: A 17-Year Epidemic."

212–13 *It cited . . . care:* Joint Commission inspection report.

213 *Had its accreditation . . . hospital:* Under federal law, an accredited hospital is deemed to be in compliance with Medicare's standards. Unaccredited hospitals must submit to a federal inspection if they

wish to receive Medicare reimbursements. It is virtually impossible for a hospital to survive any length of time without Medicare money.

213 *They could hardly . . . leg:* New York State Health Department, "Statement of Deficiencies" (survey date: January 25, 1988).

213 *In the final . . . care:* Island Peer Review Organization.

213 *At 8 A.M. . . . license:* Madin interview; Flushing, Madin's hospital, ultimately took over Parsons.

213–14 *At its fashionable . . . lightly:* The Joint Commission has since moved to the Chicago suburbs.

214 *Yes . . . week:* The Joint Commission said it voted to remove accreditation for Parsons on May 20, 1988. The commission blamed its tardiness on computer problems.

214 *According to . . . in two:* Susan FitzGerald and Steve Stecklow, "At Giuffre, Questions About Treatment and Deaths," *Philadelphia Inquirer* (April 24, 1988), p. A1.

215 *Three years . . . surgery:* Ibid.

215 *Pennsylvania health . . . inspectors:* Palley, "Giuffre Case Reveals Staff Shortage at Pa. Health Dept.," *Philadelphia Daily News* (March 25, 1988), p. 8.

215 *The Joint . . . perfect: Wall Street Journal* (October 12, 1988).

216 *The PRO subsequently . . . worse:* Testimony of Lynn J. Soffer, M.D., Public Citizen Health Research Group, Subcommittee, House Government Operations (April 4, 1989).

217 *"There's a . . . approach":* Ron Winslow, "Study Finds 4% of New York Patients in '84 Were Injured by Hospital Care," *Wall Street Journal* (February 7, 1991), p. B5.

217 *"I couldn't . . . go":* Vazquez interview.

CHAPTER 14: WAITING

221 *For that . . . read:* The American Society of Cytology recommends that no full-time Pap analyst should examine slides from more than 12,000 patients a year.

221 *Unfortunately . . . government: Robert C. Johnson v. Northern Virginia Doctors Hospital, et al.,* Case No. 56682, Circuit Court of Fairfax County, State of Virginia. Johnson accepted a settlement of $600,000. The hospital declined to comment. *The Wall Street Journal* first reported details of this case: Bogdanich, "Medical Labs, Trusted as Largely Error-Free, Are Far from Infallible" (February 2, 1987), p. A1.

221 *In the absence . . . time: Johnson v. Northern Virginia Doctors.*

222 *Other derelict . . . supervision:* Interviews conducted in 1987 with hospital officials and cancer screeners.

222 *A Los Angeles . . . lab:* Gary Webb, "Medical Test Labs: Scary Errors and Hardly Any Regulation," *San Jose Mercury News* (April 28, 1991), p. A1. Webb said in an interview that the state didn't move promptly to stop the hospital from testing.

222 *At 9 A.M. . . . Park:* Author's observation.

222–23 *Years ago . . . down:* Interview with Terrence S. Norwood, archivist, Cook County Hospital.

223 *The tour . . . history:* The author went along on the tour.

224 *Up on . . . away:* Author's observation.

224 *Several months . . . force:* Gilbert M. Gaul, "How Blood, the 'Gift of Life,' Became a Billion-Dollar Business," *Philadelphia Inquirer* (September 24, 1989), p. A1.

225 *And so it . . . necessary:* Details on Mendoza's hospital stay are from reports prepared by the Health Care Financing Administration, the Joint Commission on Accreditation of Healthcare Organizations, and the Cook County Medical Examiner's Office.

225 *Cook County was . . . group:* The College of American Pathologists said Cook County's blood bank operation has been accredited since 1981.

225–26 *Soon after . . . present:* Joint Commission.

226 *Exactly 26 . . . floor:* Interview with Augustine Mathews.

226 *"Possible . . . Misadventure":* Medical examiner's case report.

226 *The hospital . . . recalled:* Howard Wolinsky, "County Patient Gets Wrong Type of Blood, Dies," *Chicago Sun-Times* (May 19, 1988), p. 26.

226 *Meanwhile, as . . . quickly:* Memorandum written by Joint Commission official Donald W. Avant, for internal circulation at the Joint Commission (March 16, 1989). This document was obtained through sources at the commission.

227 *"Housekeeping in . . . trained":* Ibid.

227 *"It consistently . . . hospitals":* Dr. Soffer no longer works for the Health Research Group.

228 *If this . . . worst:* The Joint Commission would finally pull Cook County's accreditation early in 1991. "JCAHO Withdraws Accreditation of Cook County Hospital," *Modern Healthcare* (January 28, 1991), p. 8.

228 *It also . . . hospitals:* These are main laboratories. CAP also accredits smaller, specialized-function labs.

229 *Poor lab . . . CAP-accredited:* Joint Commission statistics. These hospitals were only in partial or minimal compliance with Joint Commission standards.

229 *"These programs . . . operate":* Testimony, Subcommittee on Oversight of Government Management (March 23, 1988).

230 *In late 1988 . . . lab:* Robin Schatz, "Health Department Unit Often

Goes Undercover to Nab Unlicensed Clinics," *Newsday* (November 27, 1989), business section, p. 1.

230 *Its president . . . deep end:* Interview, *Internist* (August 1989), p. 19. The rest of the quote, picking up with the words "deep end": ". . . with a piece of legislation for which the Health Care Financing Administration virtually does not know how to write regulations."

231 *"Women are . . . ago":* "Senators Hit HCFA Delay on Issuing Lab Standards," *American Medical News* (March 23–30, 1990), p. 1.

231 *Some 60,000 . . . rules:* "Physician Outcry over Labs Heard in Washington," *American Medical News* (December 14, 1990), p. 19.

231 *This enormously . . . organ:* Associated Press (October 1990).

CHAPTER 15: DEAR ANN LANDERS:

233 *One Michigan . . . rationalized":* "Power Shifts Lead to Moral Twilight Zones," *Hospital Ethics* (January/February 1989), p. 1. Fleck is associated with the Center for Ethics and Humanities at Michigan State University.

234 *Soon after . . . capital:* Column by Peter W. Stauffer, "Anonymous Charges in Landers Column Unfair to Stormont," *Topeka Capital-Journal* (April 30, 1989), p. 5G.

234 *Its corporate . . . services:* Interview with John Glassman, vice president, Stormont-Vail.

234 *Stormont-Vail, no . . . employers:* Ibid.

235 *A friendly . . . inquiries":* Internal documents prepared by Stormont-Vail.

235 *Meanwhile, more . . . observed:* Stauffer column.

235 *The bad . . . officer:* Stormont-Vail internal documents.

236 *Topekans owned . . . for it:* Stormont-Vail Centennial Edition, 1984–1985, and "Finance a Key to Health Care," *Topeka Capital-Journal* (July 9, 1989). Most of the background that follows on Stormont-Vail is from the Centennial Edition.

236 *Hospitals quickly . . . construction:* Paul Starr, *The Social Transformation of American Medicine* (New York: Basic Books, 1982), p. 349.

236 *Stormont-Vail . . . director:* Centennial Edition.

236 *Stormont-Vail went . . . financing:* The Centennial Edition stated, "Building plans called for $1.8 million to be paid by the city and $1.2 million by Federal funds," p. 41.

237 *Some disturbing . . . public: Canadian Medical Association Journal* (Ottawa, Ontario) (May 1, 1989), p. 1081.

238 *Aggressive coverage . . . said:* Goldsmith, "Viewpoint," *Modern Healthcare* (June 23, 1989), p. 45.

239 *"They said . . . pay":* Interview with Linda Quick.

239 *"Look at . . . yourself":* Interview with Gloria O'Dell.

239 *The* Capital-Journal*'s . . . 1980s:* The news articles and dates mentioned in this paragraph and the following paragraph were supplied by Stormont-Vail.

239 *The hospital . . . agencies:* The request for these reports was made by the author.

240 *Weeks later . . . headlines:* The headlines quoted here are from a reprint of articles published by the *Capital-Journal.*

240 *Not only was . . . board:* Centennial Edition, pp. 2, 70.

240 *One publisher . . . hospital:* "ACOG Program Reviews OB-GYN Departments," *American Medical News* (June 23–30, 1989), p. 8.

240 *John Stauffer . . . wore:* John Stauffer said in an interview that he was happy with the way his paper has covered Stormont-Vail. He said reporters shouldn't be allowed to cover hospital board meetings, because the hospital is "a private corporation."

241 *Why the . . . poorly:* The $241,000 figure covers 1986 and 1987. All figures in this paragraph are from 1986 and 1987 IRS Forms 990, Return of Organization Exempt from Income Tax. Their respective fiscal years ended September 30, 1987, and September 30, 1988. The hospital said the $69,275 was spent on direct mail solicitations.

241 *Why the hospital . . . 1988:* The $210,000 figure is from 1987 Form 990, fiscal year ending September 30, 1988. Comparative figures are contained in a May 1989 survey by TPF&C, a Towers Perrin company. New York's figure is from New York City's Health and Hospital Corporation. The hospital said its board, in setting executive salaries, was merely following the recommendations of an outside consulting firm. The hospital also said the salaries were not out of line with the industry norm.

241 *Both did . . . underused:* John Glassman, in an interview, said that in 1988, Stormont-Vail had done about 180 open-heart operations and St. Francis about 150. According to Cleveland Clinic, some organizations say an open-heart unit should perform 200 to 300 operations a year.

241 *About a month . . . filling: Vital Signs* (June 1, 1989), a Stormont-Vail employee newsletter. The jobs were listed under the section "Positions Available at S-V."

242 *"It was . . . story":* Interview with Clarence Pennington.

245 *"It's cost . . . it":* Interview with Wayne Moore.

CHAPTER 16: LESSONS FROM THE GRAVE

246 *Police sergeant . . . pleasant:* Interview with Robert Edgar.

247 *One federal . . . ignored:* Interview with Dr. Jeffrey J. Sacks, Centers for Disease Control.

247–48 *It all began . . . Department: State of Maryland* v. *Jane Frances Bolding,* Case No. 86-1757, Prince George's County Circuit Court. Opinion and Order of Court (January 25, 1988).

248 *The evidence thus . . . time: Maryland* v. *Bolding,* Opinion and Order of Court, June 21, 1988.

249 *Even the hospital . . . fluid:* Ibid.

249 *Shortly after noon . . . it out: Maryland* v. *Bolding,* Opinion and Order.

250 *"A lot of . . . stake":* Edgar interview. Complaints by Edgar and Hatfield that the local medical establishment was reluctant to investigate itself were also voiced by another key investigator, who requested anonymity.

250 *David Hatfield . . . in:* Interview with David Hatfield. He has since retired and lives in Kentucky.

251 *"The epidemiologist . . . random": Maryland* v. *Bolding,* testimony of Dr. Sacks (June 6, 1988). Unless otherwise noted, quotes from Dr. Sacks and descriptions of his activities are from his testimony on June 6 and June 7, 1988, and from an article coauthored by Sacks, "A Nurse-Associated Epidemic of Cardiac Arrests in an Intensive Care Unit," *JAMA* (February 5, 1988), p. 689.

252 *The idea . . . Hatfield:* Edgar and Hatfield interviews.

254 *"[On] the evening . . . earth":* Sacks testimony, trial transcript, p. 120.

255 *"Such conferences . . . forests":* Sacks interview.

255 *On July . . . patients:* Gregory R. Istre, Tracy L. Gustafson, Roy C. Baron, Deborah L. Martin, and James P. Orlowski, "A Mysterious Cluster of Deaths and Cardiopulmonary Arrests in a Pediatric Intensive Care Unit," p. 205, and James W. Buehler, Lesbia F. Smith, Evelyn M. Wallace, Clark W. Heath, Jr., Robert Kusiak, and Joy L. Herndon, "Unexplained Deaths in a Children's Hospital," p. 211.

255 *That nurse . . . patients:* For an excellent look at the Jones murder case, see Peter Elkind, *The Death Shift* (New York: Viking, 1989).

255–56 *In February . . . patients":* "A Nurse-Associated Epidemic," p. 695.

256 *More recently . . . Island:* Associated Press (December 14, 1989).

256 *"My impression . . . much":* Sacks interview. He based this statement not on any scientific study but on conversations with various hospital personnel.

256 *At decade's . . . units:* "Hospital Accreditation Statistics, 1986–1988."

256 *In the aftermath . . . deaths:* Joshua Quittner, "Hospital Fined After Deaths Inquiry," *Newsday* (January 27, 1989), p. 40.

257 *The Texas . . . police:* Elkind, *The Death Shift.*

257 *"The unusually long . . . evidence":* Edward W. Morgan, "Report to the Prosecuting Attorney, Franklin County, Ohio, Regarding Incidents Related to . . . Dr. Michael J. Swango," p. 57.

257 *Dr. Swango later . . . fellow paramedics.* Associated Press (May 3, 1985).

257 *A top hospital . . . upset:* This story and others about Swango were written by Gary Webb and Mary Anne Sharkey. The hospital report-

edly told medical investigators looking into the Swango affair to leave the hospital because they were disrupting the hospital and interfering with patient care.

EPILOGUE: SHOWDOWN

259 *On September . . . earlier:* For more details on how the data bank works, and problems that delayed its implementation, see "National Health Practitioner Data Bank Has Not Been Well Managed," GAO (August 1990).

259 *Usually, however . . . them:* Interviews with state medical board investigators in various states.

260 *"They . . . us":* "Chrysler Challenges Quality of Medical Care in Wi.," *Hospitals* (September 20, 1989), p. 98.

260 *The society . . . turned:* Interview with Mark Adams, corporate counsel, State Medical Society of Wisconsin. Also, Dr. James Todd, executive vice president of the AMA, said in an interview that medical societies generally won't divulge disciplinary actions.

261 *The clinic . . . one:* Interviews with two clinic officials. Also, the clinic, in its IRS Form 990, indicated that it did business in Iraq.

261 *That many . . . machines:* According to the *Plain Dealer,* AmeriTrust Corporation chairman M. Brock Weir, in a 1982 letter to former Governor James A. Rhodes, warned, "Northeastern Ohio already supports one of the costlier medical establishments in the nation, and faces the ominous prospect of having health care as its only growth industry" (June 5, 1983), p. A26.

261–62 *When an outside . . . contents:* Thomas J. Quinn and Walt Bogdanich, "PD Probe Reveals Waste, Overuse in Area Hospitals," Cleveland *Plain Dealer* (June 5, 1983). p. A1. In ordering the destruction of the study, the hospital association said it was flawed.

262 *"These are . . . people":* The author worked with Quinn on this investigation and participated in many interviews with this source. All conversations involving this source are based on the author's recollection.

262 *Although perhaps . . . notes:* Sore Throat was a mocking reference to Watergate's Deep Throat.

262 *It would be . . . 1983:* Quinn and Bogdanich, "PD Probe Reveals Waste."

263 *When one . . . you:* Interview with corporate executive who sat in on the meeting.

263 *Like other . . . Sputnik:* McClure's background, along with his quotes, are from an interview.

264 *Only years later . . . profits:* There have been many newspaper investigations of poorly run HMOs, including ones by the Cleveland *Plain Dealer* and the *Sun-Sentinel* in Fort Lauderdale, Florida. Also see Alan L. Hillman, Mark V. Pauly, and Joseph J. Kerstein, "How Do Financial Incentives Affect Physicians' Clinical Decisions and the Financial Performance of Health Maintenance Organizations?" *New England Journal of Medicine* (July 13, 1989), p. 86.

265 *"I don't use . . . Cleveland":* Interview with Powell Woods.

266 *Thus it . . . Club:* The description of this meeting is based mostly on minutes of the meeting, supplemented by interviews with several people who attended.

267 *But he did . . . campaign:* Woods didn't specifically use the term "war chest," but that was his implication.

268 *The idea . . . Nestlé:* Both Flagg and Shaller were interviewed for this chapter.

269 *By then . . . care: Journal of Occupational Medicine* (March 1991), p. 301.

269 *Moreover, corporate . . . year:* Shaller interview.

270 *Earlier, when . . . hospitals:* Medical claims from Cleveland employers were compared to those of the 90,000 residents of Minnesota's Olmsted County, almost all of whom receive medical care from two sources: the Mayo Clinic, with its 800 or so salaried physicians, and the Olmsted Medical Group, with more than 50 physicians.

270 *"Let's see . . . again":* The exchange involving Price is based on interviews with people attending the meeting.

271 *"When we decided . . . losers' ":* Interview with C. Wayne Rice.

271 *Then, they . . . employees:* The name of the program is Greater Cleveland Health Quality Choice.

271 *"I don't . . . them":* From a question-and-answer session following a speech by Woods, Citizens League, Minneapolis, Minnesota (February 12, 1991).

272 The Washington Post . . . *1991:* February 26, 1991, p. A19.

272 *The American Hospital . . . public:* The American Hospital Association confirmed this fact, first reported in *The Washington Post.*

274 *They should . . . studies:* For a number of years now, HCFA has been releasing hospital mortality statistics. With some justification, the statistics have been criticized for, among other things, failing to render a true picture of the quality of care at certain institutions. Nevertheless, the reports can be used as a basis for asking questions.

Acknowledgments

The Wall Street Journal has been extraordinarily helpful to me in writing this book. Special thanks to Paul Steiger for his unwavering support, Barney Calame for his friendship and wise counsel, and, of course, Norman Pearlstine. Albert Hunt's hospitality in giving me a base of operations was more than I deserved.

My friends Hank Gilman, Jolie Solomon, and Rich Jaroslovsky made major contributions to this book, as did Michael Waldholz, from whom I've learned so much. Others who were there when I needed them include James Neff, Ken Paul, Margaret Engel, Kevin Salwen, Jeff Tannenbaum, Rick Tulsky, Barry Meier, Tom Petzinger, Tom Ricks, Ken Bacon, and Alan Otten. Over the years, no one has been a better friend to hospital patients than Dr. Sidney Wolfe. His work will always be an inspiration.

I was blessed with two of the ablest researchers any author could hope to find: Helaine Olen and Jeffrey Daeschner. I also want to thank my brother George, who has opened so many doors for me throughout my life. His suggestions were particularly helpful in shaping this book.

My decision to explore the murky world of hospitals really began with Jane Dystel, my peerless agent and friend. Among her many contributions was to put me in touch with Fred Hills, a superb editor and consummate professional. His manuscript editor, Burton Beals, was a delight. And Daphne Bien held everything together.

The biggest contributor to this project was my wife, Stephanie, the best reporter I know. I can never thank her enough for her editing, research, and overall support. And last but not least, my son, Nicholas, did the impossible—he kept me smiling and happy through the most difficult of times. Mercifully, he shows no sign yet of becoming a Cleveland Indians fan. One in the family is more than enough.

Index

abortion, 230
admissions, 200, 246
advertising, 66, 160, 164–65, 211, 233
Agrillo, Mary, 95
Ahmed, Naymat, 36
AIDS, 22, 23, 24, 222, 225, 229
Albert Einstein Medical Center (Philadelphia, Pa.), 84
alcohol abuse, 33, 194
All Care Nursing Service, 38, 41, 42–60
  documents forged at, 53–55, 56
  investigations of, 53–60
almshouses, 197
Amatayakul, Margret, 147
ambulance crews, 23, 199
American College of Radiology, 186
American College of Surgeons, 205
American Healthcare Management, 179, 180, 181
American Hospital Association (AHA), 63, 84, 126, 139, 189, 206, 216, 272
American Journal of Nursing, 61
American Medical Association, (AMA), 10, 104, 121, 125–26, 136, 189, 204, 206, 216, 228, 231

American Medical News, 240
American Medical Record Association, 147, 152
Amick, William, 67, 68–69, 71, 77, 78, 79, 81, 82
amputation, 199
analysts, laboratory, 220–22, 228, 231
Anders, Kerry, 173–74
Anderson, Gerard, 97
Andres, Mona, 144–45
Andrulis, Dennis, 22
anemia, 224
anesthesiologists, 72, 79
Angelo, Richard, 256
antibiotics, 36
Arishita, Michael, 151
Arkansas Democrat, 37
Armstrong, Ralph, 166–67
Arrington, Lucille, 85–86, 88–89, 91, 93
Arthur D. Little, 29, 63
Associated Press, 242, 245
attorneys, 97, 150, 178, 250
  legal system and, 178, 179–84
  money spent on, 245
auditors, audits, 111
  cheating undetected and ignored by, 120, 121, 155–56
  coding abuses by, 155–56
  distracting of, 116–17

auditors, audits *(cont.)*
  incomplete records provided
    in, 117, 151–52
  training of, 118, 119, 124
Aussler, Sharon, 36–38, 41,
    42–45, 46–47, 48–50,
    55–56, 59–60
autopsies, 18, 19, 220
  substances undetectable in,
    248, 249

babies, 21, 22, 26, 89
Bacon, Ken, 91
Bailey, Chandler, 39
Baker & Hostetler, 244
Bakker, Jim and Tammy, 81
balloon angioplasty, 106, 132
barbiturates, 194
Bassett, Lisa, 56
Beaver, J. T. Eager, 126
Beckler, Richard, 179
beds:
  empty, 136, 159, 160, 178, 181,
    185, 186, 262
  patient falls from, 61
Bellevue Hospital Center (New
    York, N.Y.), 13–15, 114
  psychiatric care at, 14, 17, 18,
    21
  violence in, 14–15, 19–22
Bethesda Hospital (Boynton
    Beach, Fla.), 43, 44, 51–52
bile duct procedure, 134
biopsies, breast, 14
Birnbaum, Beth, 207–8
blood, 228
  cleaning of, 215
  storage of, 212, 224–25
blood banks, 72, 224–25
blood tests, 170, 225, 229
blood transfusions, 224–27
blood-typing, 225–27
Blue Cross and Blue Shield, 118,
    119, 121, 149, 153, 156,
    188, 263
Blutstein, Sheila, 22
Bly, Nellie, 17
Bolding, Jane, 249, 254–55
Booth, Charles, 119, 127
Boston Business Journal, 62

Bowen, Otis, 36
Bradford, Sue, 40
Brake, Ken, 114, 115–16, 123–24
breast biopsies, 14
breathing tubes, disposable, 227
Bromberg, Michael D., 126
Bronner, Sadie, 199–200
Bronson Methodist Hospital
    (Kalamazoo, Mich.),
    187–88
Brooks, Norman, 88, 89
Brooks, Patricia, 129–35, 137
brown-lung, 81
Brubaker, Sheila Ripley, 50–52,
    53–55, 59
burn victims, 224
Burt, James C., 204
Bush, George, 27, 84, 189
Butcher, Sandra, 90, 96
Buy Right, 264–71

California, University of, at San
    Francisco, 105
cancer, 176
  cervical, 219–22
  detection of, 220–22, 226
  lung, 167–68
cardiac catheterization, 96
cardioplegic solution, 67–68,
    78–79, 80, 84
cardiopulmonary resuscitation
    (CPR), 53, 255
Carolinas Heart Institute, 66, 67
Carter, Jimmy, 110, 272
Casula, Joseph S., 255
Cates, Dorothy, 26
Catholic Health Corporation,
    143–46, 156
Cawthorne, Ken, 74–78, 79–80,
    81, 82
Center for Medical Consumers,
    216
Center for Policy Studies, 264
Centers for Disease Control
    (CDC), 67, 139, 249–50,
    252, 254
Central Arkansas, University of,
    37
Central Intelligence Agency
    (CIA), 28, 102, 104

certificates of need, 171
certified nurses' aides (CNAs), 35,
    49, 53, 54, 62, 94, 156,
    200, 256
cervical cancer, 219–22
cesarean section, 273
Chapman, Thomas W., 28
Charity Hospital (New Orleans,
    La.), 228–29
Charlotte Memorial Hospital and
    Medical Center (Charlotte,
    N.C.), 65–72, 74–84
  hospital-induced deaths at,
    68–69, 70–72, 76–81,
    82–83
  pharmacy at, 71–72, 74–78,
    79–80, 82–83
  weekend surgery at, 71–72,
    80–81
Charlotte Observer, 70, 71, 81
Chase, Howard, 225, 239
chemical abuse centers, 88
chemotherapy, 219–20
CHEST, 167–68
chest pain, 94
Chicago Tribune, 188
cholera, 251
Christ's Hospital (Topeka, Kans.),
    236
Chrysler Corporation, 260
Clayton General Hospital
    (Riverdale, Ga.), 73
Cleveland Academy of Medicine,
    269, 270
Cleveland Clinic (Cleveland,
    Ohio), 72, 199, 261, 266,
    267
Cleveland Plain Dealer, 257,
    261–63, 266, 269
Cleveland Press, 198, 203
Clinical Laboratory Improvement
    Amendments of 1988, 222,
    230
clinics, 160, 165–66
cocaine, 24, 34, 72, 193, 194, 198
Codman, Ernest A., 205
Cohen, William, 222
Colella, Joseph, 248, 249
College of American Pathologists
    (CAP), 225, 228–29

colostomies, 61
Columbia Hospital Corporation,
    187
Combs, Doris, 199
community hospitals, 108, 200,
    243
computerized axial tomography
    (CAT) scan, 172, 181, 185
computers, 74, 137
  errors with, 113, 253–54
  Medicare exploited through,
    105–8, 115, 132–34, 144
Conference Board, 189
Congress, 24, 27, 66, 85, 94, 96,
    103, 104, 108, 111, 118,
    123–24, 125, 126, 128, 129,
    135, 187, 236
Connerton, Rose, 122
Constitution, U.S., 242
consultants, consulting, 134, 142,
    160, 166, 170, 261–62
  patient-buying disguised as,
    182
  from regulatory bodies, 212
consumerism, 10, 104, 202, 206,
    216, 220, 273–74
Cook County Hospital (Chicago,
    Ill.), 27, 36, 222–28
  blood transfusions at, 224–27
  unsanitary conditions at, 226,
    227
Cooper, E. Shannon, 225
coronary angioplasty, 106,
    132
coronary bypass surgery, 9,
    65–72, 76–81, 84, 87, 132,
    262
  cardioplegia induced in, 67–68
  on weekends, 71–72
corporations, 237, 241
  health benefits provided by,
    260, 268, 271, 272, 274
  physicians as owned by, 164,
    167–69, 170–71, 174, 175,
    176
  standardized quality demanded
    by, 260, 262–63, 264–71
Cosgrove, Delos "Toby," III, 72
Covington, Janet, 140–57
  settlement received by, 156–57

Covington, Janet *(cont.)*
    whistle-blower suit filed by,
        149–55, 156–57
crack abuse, 22, 24, 193
Creech, Jay, 247
critical-care units, 36
cystoscopy, 200
cytology, kitchen, 222
cytopathology, 18

Dallas Morning News, 127
Davis, Carolyne K., 133–34
D.C. General Hospital
        (Washington, D.C.), 22
death:
    hospital-induced, 23, 25, 81,
        213, 214, 217, 225–27
    rates of, 9–10, 27, 161, 213,
        261, 262, 269, 270, 273
    see also murder
Defense Department, 84, 127
de Guzman, Flor, 62
Delray Community Hospital
        (Delray Beach, Fla.), 40
Demerol, 33, 34
Dempsey, Veleria, 85, 86, 88, 91,
        92–93
deregulation, 103–4, 106, 108,
        135, 176, 185, 188, 204
Detroit Receiving Hospital
        (Detroit, Mich.), 27, 63
diagnostic-related groupings
        (DRGs), 88, 93, 97, 106–8,
        109–10, 113, 126
    administrative handling of,
        146–48
    base payment rates set for, 11,
        113–14, 119, 122–23, 127,
        128, 148
    hospitals favored by, 120, 127,
        139
    maximizing returns on, 115,
        120, 131–35, 136–39,
        144–57, 188, 262
    outdated classification of, 130,
        131
    physician attestation to, 136,
        146–58, 152
    primary vs. secondary

    diagnosis in, 106–7, 136,
        144, 152
    rushed passage of, 118, 135,
        137, 262
    splitting profits from, 121–22
    see also Medicare; prospective
        payment
Dickerman, Herbert, 229
dietitians, 26, 87, 89, 212, 227
Dilaudid, 193
DiMaggio, Joe, 209–10
discharge planners, 89–92, 198
    written plans provided by,
        95–96, 213
Doctors Hospital (now called
        Palm Beach Regional
        Hospital); (Lake Worth,
        Fla.), 54
donations, 117
Dowdal, Thomas G., 112–13, 123
Drake Memorial Hospital
        (Cincinnati, Ohio), 245
Drexel Burnham Lambert, 186
"DRG Creep: A New Hospital-
        Acquired Disease"
        (Simborg), 107, 138
drug addiction, 22, 24, 73, 259
drug-dealers, 86, 193
drugs, 21, 89, 207
    compounding and packaging
        of, 73, 76–79, 249
    dispensing of, 75, 193–95, 196,
        212–13, 217
    expiration of, 74, 212–13
    lethal doses of, 248–49, 253, 255
    mishandling of, 33, 34, 47, 61,
        79–80, 81–84, 233
    painkilling, 33, 220
    surgery vs., 214
    see also pharmacies,
        pharmacists
Dugger, Barbara, 34
Dumenigo, Fred, 187
Dunaj, William, 58, 60
Durbin, Richard, 15
Dyer, Gordon, 116–17

Easton Hospital (Easton, Pa.), 61
Edgar, Robert, 246–50, 253

Edwards, Edwin, 171
elderly patients:
  boarder, 89–90, 92, 93
  hospital bills of, 24, 189
  Medicare and, *see* Medicare
  mental condition of, 207–8
  nursing homes sought for,
    88–94
  premature discharging of, 22,
    89–92, 93–97
  profits gained from, 106,
    198–99
Elvis Presley Memorial Trauma
    Center (Memphis, Tenn.),
    61
emergency rooms (ERs), 14, 24,
    87, 174, 212, 213, 214,
    257
  overcrowding of, 188
  patient referrals from,
    172
epidemiology, 106, 251, 255–56
esophagus, 214
ethicists, medical, 171, 178,
    179–80, 186

families, 9, 69, 89, 90, 259,
    274
family practitioners, 171
Fantus, Bernard, 224–25
Faron, Peter E., 36, 38, 40
Faymore, Leonard F., 194–95,
    197–99, 201, 203
  addictive drugs dispensed by,
    193–95, 197, 198
  elderly patients seen by,
    198–200
Federal Bureau of Investigation
    (FBI), 28, 101–2
Fields, Larry, 209–10
First Amendment, 242, 243
First Amendment Award, 244–45
Flagg, Don, 268–69
Fleck, Leonard M., 233
Flemming, Wallace, 143–47, 150,
    154–55
  severance of, 143
  summaries reviewed by,
    147–48

Florida Board of Nursing, 56–58,
    59–60
Florida Hospital (Orlando, Fla.),
    156
Flushing Hospital (Flushing,
    N.Y.), 208
food supplements, 89
Ford, Susan, 238
Ford Motor Company, 196
Forrest, Kathy C., 92, 96
Fostoria City Hospital (Fostoria,
    Ohio), 242–45
Franklin General Hospital (Long
    Island, N.Y.), 230
Freedmen's Hospital
    (Washington, D.C.), 86,
    88
Fresno Community Hospital
    (Fresno, Calif.), 141, 142
Frist, Thomas, Sr., 162
Fruth, Terence M., 186
Fulbright & Jaworski, 179
fundraising foundations, 241
Furth, Russell, 178–84
  acquittal of, 184
  joint ventures suggested by,
    181–83

gallbladder surgery, 134, 176
Gandy, Pat, 160–65, 170
gangrene, 199
Garcia, Daniel R., 111–28
  counterattack on, 127–28
  investigation conducted by,
    112–28
Garloch, Karen, 71, 81
gastrectomies, 214
gastrointestinal bleeding, 97
Gellman, Sidney, 230
General Accounting Office
    (GAO), 71, 103, 111–25,
    126–28, 189
  auditors for, 123–25
  "congressionals" received by,
    123–24, 125
  data collection in, 124–25
  Medicare investigated by,
    112–28
genetics tests, 222

Georgetown Hospital
(Washington, D.C.), 90
George Washington Hospital
(Washington, D.C.), 90,
96
geriatric rehab centers, 96
Gill, Sterling, 203
Girard Medical Center
(Philadelphia, Pa.), 217
Giuffre, James C., 209, 210–11,
215. See also James C.
Guiffre Medical Center
Glassman, John, 237
Glenwood Hospital (Monroe,
La.), 171–72
Goldsmith, Jeff, 238, 239
Good Samaritan Hospital (West
Islip, N.Y.), 256
Gotsis, George, 195–96, 197, 201,
202, 203
government, U.S.:
buck-passing by, 228
hospitals left unpunished by,
119–20, 139, 140, 145, 153,
154, 176, 178–79, 201, 203,
230, 272
indigent neglected by, 97, 110
self-protecting regulations
established by, 115, 131,
139; see also regulation,
regulatory bodies
unreliable records of, 121
Greater Cleveland Hospital
Association, 261–62, 269,
271
Greater Southeast Community
Hospital (Washington,
D.C.), 28
Green, Laura, 77–78
Greene, R. W., 26
Gruninger, Carl, 120
gynecologists, 221

Hagan, Mary Genevieve, 90
Haikalas, Susan, 96
Hamilton/KSA, 187
Harding, George, IV, 186
Harlem Hospital Center (New
York, N.Y.), 27, 62
Harper's Magazine, 15

Harvard Medical School, 25, 217
Harvey, Donald, 256
Hass, Don, 116
Hatfield, David, 250, 253
Health and Human Services
Department (HHS), 27, 28,
36, 61, 81, 94, 101–4, 131,
149, 177, 178, 187, 216,
272
inspector general (IG) of,
101–3, 117, 120, 121, 133,
137, 152, 154, 155
Medicare investigated by,
120–22, 130–39
Sacred Heart Hospital
investigated by, 149–55,
156–57
health care:
cost of, 22, 25, 188, 238, 241,
260, 261, 263, 264, 268–71,
272, 274
efficiency of, 264, 274
home, 40–41, 113, 185
national, 25, 86
quality of, 137, 161, 169, 176,
205–7, 240, 241, 260,
263–64, 267, 270–74
rationing of, 22
see also hospitals; medical
community
Health Care Financing
Administration (HCFA),
27, 84, 114, 119, 127, 131,
133, 137, 230–31
health maintenance organizations
(HMOs), 90, 187–88,
263–64
Health Research Group, 227
heart attacks, 9, 65, 72, 82, 97,
132, 138
in ICU, 248, 251, 253–54, 255
heartbeat:
disruption of, 248–49
irregular, 94, 207, 249
heart disease, 95
heart-lung machine, 65
heart medicine, 213
heart transplant, 69
Heckler, Margaret, 155
helicopter landing pads, 66

Hemet Valley Hospital
    (Hemet, Calif.), 26
hemorrhoid surgery, 95
Hennepin County Medical
    Society, 185
Henry, Nancy, 26
hepatitis, 225
heroin, 193, 194
Hiatt, Howard, 217
Hicks, Fred, Sr., 77
Hicks, Rosalind, 117
Hill-Burton program, 236
Hinnant, Kathryn, 13, 15–16,
    17–22, 28
Hoffa, Jimmy, 142–43, 200
Holland, Yolanda, 34
home health care, 40–41, 113,
    185
hospital bills, 26, 138
    increase in, 188, 238, 241, 263,
        268
    insured payment of, *see*
        insurance companies
    patient-buying and, 180
    prospective payment of, *see*
        prospective payment
Hospital Corporation of America
    (HCA), 160
    lump sums paid by, 162, 164,
        166, 167, 168, 171, 176
    patients solicited by, 161–76
    private records invaded by,
        173
    property purchased by, 162,
        172
hospital industry:
    advertising in, 66, 160, 164–65,
        211, 233
    changing values of, 35, 83, 88,
        89, 90, 97, 158–59, 233
    competition in, 27, 29, 90,
        158–59, 163, 168–69, 171,
        180, 185–86, 187, 204, 241,
        245, 271
    construction and building
        acquisition in, 24, 66, 84,
        141, 159, 171, 180, 223,
        233, 236–37
    corporations and, 260, 262–63,
        264–71

financial distress in, 18, 25–26,
    27, 28, 105–6, 110, 136,
    140, 159, 188, 227, 245
hospital-induced deaths as
    viewed by, 81
lobbying by, 84, 125–26,
    272
media coverage of, 233–34,
    235, 237–45, 266, 273
postwar, 236
self-regulation of, 104, 189,
    204, 205–18, 247
see also hospitals; medical
    community
hospitalizations:
    lengthy, 89–90, 92, 93, 262
    unnecessary, 152–53, 163–64
hospital management, 18, 197
    callousness of, 22, 29
    empty beds and, 136, 159, 160,
        178, 181, 185, 186
    entertainment perks and,
        108–10, 136, 233
    see also hospital staff
Hospital of the University of
    Pennsylvania
    (Philadelphia, Pa.), 92,
    96
hospitals:
    accountability of, 135–36,
        236–38, 240–45, 273
    accreditation of, 14, 74, 81, 82,
        203, 206, 211, 213–14,
        215–17, 229
    board meetings at, 237, 241,
        243–45
    Catholic, 163
    civic pride in, 208, 239, 260
    community, 108, 200, 243
    community relations with, 88,
        164–65, 208, 236–45, 260,
        261
    consultants to, 134, 142, 160,
        166, 170, 182, 212, 261–62,
        272
    cost disparities between, 260,
        261, 268–71
    cost reports filed by, 108–10,
        113, 114–19, 122–23, 124,
        127, 135–36, 188, 216

hospitals (cont.)
  death rates in, 9–10, 27, 161, 213,
      261, 262, 269, 270, 273
  entertainment perks provided
      by, 108–10, 136, 180
  hidden income of, 117
  infection control in, 14, 22, 27,
      63, 67, 195, 212, 227
  internal-review committees in,
      247
  legal obligations of, 70–71
  management of, see hospital
      management
  murder in, 19–22, 28, 245,
      246–57
  nursing home "buyers" in, 92
  overcrowding in, 13, 23, 24,
      188, 200
  patients in, see patients
  physician referrals to, 161, 169
  as private corporations, 237
  profits sought by, 24, 106, 116,
      126, 156, 181, 236–37
  psychiatric care in, 14, 17, 18, 21
  qualitative differences between,
      161, 169, 176, 187, 260,
      263–64, 267, 270–74
  regulators of, see regulation;
      regulatory bodies
  security in, 14–15, 18, 20, 21,
      23, 26, 247, 255–57
  staff of, see hospital staff
  supplies in, 13, 212
  teaching, 87, 156
  unnecessary admissions to, 200
  see hospital industry; medical
      community
hospital staff:
  background checks on, 256
  communicable diseases in, 53
  compressed work week of, 75
  meetings of, 200
  overtime worked by, 22, 61
  overworking of, 22, 25, 26, 35,
      36, 44, 60–62, 75, 96
  part-time, 71–72
  shortages of, 13, 14, 22, 24, 35,
      62, 75, 84, 188, 227,
      232–34, 256

  temporary, see temporary help
  see also specific staff positions
housekeepers, 26, 27, 87, 89, 227
House Ways and Means
    subcommittee on health,
    125–26
Housing and Urban
    Development Department,
    103
Howard University Hospital
    (Washington, D.C.), 85–93
  elderly patients discharged
      from, 89–90, 91–93
  historical mission of, 86–87
Hudson, Steve, 70, 72, 81, 82, 83
Hussein, Saddam, 261
hydrochloric acid solution, 82
hyper-al, 76, 80

Illinois Hospital Association, 126
infection control, 14, 22, 27, 63,
    67, 195, 212, 227
inflation, 188
injections, 198
inpatient rehabilitation, 185, 212
inspections, 206, 212, 213, 226
insurance companies, 54
  coding abuses and, 155–56
  complexities of, 26, 121
  DRGs and, see
      diagnostic-related
      groupings
  early discharge and, 90, 93
  government regulators and,
      118–19
  inexperienced auditors
      employed by, 119, 124
  premiums for, 260, 268, 269
  prospective payment by, see
      prospective payment
  see also hospital bills; Medicare
intensive-care units (ICUs), 25,
    36, 62, 113, 207, 213
  drugs kept in, 248–49
  heart attacks in, 248, 251,
      253–54, 255
  murder in, 247–56
Internal Revenue Service (IRS),
    150

International Classification of Diseases, 130
interns, 136
Interstudy, 263
intravenous (IV) lines, 24, 49, 68–69, 76, 78, 84, 253, 256

Jamaica Hospital (Queens, N.Y.), 26
James C. Giuffre Medical Center (Philadelphia, Pa.), 207
   celebrity patients at, 209–10
   closing of, 214–15
   Committee of 55 at, 211–12, 214, 215
   renovation of, 217–18
Jeffrey, Balfour S., 236
JFK Medical Center (Atlantis, Fla.), 46
Johns Hopkins University, 105
Johnson, Eric, 20
Johnson, Janice, 219–22, 229
Johnson, Robert, 219–22, 231
Joint Commission on Accreditation of Healthcare Organizations, 73, 81–82, 215–17, 223, 227, 229, 230, 256, 273
Joint Commission on Accreditation of Hospitals, 206, 208, 211, 212–13
joint ventures, 181–82, 185–87
Jones, Gary, 172–75
Jones, Genene, 255, 257
Jones, Henry, Jr., 169–76
   lawsuit filed by, 175–76
   ostracizing of, 174–75, 176
Journal of the American Medical Association (JAMA), 206–7, 255–56
Joyner, LeRoy, 159–64, 172
   article published by, 167–68
   HCA offer accepted by, 162–63
Justice Department, 153–54, 156, 179, 187, 250

Kane, Richard, 177–78
Keller, Cheryl, 164, 165
kidney dialysis machines, 69

kidney function tests, 222
Kings County Hospital (Brooklyn, N.Y.), 23
King's Highway Hospital (Brooklyn, N.Y.), 22
Kinzer, David, 29
kitchen cytology, 222
Krushat, Mark, 137
Kucinich, Dennis, 266
Kusserow, Richard, 28, 101–4, 120, 128, 129, 132–34, 135–39, 151, 153, 155, 156, 189

laboratory procedures, 198, 201, 212, 253
   fatal errors in, 225–27
   money made through, 159, 170, 181, 199, 200–201
   quality controls in, 221–22, 225–31
   regulation of, 131, 220–31
Lancione, Peter, 202
Landers, Ann, 232–34, 235–36, 240, 241
Lansing, Michael, 64
Larkin, Brent, 266
lasers, 167–68
Lattimer, Agnes, 223–24
Lattimore, Linda, 179–80, 183, 184
law enforcement, 230, 272
   fear and, 119
   powerlessness of, 176
lawyers, *see* attorneys
Leighty, Mistee, 237, 240
Leland Memorial Hospital (Riverdale, Md.), 33–34
Lemont, Inger, 40–41
Lenox Hill Hospital (New York, N.Y.), 23–24, 256
Levin, Art, 216
Lewisburg Community Hospital (Lewisburg, Tenn.), 186
Leyden Community Hospital (Chicago, Ill.), 188
Lewis, Lynn, 90–91
licensed practical nurses (LPNs), 35, 37, 48–49, 53–54, 62

licenses, professional, 14, 23,
        48–49, 51, 202, 273
    forging of, 53–54
    illegal activities and, 194, 196,
        202
Licavoli, James T., 194
Lincoln Hospital (Bronx, N.Y.),
        64
lobbyists, medical, 84, 125–26,
        272
Lofton, Kevin E., 87
Lonardo, Angelo "Big Ange," 198
Loop, Floyd, 274
Lorain Community Hospital
        (Elyria, Ohio), 195–96
Lorain County Medical Society, 196
Louisiana State Board of Medical
        Examiners, 175
Louisiana State Medical School,
        173
Louisiana State Medical Society,
        175
lung cancer, 167–68
lungs, 69

McAfee, Helen, 58, 60
McAllen Medical Center
        (McAllen, Tex.), 97
McAuto Abstracting Service,
        151–52
McClure, Walter, 263–64, 265,
        267, 268, 272–73
McGaha, Fred, 175
McShane, Jerry, 177–78, 179,
        181–83
Madin, Ira, 108
magnetic resonance imaging
        (MRI) centers, 163
malpractice, 27, 33, 201
Marburger, David, 244
Marine Corps, 102, 246
Markley, Mary Beth, 238
Maryland Department of Health,
        252
Maryland Nurses Association,
        61–62
Maryland State Medical Society,
        273
Massachusetts Hospital
        Association, 29

Mathew, Leelamma, 33
Mathews, Augustine, 224
Mayo Clinic (Rochester, Minn.),
        269–70
media, 242–45, 266, 273
    at board meetings, 237, 241,
        243
    civic-minded, 233–34
    outside scrutiny provided by,
        233–34, 237–38
    public-relations staffs and, 235,
        261–62
    unbalanced reporting in, 235,
        239–40
Medicaid, 197, 237
    patient-buying and, 182, 184
medical bills, see hospital bills
medical community:
    consumerism and, 10, 104, 202,
        206, 216, 220, 273–74
    ethics in, 171, 178, 179–80, 186
    national data bank established
        by, 259–60
    political influence of, 103, 108,
        125–26, 216, 250
    self-regulation of, 104, 189,
        204, 205–18, 247
    trust in, 10–11, 29, 36, 218,
        243, 274
    see also hospital industry
medical records, medical records
        experts, 129, 130, 136, 137,
        212
    accuracy in, 138, 152, 153, 195,
        256
    consultants as, 134
    criminal investigations of, 248,
        249–56, 261
    growing significance of, 132
    media access to, 243
    researching questions about,
        147
    training of, 146, 152, 153
medical schools, 69, 250
Medicare, 9, 24, 28, 87, 200–201,
        203, 237, 272, 274
    auditors for, 111, 118–19,
        124
    computerized exploitation of,
        105–8, 115, 132–34, 144

cost data used by, 108–10, 113,
    114–19, 122–23, 124, 127,
    135–36, 188, 216
DRGs used by, *see*
    diagnostic-related
    groupings
hospitals favored by, 119–20,
    127, 152
investigations of, 112–28,
    130–39
overpayment of, 123, 125, 126,
    131–35, 138, 144–57, 197,
    262
patient-buying and, 182,
    183–84
prospective payment by, *see*
    prospective payment
regulations of, 111, 114, 118,
    200
medication, *see* drugs
Meese, Edwin, 250
Memorial Hospital (Topeka,
    Kans.), 234
Mendelson, Mary A., 198
Mendoza, Atanasia, 225–27, 228
Menninger Foundation, 234
mental confusion, 17, 207–8, 220
Mershon, Sawyer, Johnston,
    Dunwoody & Cole, 58–60
Methodist Hospital (Minneapolis,
    Minn.), 184–85
Metropolitan Hospital (New
    York, N.Y.), 23, 24
Meyer, Margaret, 145–46, 151
Michigan Department of Public
    Health, 63
Michigan State University, 233
Mikulski, Barbara A., 231
Miller, Scott, 156
Minnesota Board of Medical
    Examiners, 185
Modern Healthcare, 139, 216
Monahan, Julie, 36, 38, 41, 42–60
    forgery ordered by, 53–55
    intimidating language used by,
        45, 50, 59
    investigation of, 56–60
Montefiore Hospital and Medical
    Center (Bronx, N.Y.), 23,
    95

Moore, Barry, 187
Moore, Martha, 246–47, 249
Moore, Wayne, 245
Morford, Thomas, 27
Morley, John, 266
Mosely, Fred, 116
murder, 19–22, 28, 245, 246–57
    concealment of, 247, 250
    investigations of, 246–54
Murphy, Dillon, 65–66, 67–69,
    71, 76, 77, 78, 79, 81, 82
Murphy, Patricia, 61

Nader, Ralph, 273
Nassau County Medical Center
    (East Meadow, N.Y.), 22,
    229
National Association of Public
    Hospitals, 22
national health care, 25, 86
Nedermier, Ruth, 40–41
Nestlé Enterprises, 264, 268
Neurosurgery, 19
New England Journal of Medicine,
    29, 105, 107, 128, 132, 138,
    187, 217, 255
Newhall, David, 101
New London Hospital (Elyria,
    Ohio), 195–204
    equipment at, 199–200
    hiring practices of, 195, 196,
        197–98
Newsday, 62, 95, 216, 229
New York City Health and
    Hospitals Corporation, 15,
    82, 241
New York *Daily News,* 22, 24
New York Post, 20, 23
New York State Health
    Department, 256
New York Times, 13, 64, 127
Nicholson, Don, 129–30, 136
North Carolina Board of
    Pharmacy, 70–74, 81, 82
North Carolina Department of
    Human Resources, 83
North Carolina Society of
    Hospital Pharmacists, 83
North Central Bronx Hospital
    (Bronx, N.Y.), 23

Northern Virginia Doctors
    Hospital (Arlington, Va.),
    221–22
North Monroe Community
    Hospital (Monroe, La.),
    160–76
  emergency room of, 172, 174
  patients solicited by, 161–76
Nurkin, Harry, 82
nurses, 9, 33–41, 89, 137, 212,
    213, 248
  consecutive shifts worked by,
    44, 46, 61
  equipment used by, 35, 63
  float, 61–62
  foreign, 62–63
  home, 40–41
  out-of-work, 234
  overworking of, 25, 26, 35, 36,
    44, 60–62, 75, 96
  patients abandoned by, 33, 34
  physical exams required of, 55
  powerlessness of, 35, 61
  professional commitment
    made by, 56, 60
  shortages of, 24, 35, 62, 75,
    188, 227, 232–34, 256
  substance abuse among, 33,
    61
  temporary, see temporary help
  weekend shifts worked by, 72,
    75
nursing homes, 25, 37, 86, 88–94,
    208
  competing for space in, 90–92,
    93
  conditions in, 94, 198–99, 251
  cost of, 93
  hospital patients discharged to,
    89–94
  regulation of, 131
nursing programs, 63

O'Dell, Gloria, 239
Oder, Donald R., 126
Office of Management and
    Budget (OMB), 272
Ohio Hospital Association, 243
Ohio Medical Board, 202, 257

Ohio State Health Department,
    199, 201, 202, 203–4
Ohio State Medical Association,
    202
Ohio State University Hospitals,
    257
Ohio Supreme Court, 242, 244
O'Leary, Dennis S., 216, 230
Olenick, Paul, 120
open-heart units, 25, 27, 160, 241,
    268, 274
  deaths in, 70, 161
organized crime, 194, 198, 210
Orlovsky, Donald, 57
O'Shaughnessy, John J., 133–34
Ouachita Medical Society, 175
outpatient surgery, 96, 185
Owen, Jack W., 126, 139
oxygen, 69, 88

pacemaker implants, 14, 113
painkillers, 33, 220
Palley, Robin, 211
Palm Beach Regional Hospital
    (formerly Doctors
    Hospital; Lake Worth,
    Fla.), 38, 40
Pap smears, 220–22, 228, 230
  analysis of, 221–22, 229, 231
Paracelsus Healthcare
    Corporation, 121–22
Parsons Hospital (Queens, N.Y.),
    23, 207–8, 215
  accreditation lost by, 213–14
  Joint Commission inspection
    of, 212–13
Pasadena General Hospital
    (Houston, Tex.), 178–84
  advisory committee at, 181–82
pathology departments, 18, 221,
    230
patients:
  advocates for, 90, 185, 227, 259
  buying and selling of, 159,
    160–76, 178–89
  deception of, 35, 198, 212, 213,
    221, 226, 259–60, 261–62
  discharging of, 22, 25, 27, 87,
    89–92, 93–97

inhospital injury of, 71, 81
overcrowding of, 13, 23, 188, 200
overtreatment of, 198
privately insured, 155–56; *see also* insurance companies
recruiting of, 136
stealing from, 34, 40–41
temporary nurses as threat to, 35, 40–41, 47, 60–61
uninsured, 22, 87, 97, 165, 272
unwanted, 17, 86, 89–97, 159, 165
Pat Joyce Tavern, 261, 262
Paulo, Walter, 202
Paxton, Jim, 260
Pearson, John, 18
peer review organizations (PROs), 27–28, 135, 149, 155, 212, 216, 225
Pennington, Clarence, 241–45
Pennsylvania Health Department, 214
perfusionists, 72, 79
Persian Gulf war, 85, 86, 261
pharmacies, pharmacists, 35, 70–79, 89, 131, 212, 249
covering shifts in, 70, 74–75
mismanagement of, 70, 71, 73–75, 77–79, 80, 82–83, 84
responsibilities of, 72–73
training of, 73, 77
uncontrolled substances in, 78
unlicensed, 70, 77, 79
pharmacy technicians, 77, 78–79, 80
Philadelphia County Medical Society, 215
Philadelphia Daily News, 209, 211
Philadelphia Inquirer, 214, 224
Philippine Center for Immigrant Rights, 62
Phillips, Ernest, 71
Phipps, Bonnie, 57
physical therapy, 198
physician assistants, 214
physician bonding, 28, 185, 188

physicians, 137
as corporate-owned, 164, 167–69, 170–71, 174, 175, 176
diagnosis assigned by, 107, 136, 138, 146, 152, 195, 217
disciplinary actions against, 27, 104, 121, 202, 259, 260
drugs prescribed by, 73, 75, 93–94, 196, 197, 198
honesty of, 103–4, 259
hospitals buying patients from, 160–76, 178–89
incompetence tolerated by, 104, 189, 204
life-styles attained by, 177–78, 179, 233
money-making schemes of, 121, 126, 159
professional and business interests as balanced by, 169
specialties of, 133
staff, 136; *see also* hospital staff
unlicensed, 74, 197, 202, 207, 211
unread documents signed by, 147
Physicians and Surgeons Community Hospital (Atlanta, Ga.), 62, 73
plasma, 224
platelets, 224
podiatrists, 202
Poindexter, John, 179
politics, 171
media and, 242–45
medical community in, 103, 108, 216, 250
potassium chloride, 248–49, 250, 255
Powell, Jody, 272
Price, Ronald, 270
Prince George's County Police Department, 247, 248
Prince George's General Hospital (Cheverly, Md.), 246–56
murders at, 247–56

Prince George's *(cont.)*
  police investigation frustrated
    by, 250
"Product of a Hospital, The"
    (Codman), 205
Professional Standard Review
    Organization (PSRO), 204
prospective payment, 24–25, 28,
    41, 88, 89, 90, 93, 96,
    105–8, 110, 125, 129, 132
  acceptance of, 120, 156
  recordkeeping emphasized by,
    138
  see also diagnostic-related
    groupings
psychiatry, 14, 17, 18, 21
Public Citizen Health Research
    Group, 273
Public Health Service, 129, 130,
    137
public relations, 233, 272
  media and, 235, 261–62
pulmonary edema, 69

quality assurance, 142, 147,
    205–7, 215, 218, 221–22,
    225–31, 260, 262–63,
    264–71
Quick, Linda, 239
Quilty, Mary, 147, 150
Quinn, Thomas, 261–62

Radefeld, Denis, 195
radiation therapy, 96, 171–72,
    185, 186, 212, 219–20
Rand Corporation, 27, 94
Rather, Dan, 242
Reagan, Ronald, 27, 101
  administration of, 22, 28, 247
  budget-cutting under, 104, 126,
    135, 188
  deregulation under, 103–4,
    106, 108, 135, 176, 185,
    188, 204
recovery departments, 14,
    74
red blood cells, 69, 224
Redi-Nurse, 40
Regional Medical Center
    (Memphis, Tenn.), 97

registered nurses (RNs), 37, 213
  LPNs posing as, 48–49, 53–54,
    62
regulation, regulatory bodies, 70,
    271
  compliance vs., 95, 185
  enforcement of, 119–20, 201–4,
    212–17, 230, 272
  first attempt at, 205–6
  gaining knowledge of, 118–19
  inspections conducted by, 206,
    212, 213
  of laboratories, 220–31
  under Reagan, 103–4, 106, 108,
    135, 176, 185, 188, 204
  self-, 205–18, 247
rehabilitation, inpatient, 185, 212
Reliance Electric Company, 266
Relman, Arnold, 187
Republican party, 250
Republic Health Corporation, 186
residents, 136
Respess, Walter, Jr., 80–81
respiratory arrest, 77
respiratory therapy, 37, 89, 113
Review Times, 242–43
Reynolds, Arlen, 165–69, 170,
    172
Rhodes, James, 201–4
Rice, C. Wayne, 271
Richmond Heights General
    Hospital (Cleveland,
    Ohio), 108–9, 110
Rinehart, Wayne, 81, 83
RN, 60
Robicsek, Francis, 66–69, 76–77, 78
Ronstrum, Steve, 176
Roylance, John, 39, 45, 51, 59

Sacks, Jeffrey J., 250–56
Sacred Heart Hospital (Hanford,
    Calif.), 140–57
  Medicare defrauded by, 144–57
  multiple summaries prepared
    at, 146–49, 152
  reviews of, 145, 149–55
  unnecessary hospitalizations at,
    152–53
  whistle-blower suit against,
    149–55, 156–57

Sadowsky, Melvin, 95
St. Francis Hospital (Topeka,
    Kans.), 241
St. Francis Medical Center
    (Monroe, La.), 160
  patients diverted from, 161–76
St. Luke's Hospital (Newburgh,
    N.Y.), 26
St. Luke's Roosevelt Hospital
    (New York, N.Y.), 23
savings-and-loan industry, 22,
    103, 109
Schaffer, Randy, 183–84
Schultz, Daniel, 220, 221
Schweiker, Richard, 101, 103
security guards, 14–15, 18, 20, 21,
    23, 26, 247, 255–57
Seibert, Becky, 45, 47–50, 56, 59
seizures, 33, 88, 97
Semmelweis, Ignaz Philipp, 176
Senate, 219, 220–22, 230, 231
senility, 207–8
Shaller, Dale, 268–70
Sidicane, Stanley, 142–43, 149
Siffring, Connie, 142
Simborg, Donald W., 105–8, 128,
    132, 138
Simmons, Larry, 136–37
Skinner, Julianne, 15, 16
sleep disorder clinics, 88
Slocum, Peter, 64
Smith, Steven, 16–17, 19–22
Snow, John, 251
Social Security Administration,
    84, 129, 131, 139, 150
social workers, 26, 87, 212
  caseloads carried by, 90, 95–96
  discharge-planning by, 89–92
Society for Hospital Social Work
    Directors, 96
Soffer, Lynn J., 227
South Florida Hospital
    Association, 39, 58
Spinks, Michael, 179, 181–83
Stark, Fortney H. "Pete," 125–26,
    127, 128, 187
Starr, Paul, 237
statisticians, 137
Stauffer, John, 240–41
Stauffer, Peter W., 234, 239–40, 241

sterilization, elective, 196
stomach pains, 219, 225
Stormont-Vail Regional Medical
    Center (Topeka, Kans.),
    234–41
  construction projects of, 235
  corporate success of, 234, 243
  in media, 233–34, 235, 237–38,
    240–41
  public interest in, 236–37
strokes, 97, 131, 150
Summit County Welfare
    Department, 199
surgeons, 79
  incompetent, 194, 195, 274
  personality traits of, 18, 66
  weekend shifts worked by, 72
surgery, 95, 113, 134, 176, 200,
    212, 236
  blood in, 207, 215
  coronary-bypass, 9, 65–72, 262
  drugs vs., 214
  elective, 14, 196
  infection after, 195, 214
  outpatient, 96, 185
  reviewing of, 25, 214
  team in, 79, 214
  unnecessary, 195, 199, 211,
    214, 215
  on weekends, 71–72, 80–81
surgical consent forms, 200
surgical debridement, 131, 134
surveillance, epidemiologic, 256
Swango, Michael J., 257

TB testing, 229
technology, 89
  growing complexity of, 35, 63,
    131, 205, 238, 243
  money-making opportunities
    through, 159, 268
  see also computers
television, see media
temperature, taking of, 225, 227
temporary help, 25, 42–60, 72, 74
  demand for, 35, 46
  evaluation of, 36, 38–39, 47,
    51–52
  forged documents of, 53–55, 56
  money earned by, 46, 49, 54

temporary help *(cont.)*
  patients endangered by, 35,
      40–41, 47, 60–61, 256
  phantom-booking of, 40
  private hiring of, 63–64
  unqualified, 48–49, 51, 53–60,
      62
Tender Loving Greed
      (Mendelson), 198
terminally ill patients, 22
Tharpe, Dorothy, 227, 228
Tikker, Bessie, 57, 59
Tillman, Jacqueline, 89–90, 91–92
Time, 242
Topeka Capital-Journal, 234–36,
      238–41
Topeka Metro News, 239
Trandate, 75
tranquilizers, 88
transient ischemic attacks, 131
transplants, 69
trauma units, 17
Trental, 75
tube feeding, 88
Tuma, Joe, 119
Tweed, William Marcy "Boss," 15

ulcers, 214
Union Club (Cleveland, Ohio),
      265–67, 269–71
United Hospital Fund, 22, 29
United Network for Organ
      Sharing (UNOS), 69
United States:
  government in, *see*
      government, U.S.
  postwar, 236
University Hospitals (Cleveland,
      Ohio), 266, 267
urinary tract problems, 200

Vanderbilt University Medical
      Center (Nashville, Tenn.),
      77
Vazquez, William L., 217, 218
ventilatory assistance, 62, 88–89
Veterans Administration
      hospitals, 154
Victoria Hospital (Miami, Fla.),
      187

Vigorito, Nick, 207
vital signs, 49, 54, 213
Vladeck, Bruce, 29

Wagner, Virginia, 94
Walker, Jimmy, 17
Wall Street Journal, 81–82, 91,
      97, 180, 215–16, 222, 229,
      238
Walter Reed Army Medical
      Center, Washington, D.C.,
      250
Warhol, Andy, 64
Washington Post, 127, 272
waste, illegal storage of, 24
weekend surgery, 71–72, 80–81
weight-loss programs, 88
whistle-blower suits, 149–55,
      156–57
Whiteman, Thomas, 59
Wilensky, Gail, 84
Winston, Donald S., 180
Winters, Fred, 64
Wisconsin State Medical Society,
      260
Wolfe, Sidney, 273
Wolff, James, 166
Woods, Powell, 264–66
Work, David R., 70–74, 78, 81,
      83
workers:
  health benefits of, 238, 260,
      268, 271, 272, 274
  injuries to, 180, 238
  medical excuses written for,
      196
World War II, 236, 242
Wybaillie, Edmond, 150–52,
      153–54, 155

x-rays, 117, 170, 201

Yale University, 105
Young, Ward V., Jr., 195

Zapata, Cleo, 114
Zimmerman, Michael, 126–27